An introduction to dance movement therapy in psychiatry

Dance Movement Therapy (DMT) is newly recognized as a safe and effective therapy for psychiatric clients in community mental health care. *An Introduction to Dance Movement Therapy in Psychiatry* provides the first full-length study of this innovative approach, tracing it from its American roots to its current development in Britain and elsewhere. The book will be of great interest to all mental health professionals working in psychiatry, including occupational therapists, art therapists, psychiatric nurses, social workers and psychiatrists, as well as dance movement therapists.

Kristina Stanton-Jones gives detailed clinical descriptions of the techniques of DMT, drawing on her own professional experience working with long-term patients, adult out-patients, and with children and their families. She offers a theoretical account of different forms of DMT – psychodynamic, Jungian, ego-psychoanalytic and Gestalt – and also covers group DMT approaches, such as psychoanalytically-informed work and methods derived from Irvin Yalom's humanistic perspective. She outlines a new 'symbolic' school of DMT theory and practice, which combines traditional DMT methods with the theories of W.R. Bion and D.W. Winnicott, and which stresses how the imagery and metaphor that arise during DMT can be used to provide a safe, contained structure for exploring psychiatric patients' emotional problems.

The book explores movement and meaning in general, and examines the non-verbal communications research and choreographic movement analysis systems that underlie DMT. It also gives a survey of recent research into the movement profiles of specific diagnostic categories such as schizophrenia, depression, eating disorders and sexual abuse. In conclusion, Kristina Stanton-Jones assesses the current professional status of DMT, and gives helpful information on training institutes and related organizations which will be invaluable to both students and mental health professionals interested in new approaches to therapeutic work in psychiatry.

Kristina Stanton Jones studied Dance Movement Therapy at the Laban Centre for Music and Dance, London. She spent five years working as a dance movement therapist in child and adult psychiatry settings in the National Health Service in the UK.

An introduction to dance movement therapy in psychiatry

Kristina Stanton-Jones

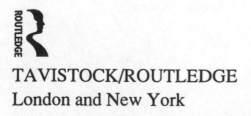

TAVISTOCK/ROUTLEDGE

London and New York

First published 1992
by Routledge
11 New Fetter Lane, London EC4P 4EE

Simultaneously published in the USA and Canada
by Routledge
a division of Routledge, Chapman and Hall, Inc.
29 West 35th Street, New York, NY 10001

© 1992 Kristina Stanton-Jones

Typeset in Times by Michael Mepham, Frome, Somerset
Printed and bound in Great Britain by
Mackays of Chatham plc, Chatham, Kent

British Library Cataloguing in Publication Data
Stanton-Jones, Kristina, 1962–
   An introduction to dance movement therapy
   in psychiatry.
   I. Title
   616.891655

Library of Congress Cataloging in Publication Data
Stanton-Jones, Kristina, 1962–
   An introduction to dance movement therapy in psychiatry/by
   Kristina Stanton-Jones.
   p.   cm.
   Includes bibliographical references and index.
   1. Dance therapy.   2. Psychiatry–methods.   I. Title.
   [DNLM: 1. Dance therapy.   2. Psychiatry–methods.   WM 450.5.D2]
   RC489.D3S73   1992
   616.89'1655–dc20
   DNLM/DLC
   for Library of Congress   91–36875
                                                                    CIP

   ISBN 0–415–06101–6
       0–415–05983–6 (pbk)

For M and L and the ones who came to try it

Contents

Preface

This book is an introduction to the use of dance movement therapy in psychiatry. It is intended for postgraduate students in dance movement therapy (DMT), as well as for other mental health professionals interested in innovative therapeutic approaches. I hope that it will therefore be of interest to psychiatric nurses, social workers, occupational therapists, psychologists, art, music and dramatherapists, verbal psychotherapists and psychiatrists, and it may be of interest to those involved in dance and the arts. The book is not a substitute for a professional training in dance movement therapy, and is in no way intended as a dance activities manual. DMT is a relatively recent addition to the spectrum of therapeutic work with patients who suffer from mental illness. This book will therefore elaborate the theory underlying DMT, as well as provide a guide to clinical practice. It is surprising that there are so few full-length books on DMT, and none that focus on DMT in psychiatry, given that a survey of the journals *The Arts in Psychotherapy* and the *American Journal of Dance Therapy* reveals an increasing interest in work with psychiatric patients, with as much as 40 per cent of the newer issues being devoted to work in this area. I have made extensive use of a recent full-length study of the history of DMT, Fran Levy's *Dance/Movement Therapy: A Healing Art*, which would provide excellent background reading for those interested in the early development of DMT, particularly in America.

This book begins with a delineation of DMT in contrast to therapeutic physical activity. This is followed by a short history of the development of dance movement therapy in psychiatry in Chapter 2. This history is complex, largely because it consists of a heterogeneous group of individuals creating their own forms of DMT along the lines of their adherence to different psychological models. Chapter 3 describes and differentiates several current schools of dance movement therapy being practised in psychiatry with individuals and groups. While the great majority of dance movement therapists are probably eclectic in their approach, borrowing insights from many traditions, four major schools can be delineated. These are: psychodynamic, Jungian, ego-psychoanalytic and group dynamic in focus. I hope to clarify for the reader the differences between these approaches by comparing the way each employs movement in keeping with its therapeutic aims.

Chapter 4 is an overview of the many ways that movement carries meaning. The fifth chapter addresses the crucial issue of appropriate therapeutic goals for DMT in psychiatry, and suggests some criteria for choosing clients who are appropriate for the DMT approach. This is followed by a discussion of some of the problems surrounding the use of therapeutic ideas in psychiatry, and a short introductory section giving a psychodynamic perspective on two of the major diagnostic categories of mental illness encountered in psychiatry, namely depression and schizophrenia.

The first clinical section of this book is found in Chapter 6, which describes work with an adult outpatient group, giving actual examples of case material to support the theoretical and technical aspects of DMT. Chapter 7 does the same thing for chronic or long-term hospitalized patients, while Chapter 8 gives examples taken from child and family psychiatry, including clinical examples of children in foster care, sexually abused children, and the use of DMT with a family group. Work with individual adult psychiatric patients is not described in this book. Such work is generally supervised by qualified dance movement therapists or by dance movement therapists also training as verbal psychotherapists, and is therefore slightly beyond the scope of this introductory book.

In Chapter 9 an attempt is made to articulate a new tradition in DMT in psychiatry, which is largely the result of my own experiences and experiments, and which reflects my own particular mixture of psychodynamic theory and movement improvisation. Unlike many dance movement therapists, my background is not in modern dance or ballet, but in movement improvisation, physical theatre, and contemporary dance and dance theatre. In order to articulate the theoretical basis of my own approach, I will relate my ideas to current DMT, and attempt to articulate how I think that the object relations tradition (including the work of W. R. Bion, Melanie Klein and D. W. Winnicott) may be fruitful in the development of a new dance movement therapy that is unique to Britain. Central to my approach is the use of metaphor and imagery as a way of connecting the experience of body and psyche, and so, because of this emphasis, my work can be termed a symbolic approach to DMT.

Chapter 10 concludes the book, with some final remarks on dance movement therapy in psychiatry, particularly on schizophrenia and factors contributing to the success of DMT in a specific setting based on relations with the staff and institution in which it is being practised. This will underline the necessity of proper training, supervision and support for the dance movement therapist undertaking the arduous but rewarding task of contributing to the treatment of psychiatric patients. The appendices that follow provide a model for an information sheet that could be made available to day hospital staff, and a summary of DMT child psychiatry assessment parameters that dance movement therapy students may find useful. Addresses of professional training institutions in DMT in the UK are also given. The extensive reference section presents a survey of literature into the movement profiles of several specific diagnostic criteria, namely, schizophrenia, depression, eating disorders and sexual abuse.

I have used both the terms 'patient' and 'client' throughout the book, which reflects current usage by people working in the field. Both words are a shorthand for *people* suffering from mental illness, and are not meant to be disparaging in any way. I have retained the term 'patient' to denote the fact that most people who are described in the clinical section suffer from serious mental illness, and are under the treatment of a psychiatrist. I recognize that there are problems with this term, and that some find it condescending, but I work in tandem with, and not in opposition to, the medical model that uses the term 'patient'. In my view, there are also problems with the term 'client', which is derived from the language of commerce and business; surely the people seen in clinical settings are more than simply 'customers' who utilize a 'service'. I have tried to avoid using the phrase, 'the schizophrenic'. In the same way as we would never call a person suffering from cancer a 'canceric', we must remember that the person in our group is a human being enduring what is often a terrifying and debilitating condition, and not simply a walking 'case' or instance of a disease. While I offer apologies to those in mental health services who find the old term 'patient' abhorrent in favour of the more current usage of 'client', I hope that my use of terminology will remind the reader that the aims for hospitalized and outpatient psychiatric groups are different from those of private clients who are not diagnosed as mentally ill, and who seek therapy voluntarily as a means to personal growth. Such work may aim at elucidating and understanding the inner emotional world in order to enrich the life experience and relationships of the client, whereas work with psychiatric patients has a different function. Although it also works with unconscious processes, DMT with psychiatric patients primarily seeks to support the patients, to aid them in forming and maintaining more satisfactory relationships with those around them, and to help integrate fragmentary emotional experiences.

Although almost all of the clinical material presented in this book is my own, I have, in the description of work with groups, not reported dialogues using the personal voice, 'I said to the patient', but rather have chosen a more distanced approach, and used 'the dance movement therapist said to the patient'. This was chosen in order that student dance movement therapist readers might more easily put themselves into the shoes of the dance movement therapist's role. As well, it seems important to step back and look at the practice of DMT in psychiatry in general, rather than my personal experiences in particular. By using the impersonal voice in the majority of the clinical sections, I in no way wish to disguise the fact that the clinical experiences are my own, though the patients and their situations have of course been altered for reasons of confidentiality. Rather, I hope that my clinical descriptions will be queried, questioned, and pulled apart by subsequent generations of dance movement therapists as they strive to evolve more effective ways of working in psychiatry.

I recognize that there are limitations to a book that represents the author's clinical experience alone; a comparison of my experiences with other dance movement therapists in psychiatry revealed that the patients I encountered were on the more 'heavy' end of mental illness, and therefore my group examples include rather more schizophrenic and personality disordered patients than depressed ones, though this is evidently not the case in many hospitals (particularly teaching hospitals), where there is a greater mix of depressed and schizophrenic patients. I hope that this slightly skewed patient population will not fundamentally alter the applicability of my ideas to work with groups of psychiatric patients. Additionally, in reviewing literature on mental illness and movement, my own research has involved a detailed study of movement pathology in schizophrenia, and so the description of movement profiles of specific diagnostic criteria found in Chapter 10 is heavily weighted towards this condition.

Readers may notice that the term dance movement therapy is sometimes written as dance/movement therapy, that the 'arts therapies' are sometimes referred to as the 'creative arts therapies', and that dramatherapy is sometimes spelt as drama therapy. The first of these sets of terms are current British spelling and usage, and the second set an American one. British usage is employed throughout the text, but quotations from American authors retain the American convention.

I have written this book to articulate what is largely an unwritten body of knowledge passed on from dance movement therapist to dance movement therapist working in this fascinating area. I hope that my ideas will not form any new orthodoxy, but rather provide a position against which dance movement therapists can define themselves, and to stimulate therapists to think about what they are really trying to do, and the techniques that best fit their goals. In terms of the development of the field of DMT, particularly in Britain, I hope that this book will motivate practitioners to formalize their own conceptualizations of their work. This would hopefully enable them to be able to say what the particular contribution of DMT can be to the treatment of mental illness, and how it works alongside psychiatric nursing, occupational therapy, psychotherapy and psychiatry. I hope, therefore, that this book will be only the first among many which attempt to articulate the complex and fascinating process of DMT as a therapeutic approach to the treatment of mental illness.

Acknowledgements

To a large degree, this book represents the setting down of an oral tradition, the articulation of knowledge shared among a group of people practising dance movement therapy. Because of this, my list of thanks is very long.

I owe a debt to the people who trained me: Dr Dianne Dulicai, Rachel Melville-Thomas and Sherry Goodill, at the Laban Centre for Movement and Dance, London, and at Hahnemann University and Medical School, Philadelphia. I am particularly grateful to Dr Marion North, director of the Laban Centre for her support of my research. This book is largely the result of my studies supported by the Laban Centre which were to have become a doctorate, but which ended prematurely when I gained acceptance to medical school. I must also thank Dr Martha Davis for reviewing my pilot study tapes in New York.

I owe an especial debt to the training group of fellow students who put up with my endless efforts to articulate what we were doing: Sheila Murphy, Irmgard Kästner, Tricia Dickinson, Barbro Wilson-Hagen, Carola Gross, and especially Konrad Noebel, who taught me that one could sustain intellectual inquiry without sacrificing emotional and aesthetic sensitivity.

The possibility to experiment and develop my work with patients was made possible by a number of people within the Canterbury and Thanet Health Authority, to whom I wish to express my gratitude. Angela Wilson, District Occupational Therapist, created my post by arguing for National Health Service (NHS), Whitley Council and Secretary of State for Health recognition of DMT. She was assisted in this by our unit general manager, Peter Goddard.

Clinical support by psychiatrists for whom I have worked has been important in inspiring me to work and write about DMT in psychiatry. I must especially thank Dr Kate Cartwright of the Child and Family Therapy Centre, Canterbury, Dr Bill Bamber of St Martin's House, and the Canterbury Community Mental Health Team. I am grateful to Dr Anthony Ryle of St Thomas' Hospital, London, who introduced me to ideas about time-limited psychotherapy within the NHS. I must also mention Dr Philip Timms, who taught at the Laban Centre during my time there. I also wish to thank John Hills for introducing me to family therapy and working with me in creating movement experiences for families who were stuck for words.

Practical support and enthusiasm was provided by a number of mental health professionals who deserve my thanks: Julie Wilton, Pauline Reynolds, Eugene O'Connor, Simon Sawyer, Val Potter, Dr Colin Lanceley, Fran Wray, Des Fisher, Jean Austin, Frances Beaumont, Sally McGregor, Pat Flavill, Dr Chris Allison, Jacquie Edge, Penny Foreman, Maureen Shaw, Linda Anderson, Jenny Elliot, Kathy Allison, Sue McDonald, Keith Robinson, Marie Patton, Barry Coleman, Jean, and the other Redwood inpatient adolescent unit staff.

I must also thank the many psychiatric nurses and occupational therapists who conquered their initial embarrassment and participated in the groups, of whom Nigel, Niall, Tracey and Rosemary deserve special mention.

I am indebted to Brigidin Gorman and Jane Lloyd, the directors of the Integrated Support Project in Sittingbourne, Kent, an independent fostering organization. They, along with Elaine Holliday, have given me the space and support to develop my work with abused children.

The many patients who came eagerly to the sessions, as well as those who were cajoled, pushed or otherwise led also deserve thanks. If they had not been willing to try this new and, for them, rather odd approach, there would be no clinical material for this book. I wish to convey special thanks to the rehabilitation patients from St Augustine's hospital during the period February 1987 to October 1988, and the St Martin's House Community Mental Health Centre clients from July 1987 to May 1988, many of whom were very forthcoming in helping to articulate what they found useful about the DMT approach, and gave important ideas for modifying the form and structure.

I acknowledge my debt to supervisors and teachers on the Observational Studies course at the Tavistock clinic who introduced me to object relations theory. Although the analytical way of working is quite different from that described in this book, their teaching enabled me to conceptualize a psychodynamic and symbolic model for DMT. I must therefore thank Margot Waddell, Lisa Miller, Gianna Williams, Mirjana Renton, Rolene Szur, Ann Alvarez and Janet Bungener.

I also owe a debt to a number of psychoanalysts, psychiatrists and academics who are colleagues and friends, for their interest in what for them must have initially sounded like a fairly 'wild' form of therapy. Respectful gratitude is owed to Jean and Nadine Laplanche, Dr Robert M. Young, Professor Hugh Freeman, Sonu Samdashani, Dr Jim Gollnick, Hilde Rapp, John Southgate, Bob and Anna Hinshelwood, Bice Benvenuto, Danuza Machado, Bernard Burgoyne, Vivien Bar, Dr Marion O'Connor, Dr James Gollnick and particularly Andrew Samuels for his provocative questions about the safety of DMT for psychiatric patients.

Further thanks are due the dance movement therapists who are my colleagues. In particular, I must acknowledge my debt to Laurence Higgens for giving me intellectual comradeship, and introducing me to the ideas around metaphor in psychotherapy which have subsequently become central to my work. Thanks also to Sarah Holden, Helen Payne, Karen Callaghan, Monika Steiner, Peta Mees, Gail Liebowitz, Jessica Shenton, Jude Webster, Dr Jan Eaton, Jackie Blatt, Bonnie

Meekums, Catalina Garvie, Janie Griffiths and other members of the (British) Association for Dance Movement Therapy.

I must thank Susan Corker, who provided essential support for my studies in London. Also, I am grateful to librarians Peter Bassett and Janet Warner of the Laban Centre for Movement and Dance, London, and Joy Sharman, head librarian of St Augustine's psychiatric library in Kent. I must also express my thanks to Dr Chris Allison and Heather Nightingale who allowed me access to archival material used in Chapter 10.

Also, a personal thanks to Susan, for inspiring my attempts at a scientifically grounded humanism, and teaching me about the value of stories that make sense of experience. Finally, mega-merci to Erika, Curtis, Vicky, Pam, David, Lucy, and especially to Martin, who said, 'You must do what you want; follow your heart.'

Chapter 1

Introduction

DANCE MOVEMENT THERAPY DEFINED

Dance movement therapy is one of the arts therapies, along with music, art and dramatherapy. The American Dance Therapy Association has defined it as 'the psychotherapeutic use of movement as a process which furthers the physical and psychic integration of an individual' (Bernstein 1979: 3). DMT seeks to combine the expressive and creative aspects of dance with the insights of psychotherapy. It focuses both on the patient's relationship with the therapist as a means of nurturing change, and on understanding unconscious mental processes which lie outside our everyday awareness.

DMT draws on a multidisciplinary body of knowledge: it employs theory and method from individual and group psychotherapy (Malan 1989, Yalom 1970); draws upon research into nonverbal communication (Davis and Skupien 1982, Davis 1975, Scheflen and Sheflen 1972), developmental psychology and developmental body movement (Kestenberg 1975); and analyses the qualities of movement using choreographic and movement analysis systems (Bartenieff 1980, Laban 1948). In DMT, movement is used to facilitate change within individuals (intrapsychically) and in their ability to relate to others (interpersonally). The patient becomes aware of how emotional and bodily experience are connected, and, by free associating with words, how movement can yield images, which are then analysed as a means to psychological understanding (Bernstein 1979, Fletcher 1974, Stanton 1991). In group DMT, engaging in movement interaction enables patients to become more aware of their interpersonal behaviour, and so modify how they form and maintain relationships with others (Schmais and Felber 1977, Schmais 1981). Furthermore, group DMT yields movement, metaphor and imagery which illustrate something of the unconscious emotional life of the group (Holden 1990).

The role of DMT in the treatment of psychiatric patients is largely adjunctive, that is, it works in addition to several other sorts of treatment. For example, adult patients with depression may attend a community mental health centre, where they will be interviewed, diagnosed and followed up by a medically trained psychiatrist, who will probably prescribe anti-depressant medication. The psychiatrist may also give psychological help in the form of verbal therapy or counselling, or may refer the patient to a psychologist or psychotherapist for group or individual therapy. A psychiatric nurse may be assigned as key-worker, offering sessions of counselling, or behaviour modification therapy aimed at reducing the patient's symptoms. The patient will probably also attend some occupational therapy, which may involve structured activities aimed at raising his or her level of functioning, such as a social skills or discussion group, or perhaps a group which addresses practical and emotional issues in looking for work, particularly if the patient has been unemployed for some time. In addition to all this, the patient may attend an art, music, drama, or dance movement therapy group. The psychiatrist and nurses determine the amount and duration of the input which the mental health centre will give to the patient, and they will continually review and revise the treatment programme, excluding different elements as the patient improves. These methods of treatment apply to all of the different types of mental illness: schizophrenia, personality disorders, depression, problems with anxiety, agoraphobia and anorexia, as well as psychological difficulties encountered by people who suffer trauma or sexual abuse. Mental illness itself is defined in terms of the patient's subjective emotional distress, the degree of impairment in the patient's relations with family and friends, and his or her ability to function in social roles within the community, the family, employment or education.

In terms of the overall psychiatric treatment of the patient, dance movement therapy can contribute in several ways. Because it uses both verbal and nonverbal modes of interaction, it 'has been found to be especially effective in engaging patients whose capacity to participate in strictly verbal group therapy is limited' (Sandel and Johnson 1983: 134). DMT in psychiatry provides vital opportunities for patients to improve social functioning in a group which, because it is creative, offers a 'no fail' experience in which the patient can make small gains in functioning during the duration of the group's meetings. In the initial stages the patient may benefit most from the warmup phase of the group, which consists of therapist-led exercises aimed at reintegration of the nonverbal elements of the patient's behaviour, reconstructing an appropriate body image, and physically activating and motivating the patient. The feeling of physical well-being and alertness may also have a beneficial knock-on effect to other treatment the patient is receiving. Later, in the course of attending a dance movement therapy group, the patient may be able to use creative movement to safely release feelings of frustration and anger within the containing structure of the group (Schmais 1985: 21).

Finally, when dance movement therapy is used in a psychiatric facility, both the staff and patients develop a greater awareness of the nonverbal dimensions of health and illness. Nurses notice more in their intake observations of patients, and patients attempt to make more eye contact, or are able to self-monitor their nonverbal behaviour by using verbal reminders which can further be reinforced by staff. If a patient becomes aware of using a threatening, hunched posture and not making eye contact, and is helped to see the effect this has on others, he or she may be able to begin to develop more appropriate modes of nonverbal presentation in social situations.

Although this book will deal exclusively with psychiatric patients, DMT may also be used for people who are not mentally ill, but who wish to have therapy as a means of self-understanding and self-exploration. Work with this client group, usually seen in private practice, will not be discussed as it lies outside the scope of this book. A recent full-length study of this type of work may be found in Joan Chodorow's *Dance Therapy and Depth Psychology: The Moving Imagination* (Chodorow 1991). The focus here is quite specifically psychiatry, and so the many other client groups with whom dance movement therapists work will not be considered. Other clinical populations addressed by DMT include those with: autism, mental handicap, learning difficulties, physical handicap or illness (e.g. stroke and head injury patients); behavioural disturbances; conduct disorders including people in prison, drug and alcohol dependence; and elderly patients. For a study of DMT with these types of patients see Helen Payne's *Dance Movement Therapy: Theory and Practice* (Payne 1992).

There are important differences between dance movement therapy and other types of physical activity; and there are also differences between DMT and verbal therapy, which are important to clarify. In DMT, the aim is not to move more freely, or more perfectly, which may be the aim of therapeutic dance activities, but to use movement experimentation to explore new ways of being and feeling, and to gain access to feelings that cannot be verbalized. In therapeutic dance activities, the dance teacher uses specific dance movements to direct the patient to feel in a particular way (Lindner *et al*. 1979, Pasch 1982). The teacher may ask students to jump, or use their arms in a floating way to feel lively, or feel joyful, in contrast to the dance movement therapist who is non-directive, and neither prescribes the emotions the client is to express, nor instructs the client on how to move.

The dance movement therapist, unlike the dance teacher, has a specific knowledge of personality development, and is trained to elicit movement interaction with therapeutic benefit for the patient. Movement in DMT, aside from the warmup at the beginning, is impromptu, and is not corrected by the therapist, as it might be by a dance teacher. However, the therapist does provide a group structure in which the improvisation takes place. Marian Chace, one of the first dance movement therapists, developed a format in which patients form a circle, and follow or mirror each other's improvised movement phrases in turn (Chaiklin 1975). At the same time, the therapist may ask questions about the quality of the movement, or ask the group to put an image to the movement or to describe its quality in words. The resulting image, or metaphor, and any further movement may be evidence of unconscious processes in the group. This process is interpreted by the therapist, and discussed by the group at the end of the session. The DMT group process is essentially one that progresses from movement to image to interpretation (Stanton 1988). Clinical examples of this will be described in detail in Chapters 6, 7 and 8.

The skill of a dance movement therapist is a specialized one. It is similar to that of the art therapist who is trained to understand meaning in a patient's painting by analysing the colour, line, form, composition and symbolic meaning of the work. Most importantly, this understanding is used within the therapeutic relationship to initiate a new psychological insight for the patient. This is arrived at primarily through the special ability of the therapist to relate to the patient, and to help manage the emotional impact of the discovery of unconscious material which is revealed in part through the created art work, and in part by relating to the therapist. Similarly, in DMT, the therapist understands movement and the way it conveys meaning through its qualities in space, weight, time and flow, as well as its rhythm, shape and symbolic content. This understanding is communicated to the patient both through verbal comments and interpretations, and through the nonverbal responses of the dance movement therapist. All of this occurs in the context of the therapeutic relationship. In DMT, the aim is not to create any sort of dance; therefore, it is said to be 'process' rather than 'product' oriented: the psychological learning comes through the process of movement and interpretation within the therapeutic relationship, and not through producing a created choreographic work which would then be analysed.

Dance movement therapy versus body therapies

Dance movement therapy must be delineated from other types of activity which try to address both the psyche (meaning the soul, spirit, mind) and soma (the body). The array of movement systems which seek to effect change in people is great, including, for example, yoga, tai-chi, eurythmy (Steiner 1931, 1953), aerobics, massage, physiotherapy, kinesiology, chiropractic, rehabilitative movement, progressive relaxation, psychomotoric therapy (Pesso 1969), bioenergetics (Lowen 1976), Rolfing (Rolf 1963) and many others. The differences between these systems can be understood by asking three questions. First: What is the overall aim of the endeavour? Second: What is the underlying theoretical basis of the work? This may be spiritual, practical, existential, or psychological. Finally: What type of movement is being employed? Is it movement aimed at expression, at achieving an aesthetic ideal, or at improving the person's overall ability to do a particular movement? In the case of yoga, tai-chi and eurythmy, one might say that special forms of movement are being performed in order to reach a spiritual goal, such as enlightenment, or awareness of God. In aerobics, massage, physiotherapy, kinesiology, chiropractic and rehabilitative movement, the aims centre on being able to achieve a level or standard of performance of a specific movement, whether that would mean doing a hundred stride-jumps or strengthening damaged muscles. The psychological feeling of well-being in these systems might be seen as a secondary benefit. In the case of psychomotoric therapy, bioenergetics and Rolfing, prescribed movement is being utilized to achieve a specific psychological effect.

DMT, as described in this book, is not the same as Rolfing or bioenergetics, which has been developed by Alexander Lowen, a pupil of Wilhelm Reich, the early radical psychoanalyst. These 'body therapies' or 'bodywork systems' actively manipulate the body through prescribed movement exercises and massage designed to undo areas of muscular holding which are assumed to represent maladaptive ego defence mechanisms. For example, breathing exercises or strong massage might be applied to the chest area in order to release the muscular holding or 'armouring' thought to represent repressed feelings of need or longing (Reich 1933, Schmais 1974: 9). Such methods are not generally used with psychiatric patients, but with private clients. The adherents of Reich and Lowen claim success in their methods, though their critics say that these intensive methods smash down the defences of patients or clients too quickly. This may leave them vulnerable to the intensity of their own feelings, and without the supportive therapeutic relationship to learn other ways of coping with the strong emotions released through such methods.

In contrast, DMT works on eventually helping the person to develop more helpful ways of defending against anxiety or emotional pain, but this is achieved: by relating to others on a nonverbal level in the group movement; by gently uncovering feelings through symbols; and in the context of a longer-term relationship to the therapist, in which the effects of these changes can be worked through. Dance movement therapists are familiar with the ideas of Reich regarding ways in which the body shows evidence of emotional conflict, but their methods of addressing these issues differ greatly from those developed by the bioenergetics school. While body therapies prescribe or direct the movement, and actively manipulate the body, dance movement therapy employs self-directed movement as the type of movement most consistent with its therapeutic goals (Levy 1988: 34).

Dance movement therapy versus verbal therapy

The relation of DMT to verbal psychotherapy is complex. While dance movement therapists rely on some of the same theories of personality and interpersonal functioning as psychotherapists, the way in which they approach the patient is very different. Being a dance movement therapist does not imply adherence to any particular therapeutic school. There are Freudian, Jungian, Adlerian, Gestalt, psychoanalytic and psychodynamically influenced dance movement therapists. As Sharon Chaiklin points out, 'differences in theoretical conceptualizations may alter the style or technique [of DMT], but the underlying movement theories are inclusive. Dance therapy offers an alternative method for working within the context of any systematized theory of human behaviour' (Chaiklin 1975). Dance movement therapists believe that working creatively with body movement can address important areas of emotional functioning which would be more difficult to access using solely verbal therapy (Silberstein 1987: 147).

Some verbal therapists do occasionally employ various types of body movement, but these are seen as adjuncts to a primarily verbal intervention (Perls 1973, Pesso 1969, Weitz 1979). The relation between psychotherapy and dance movement therapy is further complicated by the fact that some dance movement therapists, many of whom later train as verbal psychotherapists, view their use of

movement as a nonverbal illustration of specific principles of verbal psychotherapy. For example, Mary Whitehouse, a dance movement therapist influenced
by her Jungian analysis, sees 'some passages of body movement as Active Imagination in sensory terms ('the flow of unconscious material coming out in physical
form')' (Schmais 1974: 9). Active Imagination is a Jungian concept in which
conscious and unconscious elements are activated during the creative experience
(Chodorow 1984). Some dance movement therapists (many of whom have no
further training in verbal psychotherapy) selectively use methods and ideas derived
from verbal therapy, and some feel that their work should be described as 'movement psychotherapy'. In the view of the present author, dance movement therapy
is not verbal psychotherapy with movement added. The integration of movement
with psychological insight makes it a different therapeutic tool, which, while
having similar aims to other forms of psychotherapy, is distinct from them. It
belongs most correctly to the category of the arts therapies, alongside music, art
and dramatherapy. DMT can be most accurately defined as psychotherapeutically
informed therapeutic work. It is not psychotherapy proper, but it is a method by
which interpersonal and intrapsychic issues can begin to be addressed.

Dance movement therapists who have not undergone verbal therapy training,
or even personal verbal psychotherapy, sometimes find themselves in difficulty
when attempting to work at the same level as those who have. This is particularly
the case when working with transference or countertransference phenomena, or
making interpretations based on these concepts. Transference reactions are 'unconscious drives, feelings, attitudes, fantasies and defences that patients have toward
their therapists. These reactions are repetitions of past relationships with significant
others' (Dosamantes-Alperson 1987: 209, Freud 1924). The issue of how deeply
dance movement therapists should work in the transference will be discussed
further in the clinical sections of this book, which show how DMT theory is put
into practice.

In general, the differences between DMT and verbal psychotherapy are as
follows. First, dance movement therapists place great importance on the value of
the patient being able to integrate the psychological and physical aspects of
experience, and they see movement as the best means to achieve that integration.
Secondly, they are committed to the view that creativity can promote psychological
health. Thirdly, dance movement therapists make different claims about what their
therapy can do for a patient. Dance movement therapy does not aim to restructure
the personality or to understand how the patient's current illness may have had its
roots in childhood. Where the psychoanalyst's role is to help patients gain insight
into their personality and relationships by allowing the patients to transfer feelings
that they had towards their parents onto the analyst, the dance movement therapist
does not use this transference phenomenon to anywhere near the same degree. In
contrast, dance movement therapy's primary aims are: first, to help patients use
movement to re-connect the psychological and physical aspects of emotional
experience; secondly, to use movement interaction in group process to raise the

level of interpersonal functioning; and, thirdly, to employ creative movement as an access to unconscious feelings within the individuals and the group.

A further difference between DMT and verbal psychotherapy is the way in which each uses the contents of the unconscious. Broadly speaking, the verbal psychoanalyst is interested in unconscious determinants of neurotic symptoms, its role in the formation of sexuality and personality, and in manifestations of the unconscious in the transference relationship to the analyst. In contrast, DMT concerns itself with the creative aspects of the unconscious; that is, with the symbolic expression of emotions through movement and imagery which arise from the patient's unconscious. DMT gains access to the unconscious through allowing the patient to free associate, using both verbal and nonverbal channels. DMT capitalizes on the propensity of the unconscious to make new and unexpected connections between ideas, movement and imagery. The awareness of the unconscious contents (such as emotions, sensations, fantasies and images) and their integration into the patient's consciousness is probably the primary psychotherapeutic type of benefit of DMT. By contrast, the psychoanalyst uncovers repressed unconscious contents through dreams, childhood memories, and the reactions of the patient to the analyst, in order to effect a restructuring of the patient's personality through the transformative potential of the analytical relationship. While there is some overlap between the therapeutic use of unconscious phenomena in DMT and in verbal psychotherapy, there is a fundamental difference of emphasis and technique in working with powerful material that can be generated by unconscious aspects of the psyche.

A further difference between DMT and verbal psychotherapy is in the depth and quality of change which each approach offers to the patient. These differences can be related to the relative length of training which each practice requires. While many psychoanalytic psychotherapists spend five or more years in postgraduate training, dance movement therapists (after finishing a Bachelor of Arts degree in Psychology or Dance) spend approximately two years training at a postgraduate level. Where personal therapy for the trainee verbal psychotherapist is seen to be an essential core of the training, personal therapy is considered to be quite important in DMT, but not wholly central to the training. There are impending changes in dance movement therapy postgraduate education (and in professional accreditation in the UK) which may make personal therapy mandatory for trainee dance movement therapists, but at present this is not the case. In the next section, in which approaches in DMT are described, it will be noted that some senior practitioners, after doing a DMT training course, then go on to train as verbal psychoanalysts or psychotherapists. This means that they are able to work on as deep a level as the longer-trained verbal psychotherapists. Finally, the amount of time a patient spends in verbal therapy is usually far greater than that spent with the dance movement therapist, at least in public service sectors, and this must influence the degree of change in the patient which is possible using DMT.

In conclusion, it will be clear that DMT is neither a verbal therapy with movement added, nor a 'movement psychotherapy', if that term implies that the therapist works to fundamentally restructure or at least change the patient's personality, or remove neurotic symptoms by working in the transference (Dosamantes-Alperson 1987). DMT represents an innovative therapeutic approach which is unique because it addresses the body/mind problem by combining movement experience and psychological theory. In summary,

> dance therapists see the attributes and dynamics of dance and movement as uniquely suited for the expression of the unconscious along with id, ego, and superego expression, in addition to providing a framework for relationship building and body image and personality development.
>
> (Levy 1988: 13)

The next section will describe the theoretical foundation which underlies the therapeutic goals of DMT.

FIVE THEORETICAL PRINCIPLES

Dance movement therapy rests on five essential theoretical principles. The first is that 'body and mind are in constant reciprocal interaction' (Schoop 1974: 44). Therefore, 'significant changes occur on the movement level that can affect total functioning' (Schmais 1974: 10). In practice, this means that the dance movement therapist is constantly encouraging patients to connect verbal insight with movement experience, both by encouraging free association and by interpreting the ongoing movement.

The second assumption is that movement reflects personality. Dance movement therapists utilize a range of psychological theories that support this point. Freud said 'the ego is first and foremost a body ego' (Freud 1923). Freud's follower, Wilhelm Reich, concluded that body posture, gesture and movement all evidence our defensive warding off of feelings of aggression, sexuality and anxiety. He further felt that the body shows the scars of childhood trauma, as though it held a memory of which the mind was unaware (Reich 1933). The psychoanalyst Judith Kestenberg has made detailed studies of how Freud's ideas about the psychosexual development of the child, through oral, anal and phallic stages, can be seen in movement (Kestenberg 1975, Stanton 1991b).

Furthermore, many psychotherapists also hold the theory that an early mother–infant interaction is crucial in the formation of the personality (Miller *et al.* 1989, Segal 1964). This first important relationship is primarily a nonverbal event (Stern 1985). Dance movement therapy capitalizes on the nonverbal dimension of personality development by using the technique of mirroring the patient's movement. Mirroring recapitulates an important developmental psychological process: 'as children, we learn who we are by experiencing ourselves through the reactions of others' (Kaplan-Westbrook and Sing 1988, Kornblum 1982, Leventhal 1980, Naess 1982, Schmais 1974: 11, Wilson-Hagen 1988).

In addition to these developmental principles, DMT uses other aspects of nonverbal behaviour which reflect personality. Research suggests that movement can illustrate psychopathology (Davis 1981), or socially conditioned elements of the personality (Scheflen and Scheflen 1972). More broadly, other writers, including those on aesthetics, dance criticism and philosophy, contend that self and the body are uniquely related, particularly in the context of the artistic process. Some argue that movement, specifically dance, may be deeply and puzzlingly related to both self-knowledge and self-transformation (Sparshott 1988).

A third principle of DMT is that the relationship of the dance movement therapist to the patient is central to the effectiveness of the approach. In DMT, 'the relationship established between the therapist and patient through movement supports and enables behavioral change' (Schmais 1974: 10). In contrast to psychotherapy in which the therapist's responses to the patient are primarily verbal, the dance movement therapist responds by mirroring, synchronizing, amplifying and interacting with the patient's movement. This means that the relationship is a powerful one, and necessitates supervision and support for the therapist (Sandel 1980). In practice, this means that DMT is a useful intervention for patients who are so ill or so regressed that they are inaccessible to verbal therapeutic intervention (Schoop and Mitchell 1979, Wilson-Hagen 1988). DMT may also be effective for those who are heavily defended in verbal therapy, since it attempts to use the body as a means to access unconscious feeling. Interestingly, trained dancers are said to be able to defend themselves in movement terms; instead of allowing movement to give expression to unconscious material, they can, through use of practised form and style, avoid such expression in the manner that patients in verbal therapy are said to defend themselves through intellectualization in words.

A fourth theoretical principle is that movement, like dreams, drawings, squiggles (Winnicott 1971), slips of the tongue and free association, can be evidence of the unconscious (Davis 1974). The 'unconscious' is defined as those contents of the mind that are not present in the field of conscious awareness, and include ideas, feelings and images that have been repressed (Ellenberger 1970, Laplanche and Pontalis 1973: 474). The contents of the unconscious are believed to represent primitive, instinctual, or infantile aspects of the personality. The approach developed by the present author in Chapter 9 stresses the central importance of the symbols and metaphors that are articulated by the patient during the movement therapy process. These symbols are essential vehicles for gaining access to the contents of the patient's unconscious, and for aiding in reintegrating unconscious feelings into awareness. The process which unfolds from movement to symbol to interpretation is a mechanism for therapeutic change.

A fifth and final principle is that the act of creating a movement through improvisation is inherently therapeutic since it allows the individual to experiment with novel ways of moving, which generate a new experience of being-in-the-world. The therapeutic value of creativity has been articulated in psychological theories of creativity, which underlie the arts therapies (Kubie 1958).

These theories support the notion that the medium of dance, like that of painting, sculpture, music and drama, draws upon the unconscious as a source of creative inspiration. As such, the arts 'afford vicarious fantasy gratification of unsatisfied [unconscious] wishes in a sublimated, that is, socially acceptable form' (Kreitler and Kreitler 1972: 7). Furthermore, art, like dreams, takes unconscious material and renders it into symbol. For example, the image of a violent thunderstorm might be used in a painting to represent rage and destructiveness. The act of painting allows the artist to create a symbol. In therapy, the patient makes symbolic communications in a similar way, and with the therapist's help comes to understand what the feelings that inspired the symbol might be. In therapy, unlike in art, the symbols are created primarily as a way to get back to their unconscious source, in the hope that the feelings from the unconscious can be brought to awareness and integrated into the personality, instead of being acted out destructively in real life. In a group dance movement therapy session in which the patients create an image, such as walking through a thunderstorm, they might use movements with strong or aggressive qualities to symbolize the lightning, thunder and wind; discussing later the feelings that doing these strong movements provoked would allow them to acknowledge both the sources and targets of their anger. This could provide a way of dealing with angry feelings more productively: rather than occasionally flying off into a rage without warning, they can be aware of what makes them angry, and release some of the energy of their unconscious anger through using the symbol of the thunder and lightning, thereby processing some stormy or unpredictable emotions.

These assumptions about the unconscious sources of creativity are important for dance movement therapy. Creativity, considered in this way, can be defined as the 'capacity to find new and unexpected connections . . . to find new relationships in time and space, and thus new meanings' (Kästner 1988, Kubie 1958: 141).

The five theoretical principles that underly DMT can be summarized as follows:

1 The mind and the body are in constant complex reciprocal interaction.
2 Movement reflects aspects of the personality, including psychological developmental processes, psychopathology, expressions of subjectivity and interpersonal patterns of relating.
3 The therapeutic relationship established between the patient and the dance movement therapist is central to the effectiveness of DMT.
4 Movement evidences unconscious processes, in a manner similar to dreams and other psychological phenomena.
5 The creative process embodied in the use of free association in movement is inherently therapeutic.

The next chapter will examine the early work of dance movement therapists with psychiatric patients. It will be evident that the early practitioners evolved methods of working which stress one or more of these five theoretical principles to a greater or lesser degree.

Chapter 2

History of dance movement therapy in psychiatry

HISTORICAL ANTECEDENTS

Dance movement therapy is a late twentieth-century phenomenon. It has been formed by concurrent developments in modern dance and psychology. This chapter will describe briefly two of the first dance movement therapists who were concerned with psychiatry, namely, Marian Chace and Francizka Boas. Brief mention will also be made of the work of Mary Whitehouse, Trudi Schoop and Alma Hawkins. Most of their work was done in the 1940s and 1950s. They were not trained as therapists, but were dance teachers, encouraged by psychiatrists to use the communicative power of their art to make contact with patients from closed wards, many of whom were not amenable to verbal therapy. Before describing each of these early practitioners' work in detail, it is important to situate their work in its historical context.

Dance is continually evolving, and changes from decade to decade as cultural shifts occur in conceptions of fine art, ritual and bodily expression. A wide variety of functions has therefore been attributed to dance. Primitive societies stress the role of dance in rituals, such as rites of passage, or ceremonies designed to appease frightening gods and to worship benevolent ones. The ancient Greeks viewed certain forms of dance as cathartic, or healing, because they allowed for a powerful release of emotion. Later, the eighteenth-century aestheticians viewed courtly dances as perfect mirrors for their conceptions of celestial order, and as supportive proof for the connection between the beauty and truth of the rule of the monarch, and that of the heavenly universe. Radical changes in popular dance, such as those which occurred in the 1960s, were a nonverbal illustration of popular culture's concerns with a new freedom from old-established codes, changes in sex roles, and experimentation in expanding consciousness through the use of drugs or meditation. Recent work on the philosophy of dance illustrates how what we understand as 'dance' is intimately connected with culturally laden concepts of intention and will, mind and body, desire and inhibition (Sparshott 1988).

At the turn of the century, dance as fine art, represented almost solely by ballet, 'had deteriorated, some believed, into empty technical display' (Levy 1988: 2). In the early part of this century, radical shifts in dance occurred in tandem with other major social and intellectual movements, such as the advent of widespread indus-trialization and the emancipation of women, as well as cultural movements such as expressionism, futurism, cubism and dadaism. The values extolled by early proponents of modern dance therefore included 'spontaneity, authenticity of indi-vidual expression, awareness of the body, themes that stressed a whole range of feelings and relationships. The great pioneers of its early years personified themes of human conflict, despair, frustration and social crisis' (Bartenieff 1975: 246).

Fran Levy, in her authoritative history, *Dance/Movement Therapy: A Healing Art*, illustrates fully the major impact which modern dance had on the early dance movement therapists. DMT would have been unthinkable without the artistic and choreographic ideas that centred on direct emotional expression and abandoned formalism. Isadora Duncan (1878–1927), viewed by some as the original founder of modern dance in America, expressed views which contemporary Jungian dance movement therapists would still find sympathetic to their approach:

> In my dance, the artifices of dancing are thrown aside, the great Rhythms of Life are enabled to play through the physical instrument, the profundities of con-sciousness are given a channel to the light of our social day. These profundities of consciousness are in us all.
>
> (Rosemont 1981: 51)

Other systems of modern dance, such as the Denishawn school, formed by Ruth St Denis and Ted Shawn, turned to Eastern culture to express ideas about spirituality. They were to inspire Martha Graham and Doris Humphrey, who in turn inspired Marian Chace, the woman commonly regarded as the primary founder of dance movement therapy (Bernstein 1979). In Europe, the dance of Mary Wigman exemplified the authenticity of personal expression and the rebellion against formal structure so essential to modern dance. Wigman's work can be seen as an example of 'inner dance', which is inspired by subjective emotion, rather than dictated by particular steps (Levy 1988: 5). Her work, and that of her contemporary, Rudolf Laban, had a formative impact on the ideas of the other major early dance movement therapists, particularly Mary Whitehouse and Francizka Boas, who will be considered presently. Laban was a Hungarian pioneer of modern dance, theory, notation and technique. He

> insisted that in the human body there is a three-fold unity: body, mind and spirit. Each of these is movement-related and interdependent and throughout there is a two-way process in operation: we feel, we think, and that affects and effects body movement; we move in a certain way and that affects and effects outlook and thought. It is well-nigh impossible to walk tall and open and feel 'down', or to move in a slovenly, round shouldered fashion and have a healthy, positive outlook.
>
> (Hodgson and Preston-Dunlop 1990: 17)

During the first half of this century, there were also new developments in psychiatry and psychoanalysis, and a continuing refinement of interest in nonverbal aspects of psychology and psychopathology. Scientific study of movement had begun in the late nineteenth century with the publication of Darwin's *The Expression of the Emotions in Man and Animals*, which examined the origins and functions of facial and bodily expression. Darwin had solicited the views of doctors at a London asylum on the facial expressions and body movements of mental patients (Davis 1975). In so doing, he tapped a trend in early diagnosis of mental illness which included looking at the shape of the patient's body, and the movements that patients made during stages of acute illness. Eugen Bleuler in Switzerland, Jean-Martin Charcot in France and Henry Maudsley in England meticulously observed their patients' bizarre movements, fits, sterotypies and gestures. They did this in the hope that they could turn these phenomena into clear diagnostic criteria that could help predict the course of the disease 'dementia praecox', now known as schizophrenia. They would then be able to differentiate it from categories such as 'mania', 'melancholia' (now known as depression) and 'hysteria' (Bleuler 1950, Manschreck *et al*. 1982, Simon-Dhouailly 1986).

In the 1920s and 1930s, in both Europe and America, studies on emotion and its physical expression continued (Davis 1975: 14). By the 1950s, such studies became more sophisticated, using analogies not of animal instinct or motor discharge to explain expressive behaviour, but rather, likening nonverbal interchange between people to structural linguistics (Birdwhistell 1970: 128).

During the same period, psychoanalytic ideas gained a wider audience, both within intellectual circles and in psychiatric practice. Freud, Jung and Adler were, of course, major figures (Ellenberger 1970). Also important for dance movement therapy were the ideas of the American psychiatrist Harry Stack Sullivan, who attempted to integrate Freudian and Adlerian ideas into the treatment of schizophrenia. Sullivan was, along with Frieda Fromm-Reichmann and others, a founder of the psychodynamic psychiatry movement (Fromm-Reichmann 1960, Karon and Vandenbos 1981, Sullivan 1940). Marian Chace found support for her work in Sullivan's ideas, in valuing the attempt to make honest and direct contact with schizophrenics, and trying to understand their bizarre behaviour as a valuable, if distorted, form of communication.

After the Second World War, psychiatric services were challenged to provide therapy for large numbers of returning war veterans. Many methods were tried and developed, including abreaction using drugs. This method involved administering drugs, such as barbiturates, while the patient was still partly conscious, so that they could, when prompted, recall repressed traumatic memories and thereby remove their influence on the personality. Electro-shock treatment, and psychosurgery, such as leucotomy, were also developed (Sargant 1957). Such drastic measures were eventually replaced by moderate amounts of medication in combination with group or individual therapy. During this period, in both England and America, the need to rehabilitate large numbers of soldiers to function socially, in family and work groups, gave rise to innovative approaches which form the basis of modern group psychotherapy (Bion 1961: 12).

There were other influences which also contributed to the continuing success of dance movement therapy, after the work of the early pioneers. The first was the dramatic increase in interest in nonverbal communications research which took place in the late 1950s and continued throughout the 1960s and 1970s (Davis 1975). This was inspired in part by developments in film technology and by cross-cultural anthropological studies which, perhaps because they lacked access to indigenous languages, focused on the nonverbal dimensions of culture. Secondly, the early 1960s saw a massive increase in popular therapies, especially encounter groups and training groups (Yalom 1970: x). Many of these were concerned with interaction, and they found that the use of nonverbal exercises involving body movement

> led to heightened awareness of themselves and others, increased their ability to express affect and engage in more empathetic relationships. Movement experience became highly valued in developing sensitivity and reducing defensive behaviour.
>
> (Schmais 1974: 8)

In conclusion, it can be seen that both societal and cultural changes, coupled with new innovations in modern dance and in psychological treatment, provided the ground which nurtured dance movement therapy.

MARIAN CHACE

Marian Chace (1896–1970) is commonly acknowledged as the founder of dance movement therapy and her theory and method have had a strong influence on subsequent generations of dance movement therapists, including Sharon Chaiklin, Dianne Dulicai, Dianne Fletcher, Susan Sandel and others, some of whom will be discussed in the next chapter (Levy 1988: 278–281). Chace studied with the Denishawn school, and taught modern dance from the early 1920s until the early 1940s, when she began experimenting with what she then called 'dance for communication' (Chaiklin 1975: 12). She was influenced by Sullivan's ideas on psychiatry which stressed that personality was formed through relationships, and so she set out to use the interactive dimension of dance therapeutically.

She worked at St Elizabeth's Hospital in Washington DC, and at the innovative Chestnut Lodge Sanatorium from the early 1940s, where Sullivan's ideas were being used and where Frieda Fromm-Reichmann developed her innovative work with schizophrenics by modifying traditional psychoanalytic practice (Fromm-Reichmann 1960, Green 1964, Greenberg 1974, Levy 1988: 23). Towards the end of her career, Chace helped organize the American Dance Therapy Association, and was its first president in 1966. She never formalized her work into a full-length study, though her papers have since been collected and published (Chaiklin 1975). Chace trained a number of important second-generation therapists, including Claire Schmais and Sharon Chaiklin (Chaiklin and Schmais 1979, Schmais and Felber 1977, Schmais 1974, 1981, 1985, 1986). She developed a number of methods that are still in use today, examples of which will be described in the clinical section of this book. Six aspects of Chace's work will be considered here: her development of a structure for group interaction, her use of group rhythmic activity, the value of movement in integration, the technique of mirroring, the importance she placed on the therapist–patient relationship, and her use of symbolism.

Chace's primary technical contribution

Chace began her sessions on the psychiatric wards by engaging patients in some small nonverbal interaction, and gradually encouraging them to group into a circle, where they would do some warmup movements together. Then, the central section would consist of a shared leadership format, in which each member of the group initiated an impromptu movement and the rest of the group mirrored or followed. This shared leadership structure forms the basis for organized group interaction and is still extremely valuable in work with psychiatric patients. Chace would comment verbally on the quality of the movement, eliciting and suggesting imagery to accompany it. She asked the group questions about the movement, in order to gain access to their ideas and impressions. This verbal intervention often had the effect of altering or enhancing the movement. This central section of the session frequently contained a few specific shared group themes, which the therapist brought to the group's awareness. The session ended with a closure section which consisted of a shared rhythmic movement and some brief communal discussion of what the group had done that day.

The power of rhythm to structure and organize a number of individuals into a group is one that Chace took from 'primitive dance'. She said that 'even primitive man understood that a group of people moving together gained a feeling of more strength and security than any one individual could feel alone' (Chaiklin 1975: 54). Rhythm fulfils two roles in movement: it structures the action of an individual, and it facilitates a feeling of connection to the group. Whether a group is rocking gently together or stamping energetically, the rhythm enables them to share a group experience. They do not need to have the same shape in space (in the manner of marching soldiers), as long as they share a common rhythm to their movement. Rhythm can enable the patient to develop and maintain his or her own integrity while accepting social influences. This special sense of belonging to a group is one of the major therapeutic factors in group psychotherapy (Yalom 1970: 70). Furthermore, the patient can channel energy within the structure of the rhythm, and gain a sense of personal vitality (Chaiklin and Schmais 1979: 21).

For Chace, movement was communicative, but it also had an effect on the patient in other respects. She wrote:

> Since muscular activity expressing emotion is the substratum of dance, and since dance is a means of structuring and organizing such activity, it might be supposed that dance could be a potent means of communication for the reintegration of the seriously ill mental patient.
>
> (Chaiklin 1975: 71)

Movement does have an integrating effect on the patient, and this can help to reduce confusion and apathy and engender a sense of mental clarity. 'Body action' of this type also helps to create a realistic body image, mobilize the patient's energy, and expand the expressive range of both movement and emotion (Chaiklin and Schmais 1979: 21). It is important to note that Chace did not achieve these goals by *directing* patients to move in a particular fashion; rather, she used the inherent organizing principles of dance (such as rhythm and the spatial arrangement of a circle) to allow the patients' *self-directed* movement to work to maximum therapeutic effect.

Chace developed the technique of mirroring the patients' movement, which became useful in achieving many goals of DMT, including establishing an empathetic relationship, engendering an interaction, and extending an unconscious theme in movement. Mirroring is not simply imitating or mimicking the patients' movement; it is a sympathetic reflection, and a structure in which interaction can take place. Chace's knowledge of dance enabled her to extract the quality of the movement and subtly extend it, or take it to a conclusion. This broadened the patients' expressive movement potential, because their movement altered as they interacted with her. Mirroring also elicits more movement, and promotes movement dialogue.

The process of reflecting the patient nonverbally in order to foster a sense of acceptance and trust is one that is paralleled in many forms of verbal therapy in which the therapist rephrases the patient's statements, or uses the patient's own words (Rogers 1951). This process also has parallels in child development, wherein the mother's nonverbal synchrony and harmony with the child fosters an early sense of identity, and is the language whereby the child comes to comprehend both self and other (Stern 1985, Winnicott 1971b).

Chace was influenced by Sullivan's views on the importance of repairing the damaged relationships of the mentally ill person, and therefore placed the patient–therapist relationship at the heart of her approach (Sullivan 1956: 361). Within this relationship, a sense of trust could be rebuilt, and possibly foster interest in other relationships. This is a crucial factor in schizophrenia, which is characterized by a general withdrawal from human contact (American Psychiatric Association 1987). Chace entered the world of the patient by recreating their movement behaviour through her own body. This was initially necessary for patients who would not or did not speak, but this movement interaction, or nonverbal relationship, remains essential to all forms of dance movement therapy.

Finally, central to Chace's approach is her use of symbolism, both verbal and nonverbal. She said that

> schizophrenics, in particular, seem at home with the symbolic language of movement, whereas they often cannot communicate through words, nor benefit from verbal interpretations. The camouflage of the movement symbol makes it easier for these patients to express needs, feelings and desires.
>
> (Chaiklin and Schmais 1979: 17)

Dance, as a physical expression of an emotional state and as a mode of interpersonal communication, is therefore, in its very essence, symbolic. Chace believed that, even when a patient was not able to verbalize the symbolic dance action that had occurred in a session, by adding verbal symbols or language, his or her problems could sometimes still be worked-through on a movement level alone. This is because the therapist mirrors the patient's movement, which allows the patient to feel understood. This, in turn, enables the patient to continue symbolic statements in movement, and, later, possibly add words. Chace would often suggest imagery to go with a patient's movement, if that imagery was not spontaneous. The understanding of the symbols, and the reintegration of their meaning into consciousness, thus provide a powerful agent for therapeutic change.

Despite the lack of formal theorization in Chace's work, she took the expressive, symbolic, integrative and interactive elements of dance, and merged them into a unique form of therapy. Her work provides an essential basis for almost all of the later work in DMT in psychiatry. In addition to being a major influence on Claire Schmais, Chace's ideas and methods have subsequently inspired many other dance movement therapists, including Susan Sandel, Diane Fletcher and Arlene Avstreih, who have integrated a more formal psychotherapy theory with Chace's techniques and systemized their use in DMT (Brown and Avstreih 1980, Fletcher 1974, Sandel and Johnson 1983). Claire Schmais is a major figure in DMT, and could easily be profiled here along with other early dance movement therapists such as Trudi Schoop and Alma Hawkins. However, her major contribution has been to group DMT, and so her work is described in the second part of Chapter 3, which considers group approaches to DMT.

DMT group approaches, as described in this book, are fundamentally based in the shared leadership format developed by Chace in her early work in psychiatry. The symbolic approach described in Chapter 9 is essentially the addition of psychodynamic group theory to Chace's methodology, with special emphasis on the symbols, imagery and metaphor which arise in that context.

FRANCIZKA BOAS

Francizka Boas taught creative modern dance to children at Bellevue Psychiatric Hospital in New York during the 1940s (Levy 1988: 107). She incorporated into her work ideas from her colleagues Lauretta Bender, a child psychiatrist, and Paul Schilder, a psychoanalyst and psychiatrist who wrote the seminal work *The Image and Appearance of the Human Body* (Schilder 1950). Although she did not work with adult psychiatric patients, her ideas are a useful inspiration for DMT with both child and adult psychiatric patients because she combined her personal experience of psychoanalysis – together with other psychoanalytic concepts – with dance in her treatment of both child psychiatry patients and other dancers in her studio (Bender 1952, Bender and Boas 1941, Boas 1989).

As a modern dancer of her time, Boas was influenced by Mary Wigman and Bird Larson. She said: 'I make no separation between dance as an art and dance as a therapy. Every art has a therapeutic effect on both the artist and on the observer' (Boas 1989: 28). She used music, specifically percussion instruments, as part of her approach, and found that rhythm was a good means to channel emotion. She speculated that 'the sensory impression of the percussive beat may have a deep psychological influence. Furthermore, rhythmic sound tends to invite even the most resistant children into a participation and often acts as a safety guard for feelings' (Levy 1988: 113).

Boas made interesting connections between psychoanalytic concepts and modern dance techniques. For example, she understood Schilder's concept of the body image and used this in her therapeutic work with children. Body image, as defined by Schilder, is the picture of the body that is formed in the mind, constituted from sensory impressions, the immediate experience of the body, and past memories of bodily sensations and experiences (Schilder 1950: 11). Boas thought that the body image, as conceived by Schilder, could be altered through movement exploration. Schilder's belief that the way people move is a direct expression of their body image prompted her to use new movement experiences to alter the distorted body image that many of her psychiatric child cases displayed by their restricted movements.

She further thought that attempts at psychophysical integration could be hampered by patients' fears of a new experience of themselves. She wrote:

The feeling of his own physical strength and the ability to control and direct it is a stage the dancer reaches after having freed himself from anxiety and fear over the dynamic violence of primitive motility and its associated emotions. For the dancer, anxiety and fear of dynamic movement spring from insecurity in the concept of his own body image and from the resistance to consecutive changes in himself. Exploration of the dynamic power of movement brings to the fore instincts of self-preservation, destructive and constructive drives, and through their mastery brings about an understanding of these elements. In the case of successful sublimation it should lead to a feeling of security through a knowledge of the emotional sources underlying these drives, and therefore to their control.

(Boas 1952: 273)

At the Bellevue psychiatric hospital at the time Boas worked there, a number of new projective psychological tests were being developed. In these, an individual's thoughts and feelings are projected onto an external object. For example, in a Rorschach test, a person is asked to state what an ink blot-type pattern might represent. This is then taken as evidence of unconscious processes of the mind, and is compared with the answers of a large number of other subjects, whose answers constitute a standard of responses against which each new respondent is compared. Boas used imagery with children to this same effect. She employed the idea of animals, for example, with which children could, in movement and words, action and story, contact their unconscious fantasy material and so reintegrate it into awareness.

Boas used movement with the disturbed children to encourage the verbalization of fantasies. Her aims were 'improved motility, integrated with the acknowledgement, acceptance, and development of the concomitant psychic fantasies' (Levy 1988: 113). Interestingly, many dance movement therapists report that the memories that come up spontaneously during dance movement therapy sessions are often very useful for patients (Bernstein 1979).

Perhaps most significant for later dance movement therapists is the fact that Boas developed the concept of 'psychomotor free association during dance' (Levy 1988: 115). In her work with adult dancers, she encouraged them to move, with eyes closed, so that they were not performing, but sensing the movement. She asked them to move only when inner impulse or thought appeared. She noted that:

> There is a logic in the development of one movement into another both in the body and in the use of space. To the trained observer any interjection of an arbitrary movement can immediately be discerned. This is a sign of a break in concentration and usually takes the form of some habitual movement pattern which the pupil considers 'safe', that is, either it covers up the externalization of a 'forbidden' fantasy or sensation, or it prevents exploration into the unknown.
>
> (Boas 1952: 273)

Finally, Boas differentiated between active, self-directed, conscious movement that could be defensive, and 'passive movement' in which the movers allowed impulses to take them over, in an openness to both internal and external stimuli, with the movement coming from the unconscious parts of the self. In her work with children she used exercises on the floor which were 'a purposeful reversal to infantile movement' (Boas 1952: 273). Noting that the adult therapist and even the child had resistances to using such movement because each 'has been taught at some time that such activity is not proper', she concluded that allowing such regression in movement, a 'block or resistance is removed and the path is open for acceptance of the psychological content through sublimation in dance form' (Boas 1952: 273). In other words, Boas felt that, through creative dance exercises, the early, primitive part of the personality could be contacted. Through the structures of rhythm and the form of dance, these early feelings of anxiety, rage, or joy could be examined and, with the help of the therapist, reintegrated into the child's consciousness, thereby reducing destructive behaviour. In the case of disturbed children, having such feelings understood and worked through had the effect that their disturbed behaviour lessened, and psychological growth could begin to occur.

In conclusion, Boas made a remarkable early contribution to DMT with psychiatric patients, through articulating four fundamental concepts: first, that of psychomotor free association; secondly, the psychoanalytic reading of fantasy material engendered by movement; thirdly, the reconstruction of a healthy body image through new movement experience; fourthly and finally, the recognition that movement could also be evidence of a *defence* against emotion, as well as an *expression* of emotion.

OTHER EARLY DANCE MOVEMENT THERAPISTS

Mary Whitehouse

Mary Whitehouse (1911–1975) was a modern dance teacher working on the west coast of the USA during the early 1950s. She studied with Mary Wigman in Germany, and was strongly influenced by her own experience of Jungian psycho-analysis. She called her approach 'movement in depth', alluding to Jung and Bleuler's terminology, 'depth psychology', which 'denotes that branch of psychology which is concerned with the phenomena of the unconscious' (Samuels *et al.* 1986: 44). Her work has an important influence on Jungian dance movement therapists today working in the private sector with non-psychiatric patients, some-times termed 'normal neurotics'. Although she did not work with psychiatric patients, her work illustrates how Jungian thought can be combined with move-ment. Her theories, if not her techniques, support the use of spontaneous movement expression as a reflection of unconscious process, which is an important element of DMT in psychiatry.

Whitehouse described her work as 'physical movement as a revelation of the Self' (Bernstein 1979: 65). The Self in this context is an 'archetypal image of man's fullest potential and the unity of the personality as a whole' (Samuels *et al.* 1986: 135). For Whitehouse, authentic movement was a means to reach wholeness, or individuation, in which one recognizes one's true relation to oneself, to others and to the collective history of mankind.

Whitehouse's most important contribution was in asserting that movement experience could be used to access the unconscious, which contains the archetypes, the transformational elements of the psyche. In using spontaneous movement, a creative process is engendered which could be used to effect therapeutic aims. She used the Jungian term 'active imagination' to describe this process. Jung defined active imagination as 'dreaming with open eyes. At the outset one concentrates on a specific point, mood, picture or event, then allows a chain of associated fantasies to develop and gradually take on a dramatic character' (Samuels *et al.* 1986: 9). Whitehouse was responsible for adding movement to this list of types of creative experiences in which conscious and unconscious elements are combined. She said that

> the inner sensation, allowing the impulse to take the form of physical action, is active imagination in movement, just as following the visual image is active imagination in fantasy. It is here that the most dramatic psycho-physical connections are made available to consciousness.
>
> (Levy 1988: 65)

Whitehouse did not try to elicit this type of spontaneous movement and fantasy experience with psychiatric patients. She felt that her dance students (many of whom were also in verbal psychoanalysis) could tolerate less therapist direction and more psychic probing, whereas with psychiatric patients, 'due to a more fragile ego structure, greater stress needed to be placed on emotional support and providing patients with more structured forms of expressive movement' (Levy 1988: 61).

Trudi Schoop

Trudi Schoop used creative movement with disturbed hospitalized patients during the early 1940s. She wrote a full-length book entitled, *Won't you Join the Dance? A dancer's essay into the treatment of psychosis*. This is one of the few full-length books on DMT, and so Schoop must be included among the forerunners of contemporary DMT, though her work, which does not have a strong psychotherapeutic theory underlying it, would probably now be termed therapeutic dance, rather than DMT.

She worked with unmedicated psychotic, deluded patients, something that would be quite rare to see today, except in the early stages of admission to an acute ward. Perhaps because of the disorganized mental state of many of the patients, Schoop concluded an initial phase of free movement with a section in which she choreographed the material that had emerged. Unlike Chace, who used verbal interpretation to organize and understand the patient's movement and its emotional content, Schoop relied on choreographic integration in movement to achieve this reintegration.

Schoop's work, although more aligned to creative dance than to therapy, was important in that it was an early attempt to work with psychotic patients. She proved that movement could be used to re-educate the mentally ill in ways of expressing emotion by giving new movement experiences; structuring affect via rhythm, and using a planned movement reformulation of material which emerged after a phase of free movement. These clinical insights, which were undertaken without reference to a psychotherapeutic system of ideas, underline those particular elements of dance that are themselves of inherently therapeutic value to disturbed psychiatric patients.

Alma Hawkins

Alma Hawkins founded the dance movement therapy programme at the University of California at Los Angeles in the early 1960s, after having studied extensively with early modern dancers such as Doris Humphrey, as well as American followers of Mary Wigman. Although her primary focus is not in psychiatry, her humanistic psychological framework and academic commitment to dance have influenced dance movement therapists who work psychoanalytically with psychiatric patients, notably Erma Dosamantes-Alperson and Diane Fletcher, who will be discussed in the next chapter.

Hawkins' foci are on understanding the nature of the creative experience, and on exploring the relation of movement experience to cognition. Hawkins states: '. . . what I am trying to do is not *dancing*; rather we are stripping the experience down to the purest approach to movement. . . . The more I work, the more I see that movement and the body are related to perception' (Levy 1988: 92).

Hawkins' therapeutic approach is based on humanistic psychology, which takes psychological growth and development as its centre; she believes that 'man seeks creative and aesthetic experiences because they enrich him . . . help him become an integrated individual and help him feel in harmony with his world' (Levy 1988: 94). Consistent with her humanistic approach is her view that the therapist's role is that of a facilitator or guide who supports the individual in his or her search for self-realization.

She also uses imagery, which connects her work with that of Chace, Boas and Whitehouse. She uses imagery that is open ended, and allows for a self-directed response by the client. She said

> I began to work with imagery in dance classes in the early 1960s. Then when I started working with dance therapy I experimented with a wider range of imagery – personal, concrete, abstract. And in recent work I have worked in greater depth, especially in the use of imagery as a means of facilitating 'inner sensing' and the creative process.
>
> (Levy 1988: 94–95)

For Hawkins, the process of inner sensing, feeling and imagery within a creative experience are the primary therapeutic principles in DMT (Hawkins 1971). The process, which Hawkins calls 'inner sensing', may be likened to Boas's concept of listening to inner movement as a way to engender psychological insight.

COMMON THEMES IN EARLY DMT

This brief overview of early dance movement therapists – Marian Chace, Francizka Boas, Mary Whitehouse, Trudi Schoop and Alma Hawkins – illustrates a number of important issues. First, all of these founders of DMT were grounded in a modern dance tradition which stressed direct expression, and in their work they moved continually away from what was formally 'dance' towards varying degrees of 'spontaneous movement', aimed at expressing the inner emotional world of a person rather than performing to an aesthetic standard.

There remains a tension in this early work between wanting to teach the patient to move, in order to expand the expressive range, and wanting the movement to be self-directed. A compromise was reached by Chace, Boas and Hawkins by using some directive movement tasks in the warmup phase of their work, and allowing the main section of their sessions to be devoted to allowing unconscious 'inner' (Hawkins), 'authentic' (Whitehouse) or 'primitive' (Boas) parts of the psyche to inspire the movement.

The use that they made of this special type of movement in therapy depended on whether it was intended for forming relationships (Chace), releasing energy (Schoop), expressing drives (Boas), or allowing the unconscious to guide the movement (Whitehouse and Hawkins). All of the early women using dance in psychiatry concurred in seeing the importance of rhythm to organize and structure group and individual emotional experiences, and in feeling that imagery could be of therapeutic value.

Chace, Boas, Whitehouse, Schoop and Hawkins laid the technical and theoretical foundations for dance movement therapy. They discovered that movement revealed the unconscious, and they extracted specific elements of dance that proved integrative for patients. Each in their own way conceived that the role of the dance movement therapist was very different to that of teacher; the therapist reflected, interpreted and supported movement exploration, and also elicited and contained emotional experience in movement, and with words.

It is interesting to speculate how these early creators of dance movement therapy evolved away from dance and towards therapy. Even today, there are artists and community organizations who take pure dance into psychiatric hospitals with the aim of providing aesthetic experiences for patients. Perhaps the early DMT can be seen as a product of a period in which cultural ideas about dance as pure expression, coupled with new psychological theories about the unconscious and its expression, as well as the benefits of interaction, were combined with the particular vision of dance as an art form that was held by these women and those around them. The interaction of social, cultural and psychological elements with the use of dance as a fine art applied to psychiatric patients seems to have given rise to a new way of viewing dance and movement in a therapeutic context. By the early 1940s, Boas was able to write that

> dance is the expression of human fantasy and emotion using as its medium the motility of the body passing through space and time. This process of formulation of movement concerns itself not only with the form and action of the joints and muscles, but also with the subjective concept of the body, and with the body as seen and interpreted by the observer.
>
> (Boas cited in Bender 1952: 258)

The next chapter will look at the work of the second generation of dance movement therapists, and how they developed the ideas that were discovered during this early period in DMT in psychiatry.

Chapter 3

Theoretical approaches and current schools of practice of dance movement therapy in psychiatry

Part I: Work with individuals

INTRODUCTION

This chapter will provide brief highlights from a number of the established schools of practice of DMT and will illustrate the diversity of psychotherapy theory applied in the practice of DMT. It may seem to a new reader that these approaches – psychodynamic, Jungian, ego-psychoanalytic, Gestalt and group psychotherapy – are too disparate to form a coherent whole. However, it is the use of movement, specifically in its expressive, symbolic and integrative qualities, which provides the unifying element.

Each section below will discuss the aims of therapy and the different ways movement is used to achieve therapeutic goals, as well as the sorts of patients or clients for whom these methods are appropriate. Not all of these are examples drawn from work with psychiatric patients, but the reader can gain an idea of the current spectrum of DMT approaches, and also understand why some therapeutic goals and techniques are more appropriate to particular clinical populations than others.

It is essential that dance movement therapists who have set themselves the difficult task of effecting therapeutic change have 'a clear understanding of what psychotherapy means, as well as dance therapy in relation to psychotherapy, and a systematized concept of theory and principles of change relating to dance therapy and dynamic developmental human behaviour' (Chaiklin 1977: 27). Each psychotherapy theory provides a framework in which to view the underlying reasons why people behave as they do, and this usually relates to a way of understanding how personality develops, from infancy to childhood, through adolescence to adulthood and on to old age. Furthermore, each psychotherapy theory provides models for understanding the aetiology or genesis of psychopathology. Finally, each school will elaborate the role of the therapist in initiating or supporting behavioural change, 'whether it is a change of choice ("to feel better"), or necessity (because of conflict with societal norms, eg. sexual exhibitionism)' (Chaiklin 1977: 26). There are varying amounts of disagreement between adherents of different schools of psychotherapy as to what should constitute therapeutic aims. Many believe that psychotherapy is 'intended to change people, to make them think differently (cognition), to make them feel differently (affection), and to make them act differently (behaviour)' (Corsini 1984: 4). Others, including the present author, would say that psychotherapy may not so much be about actually changing people, but is about facilitating psychological insight, and using the therapeutic relationship to support change, if the patient wishes to change.

PSYCHODYNAMIC DMT

The term 'psychodynamic' broadly encompasses therapies which are informed by Freudian and post-Freudian theory (Brown and Pedder 1979, Malan 1989). Psycho-dynamic psychotherapy theory includes concepts of 'defense, anxiety, and hidden feeling, and hence the existence of the "unconscious"; the "return of the repressed"; transference; and the validation of these concepts through direct observation of the response to interpretation' (Malan 1989: 254). The particular elements of psycho-dynamic theory stressed and the choice of which theorists are employed differ between psychodynamic therapies, and depend on the particular practitioner or school.

Diane Fletcher's work illustrates how psychodynamic principles can be applied to DMT (Fletcher 1979). She cites the ideas of Freud, Bion, Guntrip and Klein as influential to her thinking. She writes that in her work she employs a category which she terms '*intra-psychic reorganization through insight into meaning*, [in which] body experience is used as a tool to bring pre-verbal and undifferentiated experi-ences up to the level of conscious feelings, insight and thought' (Fletcher 1979: 134).

Further aims of her work include: enabling the person to discover new experi-ence, a physical restructuring of the body, and the use of body experience for the purpose of relating to others. She believes that 'movement operates as a medium, like language, by which interpersonal skills and relations can be developed and an initial feeling of self through relating to others can be found' (Fletcher 1979: 143).

She works with non-psychiatric clients, and occasionally with outpatients diagnosed as 'borderline', meaning that they are not schizophrenic, but may have occasional psychotic-type experiences. A patient with this borderline personality organization is said to have 'a pervasive pattern of instability of self-image, interpersonal relationships and mood, beginning by early adulthood and present in a variety of contexts' (American Psychiatric Association 1987: 346). Her work draws on DMT techniques developed by Alma Hawkins, in which the client or patient is asked to attend to inner sensation and follow these into spontaneous movement. The therapist may choose to sit and observe, or follow the client's lead and interact, usually by mirroring. Fletcher uses body movement as an opportunity for the patient or client to free associate (both verbally and in movement), thereby bringing the inner mental life into awareness. The use of psychomotor free association 'means allowing the bits of sensation, motion, impulses, body images, etc., to "come up" to consciousness, to be brought into meaningful relation to the subjective sense of self or identity and to the world' (Fletcher 1979: 138).

The inner world of cognition and emotion includes memories and images of one's parents and one's self in relation to them. Patterns of relating to one's parents are formative of personality; they are learned from infancy, and shape our behaviour towards other people as well as our view of ourselves. The pattern is repeated in the dynamics of the relation to the therapist, onto whom these dynamics are projected, or transferred. The pattern may have the quality of dependency, or often ambivalence, and is always a mixture of strong negative and positive feelings. These patterns can also be seen in movement terms. The body as well as the psyche acts out these 'object' relationships, where 'object' is taken to mean the mental image of parents or significant others. Often these inner objects are distorted, and represent how one feels towards significant others, rather than any accurate memory or repetition of actual early relationships. The dynamic interplay of fantasy and reality in psychic life has been articulated by the object relations school, including W. R. Bion, D. W. Winnicott, W. R. D. Fairbairn and Melanie Klein (Bion 1961, Segal 1964, Winnicott 1949, 1953, 1958, 1971, 1986).

Case example

Fletcher uses object relations theory in movement terms in her clinical work. She worked with a man in his early forties who sought therapy after a series of unsuccessful relationships. He had had two years of verbal therapy before beginning weekly dance movement therapy sessions. Fletcher describes the way that the man's body movement changed during a sequence that encapsulated some of his difficulties. When he moved towards a large wooden chest, which was at one end of the dance movement therapist's room, his body became less caved in, less constrained, and more relaxed. When he moved away from this wooden chest, his body became more stiff, chest sunken, shoulders raised, 'as if he were using his back to provide a cloak for himself, under which he could huddle' (Fletcher 1979: 149). This change was pointed out by the dance movement therapist. The client, while moving, said he felt protected by the chest, and he associated it with the idea of a 'home base'. He related this later to a feeling that he was lacking from his own mother, whom he felt had always been distant and cool towards him. Through these feelings gained in movement, his free association in words and further movement, and their interpretation by the dance movement therapist, he became aware of his dependent longings for emotional security. He related this to his unsuccessful attempts to obtain this security in his current relationship with his girlfriend. He then identified this pattern of behaviour, both towards her and towards the therapist, as an expression of these needs, which had been previously unacknowledged. He was then able to think about doing something towards addressing these needs more appropriately.

Fletcher's use of psychodynamic ideas in her work raises two further interesting points. One is how movement can be used as a psychological defence mechanism.

A defence is a way of protecting oneself from consciously experiencing a painful feeling, realization, or anxiety. Fletcher argues that simple catharsis of these feelings, or simple release without thinking about the content of the feelings, is counterproductive. The feelings continue to return, and so need to be got rid of again, which takes up a lot of emotional energy. She writes that it

> might feel better to 'dance out' the threatening feelings and to make oneself feel better, at least temporarily; however by doing just this the opportunity to really discover what those unbearable thoughts and feelings *are* is passed by.
>
> (Fletcher 1979: 140)

This is not to say that release or cathartic discharge of feelings in movement is never appropriate; it is only counter-therapeutic if this release is simply left as an experience that is undigested, and not made sense of within the context of the therapeutic relationship. Fletcher believes that 'there are occasions where discharge, if accompanied by emotion, thought and memory in the context of a present experience, can then be used toward psychic reorganization and change' (Fletcher 1979: 141).

Prohibiting the use of touch

A second important point that Fletcher's work raises is the issue of touch, which she considers in the context of her psychodynamic view of behaviour. She notes that there are therapeutic dangers inherent in using the powerful tool of movement and nonverbal interaction. She feels that

> Manipulation and massage of the body, touch, overt teaching, leading, helping, demonstrating and spontaneously interacting in movement with the client may all be used counter-therapeutically by the client in his attempt to engage the therapist to fulfill unstated and often unconscious longings to be taken care of by the therapist, to be told what to do, or controlled, etc., all of which defeat the goals of therapy. The acting out and gratification of longings often keeps these feelings at an unfelt (and unconsciously gratified) level and prevents them from emerging into the therapeutic process.
>
> (Fletcher 1979: 146)

She further notes that it is easy for the therapist to project his or her own unidentified longings onto the patient, and try to fulfil them, vicariously attempting to satisfy oneself by trying to satisfy the client. This sort of attempt at satisfying one's own needs through giving to others is a particular danger for women, according to some psychodynamic thinkers (Orbach and Eichenbaum 1987).

Thinking carefully about what movement means in the therapeutic relationship, and taking care about its use are also important ideas gained from psychodynamic thinking. On the whole, touch between patients and therapists should not be initiated by the therapist, unless one is working with children, and even then it should be used carefully. Touch in an adult psychiatric group brings up issues around sexuality and power, does not help to normalize behaviour, and brings up legal and ethical issues as well (Willis 1987: 52).

Psychodynamic DMT with a schizophrenic client

Some psychodynamic concepts can also be used with schizophrenics, though it is not possible to use the same degree of patient-directed, unstructured activity as described by Fletcher. An article by another psychodynamic dance movement therapist, Sacha Silberstein, describes how she made contact with an extremely withdrawn chronic schizophrenic man (Silberstein 1987: 148). She mirrored the patient's movement in an individual session. She noted that it was necessary for her to modulate her own movement to come closer to the energy level of the patient's withdrawn and lethargic state. This ensured that the therapist's vitality and energy were not overwhelming or threatening for the patient.

Silberstein hypothesized that the integrative function of DMT is one in which 'the process moves from a sensorimotor to an imagistic to a verbal level' (Silberstein 1988: 147). This can also be described as a sequence which shifts from movement to image to interpretation (Stanton, 1988, 1991, Stanton and Stanton 1989). At first, there is the primitive level of movement experience, which generates a psychophysical feeling state. This often progresses to an image, or word, which describes that state. The therapist may then, with the help of the client, try to articulate what has been generated by the movement and to take into conscious awareness the feelings that have arisen during the therapeutic movement interaction. Changes and integration occur in the patient both internally, or intrapsychically, as well as interpersonally, in relations to the therapist or to other group members. It is important to note that for many patients, working with the verbal level alone (as in conventional psychotherapy) is not possible; there are too many distortions and defences which prevent insight or interaction. One of the main strengths of DMT is its ability to provide a primary movement experience that the client can use as material on which to work towards understanding feelings and relationships.

In addition to the verbal–movement connection, Silberstein cites research which postulates that the initial somatic work may be of great benefit to the schizophrenic: 'patients must first develop a coherent body image before they can develop an ego' (Silberstein 1987: 147). Like Fletcher, she uses movement, including structured warmup, to increase the patient's 'self synchrony', a term used by the nonverbal communications researcher Condon to describe body parts which move in harmony rather than in a disorganized manner (Condon and Ogston 1966).

Silberstein hypothesizes that 'the use of the less defended nonverbal modes of communication can, at least in some cases, lessen the amount of initial resistance encountered' in forming a relationship with a schizophrenic client (Silberstein 1987: 147). Psychodynamic theory asserts that early mother–infant interaction in the first year of life sets the crucial tone for all later relationships. Many psychodynamic dance movement therapists believe that 'the nonverbal nature of dance therapy provides its practitioners with particular access to areas of consciousness rooted in an early, preverbal time of life' (Brown and Avstreih in Robbins 1980: 170, Fletcher 1979: 136, Silberstein 1987: 147). This phenomenon was recognized by the nineteenth-century psychiatrist Charcot, and was later taken up in America in the 1950s by the psychoanalyst Felix Deutsch, who attempted to use psychomotor stimuli with his patients in order to gain access to their earliest memories and feelings (Deutsch 1952, 1962).

DMT provides a therapeutic approach which focuses on the body and bodily experience; psychodynamic thought provides a framework with which to understand the powerful emotive phenomena that arise in working with body movement and its concomitant affective experiences, imagery and interaction. The way in which psychodynamic ideas are used in DMT varies between practitioners, who may choose to stress different aspects of psychodynamic theory blended with particular aspects of the movement process. For example, where Fletcher uses movement improvisation which she interprets within a psychodynamic framework based on Bion, Fairbairn and Klein, Penny Lewis Bernstein's later work focuses on movement tasks within what she terms 'psychodynamic ego-psychology', which conceptualizes movement in developmental terms (Lewis 1986). The approach described in Chapter 9 of this book focuses on free association in movement, and the interpretation of the symbols that arise from this within the context of the group process.

JUNGIAN DMT

The work of Jungian dance movement therapists is informed by ideas drawn from Analytical Psychology, the name given to the school of C. G. Jung (Jung 1965). Although most Jungian dance movement therapists do not work exclusively with psychiatric patients, they do form a large school within DMT. Many draw on Mary Whitehouse's work, and understand both personality and movement through a Jungian frame of reference. Joan Chodorow is a Californian dance movement therapist who also trained as a Jungian psychotherapist. She has written a recent full-length study of her work entitled, *Dance Therapy and Depth Psychology: The Moving Imagination* (Chodorow 1991). For her, the goal of therapy is individuation, which is defined as 'a person becoming himself, whole, indivisible and distinct from other people's or collective psychology (though also in relation to these)' (Samuels *et al.* 1986: 76). This is achieved by recognizing one's own life struggles as parallel to those described in myth, folklore, fairytale, legend and religious imagery, all of which are evidence, by way of projection, of universal unconscious processes (Royston 1989: 52).

Chodorow relies on the use of a 'structure for self-directed movement that will enable discovery and development of themes from the unconscious' (Chodorow 1984: 195). This dialogue with the body is a form of active imagination, in which conscious and unconscious elements are united in the creative process. In contrast to a psychodynamic approach, in which movement is largely spontaneous, Jungian dance movement therapists may use improvised movement to explore diverse phenomena such as dreams, specific fantasies, early body memories, images from art (such as the mandala), life relationships, as well as transference issues directed towards the therapist. Chodorow notes that movement is a powerful experience which may

> lead toward the reduction of the theme to a personal early memory, or it may unfold toward mythological motifs and other universal experiences. Often both occur, whether the therapist watches or enters into the patient's enactments, the therapeutic relationship is the vital container.

> (Chodorow 1984: 195)

She reads movement experience using Jungian views of interrelationship and notes that with a 'deepening, mutual sense of involvement, mover and observer approach the synchronistic moment that transcends conscious–unconscious, inner–outer, self–other' (Chodorow 1984: 196). Here, 'synchronistic' refers to a meaningful psychological connection between two events which coincide in time and space (Samuels *et al.* 1986: 146).

The relationship between the client's movement and that of the therapist is important: the therapist's physical response to the client's movement can provide a sensitivity that will help the therapist to share and understand the client's experience. Jungian DMT allows a longer time for the client to engage in solo movement for self-discovery. Clearly this lack of structure would not be advisable for a more fragile patient who did not have the confidence or self-containment necessary to engage in such free exploration. Furthermore, this situation – in which, in a sense, the client performs for the therapist who serves as audience – may only be acceptable to those who are able to be essentially trusting of others. For a patient who is suspicious or paranoid or feels controlled by the power of the therapist, this situation would have a negative effect on the therapeutic process.

Jung hypothesized that there were different properties or functions of consciousness: thinking, feeling, sensing and intuiting (Jung 1923). Following this notion of a typology, Chodorow suggests that some people may use movement predominantly as *expression* and others as *impression*. Expression is the translation of an internal state into movement. By contrast, for those who use movement as impression, 'the movement may *produce* emotion or subdue it or otherwise have an effect upon internal states' (Chodorow 1984: 199). In her view, the movement process 'serves as a bridge between inner and outer worlds, each having an impact on the other' (Chodorow 1984: 199). Chodorow noted that in DMT some people experienced the movement predominantly through felt bodily *sensations*, and these may remain ineffable and not be translated into words. She suggested that those who used imagery usually made *intuitive* connections between the movement experience and their lives. She concluded that the richest movement experiences seem to involve both sensation and image, fluctuating back and forth, or occurring simultaneously. It is interesting to speculate whether, for the disoriented or disorganized person who is mentally ill, the connection of sensation to image could be an integrative experience.

Case example

In a case example, Chodorow described a woman who explored two different movement qualities, one with the left side of the body and the other with the right. While with one side the quality was quick, definite and firm, the other side was sustained, using softness, and gathering in, as though enveloping a small unseen shape. In attempting to integrate these two disparate sides, the woman had great difficulty in finding a balance. The therapist mirrored this and connected the movement to the woman's struggle to balance career and motherhood. No resolution was achieved, but recognition of these two oppositions enabled a more clear articulation of the difficulty of reconciling these two opposing forces, which had illustrated themselves in the movement.

Ways of reading movement as encompassing opposition or forming polarities or complementary pairs is unique to the Jungian DMT approach. So, too, are the elucidation and recognition of universal symbolic themes in the material that the clients may bring to the therapy sessions. Each psychological framework implies a way of understanding symbolism, as well as proposing specific psychic structures with which to understand the personality. The Jungian approach stresses wholeness, balance and integration of opposing forces, and also notes that the struggle of the individual is deeply connected with the universal human struggle. It is interesting to note that group themes in both inpatient and outpatient psychiatry do often evidence archetypal material. In these group DMT sessions, stories of intense struggle against a powerful force of evil (such as a knight against a wicked king), or the arduous quest for a valued object, place, or state (whether symbolized by the Holy Grail, paradise, or union with the beloved), often occur (Loomis and Loomis 1957).

The Jungian DMT tradition has extended Jung's essential hypothesis that 'psyche and matter are two different aspects of the same thing', and that 'the symbols of the self arise out of the depths of the body' (Chodorow 1984: 193). Jungian DMT, as articulated by Whitehouse and Chodorow, extensively uses bodily experience as a form of active imagination, and in doing so illustrates that movement is a powerful tool with which to access the unconscious and integrate its contents into consciousness. This last insight is particularly relevant to DMT in psychiatry, and underlines the idea that the creative process of making movement is, at its core, a therapeutic one.

EGO-PSYCHOANALYTIC DMT

Elaine Siegel, a dance movement therapist who trained as a psychoanalyst in the American ego-psychoanalytic tradition, has written a full-length work entitled *Dance/Movement Therapy Mirror of Ourselves: A Psychoanalytic Approach* (Siegel 1984). In this book she builds a theoretical structure for her work with psychiatric and non-psychiatric patients which relies heavily on her insights from such theorists as Heinz Hartmann, Otto Kernberg, Rene Spitz, Margaret Mahler and Heinz Kohut. Her dance influences are diverse and include ballet as well as Haitian and African dance (Levy 1989: 167). She is influenced by Marian Chace, and by Liljan Espenak, the Adlerian dance movement therapist (Espenak 1981).

Like Chace, she uses mirroring and rhythm to facilitate movement interaction. Siegel trained with Espenak, who uses directive movement and movement tests to assess patients. She takes psychoanalytic concepts and translates them literally into movement parameters; for example, being able to lift the arms into a wide, open movement is seen as indicative of relative ego-strength. The complex terminology which Siegel employs, and the way she sees movement as precisely representative of specific aspects of psychoanalytic concepts of personality formation, may be difficult for readers unfamiliar with or unsympathetic to psychoanalysis. However, many of her ideas are useful, particularly those which relate to her work with severely disturbed psychiatric patients (Siegel 1974). Siegel makes psychoanalytic interpretations of movement behaviour in which she sees evidence of underlying infantile conflicts. Such interpretations would not be appropriate for all dance movement therapists to use, but are part of the psychoanalytic psychosexual developmental framework in which Siegel understands her patients.

Ego-psychoanalytic writers such as Kohut, Mahler, Hartmann and Spitz incorporate Freudian theory, but choose to focus on the ego as the agent which integrates impulses of the id with the dictates of the superego. They view the earliest stages of infancy and childhood as crucially formative in the development of the ego or self. They see pathology developing when a person is 'stuck' or fixated in a particular stage of development. For example, they hypothesize that schizophrenia may be related to a failure to emerge from what Margaret Mahler termed the symbiotic stage of personality formation, after which the infant develops a distinct ego identity separate from that of the mother (Mahler et al. 1975, Siegel 1984: 80). The therapeutic process entails regressing to this fixation point and reworking the personality in the interaction with the therapist. Direct parallels are drawn from the relationship between mother and child to that of the role of the therapist and client or patient. The patient is thought to replay elements of early mother–child interaction with the therapist. This is then interpreted by the therapist, who provides insight into the quality of the interaction by verbal interpretations. This gives new meanings to the patient's relations with others, and as such, therapy is seen as a way to alter the patient's basic sense of self as well as patterns of perceiving others. This conceptualization is common to the psychoanalytic psychotherapies; Siegel's unique contribution lies in her bringing movement to bear on these therapeutic processes and in articulating the role of the body within them.

Psychoanalytic conceptualization of motility

Siegel has also contributed a great deal to the articulation of the role of movement and body image in personality development within the ego-psychoanalytic framework. For example, she states that 'motility itself is neither libidinous nor aggressive until other drives merge with it' (Siegel 1984: 59). Here she draws on the work of Bela Mittelmann, a psychoanalyst who discussed ideas about motility and psyche in the 1950s (Mittelmann 1954, 1957). By arguing that movement is a primary drive, and neither merely an expression of sexuality nor of aggression, Siegel addresses the fears some psychoanalysts have that using movement in therapy may be too gratifying of either of these drives, and so not a suitable medium for working through issues in the patient–therapist relationship.

Siegel believes that 'the drive constellation of the total concept "motility" has its base in the id, while the executive function of the drives are connected to motility itself in the service of the ego' (Siegel 1984: 64). Movement then, can come from the id, which is a reservoir of psychical energy, and the instinctual pole of the personality (Laplanche and Pontalis 1973: 197). Alternatively, it can be directed by the ego, that part of the personality which is responsible for the interests of the person as a whole, and which brings defence mechanisms into play if unpleasurable emotion threatens to come to the fore. The idea that movement can reflect both the id and the ego, the unconscious and the conscious, is an important one. This means that movement can express primitive emotions as well as reflect defences against them, or modulations or compromises between conflicting emotions. Siegel concludes that 'constricted motility then, is always an indicator of repression' (Siegel 1984: 70).

It is important that dance movement therapists recognize that movement can mean many things, and that if they decide to focus on spontaneous movement as an indicator of unconscious process, rather than a conscious, intentional act which reflects the ego, they are only choosing one way of reading the movement from a possible spectrum of many. Differentiating defended movement from spontaneous or unconscious movement is a difficult task which requires over one hundred hours of learning movement observation, using live and video examples of psychiatric and non-psychiatric patients. Acquiring these observational and analytical skills forms a large part of the training of dance movement therapists.

For Siegel, DMT is an adjunctive treatment to verbal therapy which can, via a working through of the transference relationship, help patients resolve conflict. At the end of therapy, the patients come to appreciate something of the real person of the therapist, and withdraw projections of their infantile objects from the therapist, in the realization that these projections reside within their unconscious. Siegel notes that 'motility creates a whole new dimension to transference that has never been examined before' (Siegel 1984: 88). However, she does not see working in the transference as feasible or desirable in the usual psychiatric hospital setting; first, because there may not be enough time available; and, secondly, because the patient may be too fragmented to make use of this type of treatment approach. Instead, she sees the 'body image distortions, lack of appropriate motor behaviour and need for tension discharge' as problems that are suitable to approach with psychotic patients (Siegel 1984: 77). This last view connects her work with the psychodynamic dance movement therapists, including Diane Fletcher and Sacha Silberstein discussed in a previous section.

Case example

Siegel's book describes DMT with various types of patient, and describes different qualities of transferences that occur in work with such patients as psychotic, autistic, borderline, obsessive compulsive and classic. She describes her reconstructive dance activities, which include using self-touch, moving each body part in a sequence, and employing forms and positions from ballet to influence the body image. She notes that 'object-relations are in turn tied to the relative state of the body image' (Siegel 1984: 92). In other words, the body images will bear traces of the developmental stages at which the clients are fixated in their personality development. For example, those with unresolved issues from the oral stage may show a cathexis or investment in the face, and specifically the mouth area. They may further show a preference for rocking-type rhythms in movement or dance (Kestenberg 1975, Lewis 1986).

Siegel uses very little free improvisation with psychotic patients, instead using Chaceian methods, such as focusing on rhythm and asking patients to mirror each other's movements. Instead of interpreting the images which arise from group movement, Siegel interprets in the transference, and concentrates on reading movement behaviour as an indication of the role the patients project onto the therapist, whether they try to imitate her completely, as in a symbiotic transference, or whether they cannot synchronize with the therapist for fear of being engulfed by her, as is the case in the transference situation with some psychotic patients.

In her book, *Dance Movement Therapy: Mirror of Ourselves: A Psychoanalytic Approach*, Siegel describes work with six adolescent psychiatric patients in a group, all of whom, at the beginning of their therapy, were very stiff and unmoving, which she understood to be an attempt to 'hold themselves together' (Siegel 1984). She noted their fragmentary communications, and hypothesized that they did not see her as a real, whole person, but as partial, and only fleetingly present. She used rock 'n' roll music to engage them, and started a simple rhythmic stamping movement which many of the teenagers could follow. This elicited fantasies of being rocked, or held, and some satisfaction was gained by some group members in using this movement. Later, they were able to fantasize about their needs to be taken care of, and these traces of early personality development were understood in their feelings towards the therapist, and interpreted as such by her.

Although Siegel noted that probing for unconscious conflicts in these patients was not appropriate (choosing instead to focus on reconstructing the body image), she did interpret some body movements as symptoms of the patient's unconscious conflicts. Just as Freud interpreted the somatic disturbances in his hysterical patients as illustrating aspects of their psychological problems, Siegel noted that one group member could not move his neck very well, and instead held his head very stiff. She asked him to perform a neck-roll exercise and, as he did so, her patient said he thought that his head would fall off. She showed him that his head was not falling off and illustrated that her head also was firmly fixed to her shoulders. It was later discovered that the patient had internalized a negative attitude towards himself which he had learned from his parents. He had 'used the symptom of the falling head to express both his wish and his fear that his mother's standard sayings, "I'm going to lose my mind if you keep annoying me," and "You're giving me a splitting headache," might become real' (Seigel 1984: 138).

In conclusion, it can be seen that ego-psychoanalytic DMT draws upon a rich and complex theoretical background. Siegel makes interpretations of behaviour based on hypotheses about unconscious infantile feelings which patients are believed to experience in the early stages of personality development. Such interpretations of the patient's behaviour towards the therapist require lengthy psychoanalytic training, including a personal psychoanalysis and supervision to carry out effectively. Ideas derived from ego-psychoanalytic DMT are useful in work with psychiatric patients, particularly by providing a rationale for seeing movement as either ego-directed, or as a defence against feelings. This tradition stresses the psychosexual nature of the body image, suggesting that specific periods in childhood development strongly colour a client's movement pattern. This provides a theoretical basis for using active, directive movement in the form of specific dance exercises to help rebuild the distorted body image of the psychiatric patient.

Lastly, the ego-psychoanalytic tradition suggests that movement can be symbolic of fantasies that patients have about the therapist, about their own bodies, or that represent early internalized messages from their parents.

GESTALT DMT

Many dance movement therapists, including Penny Lewis Bernstein, who is a major theoretician and practitioner, are informed by the therapeutic techniques and theory of the school of Gestalt psychotherapy which was developed by Fritz Perls (Clarkson 1989, Lewis 1986: 109, Perls 1973). The Gestalt approach stresses attending to present emotional experience and uses techniques of role play to clarify feelings. Gestalt psychotherapy informs much of the work done in dramatherapy because of its reliance on role play, its emphasis on immediacy of experience, as well as attention to symbolism and metaphor (Holmes and Karp 1991). Although primarily practised with people seeking therapy as a way to gain self-awareness, Gestalt-derived ideas are sometimes used in outpatient psychiatric settings, though generally in a group, and not in an individual therapy session.

Dance movement therapists Penny Lewis Bernstein and Linni Silberman-Diehl both use Gestalt ideas in different ways (Bernstein 1972, Lewis 1986, Silberman-Diehl and Komisaruk 1985). Bernstein writes that 'growth is more apt to take place if an individual is involved in the experience they are feeling, rather than just talking about it' (Bernstein 1979: 111). She notes that Gestalt theory employs basic perceptual concepts such as the figure–ground relationship, 'bringing into awareness and experience the shadowy pockets of unresolved conflicts' (Bernstein 1979: 113). She defines Gestalt dance movement therapy as

> any holistic present-oriented use of body awareness and movement directed toward the grounded integration of dissociated areas of an individual through the formation of spontaneous figure formation and organismic self-regulation towards expressive contact with the environment.

> (Bernstein 1979: 115)

Case example

Bernstein achieves these goals through structured 'movement experiments', and guided movement imagery. The client is repeatedly asked to finish the sentence, 'Now I am feeling . . .' in order to gain a 'here-and-now awareness emphasizing the experience of behaviour as it is sensed'. She also uses a technique called 'the body talks' in which the client, usually after a relaxation exercise, articulates, via body symbolism, what he or she is feeling. For example, a patient named Beth said, 'I am Beth's legs, I want to run away. I am Beth's hands, I am making a fist and I want to punch out' (Bernstein 1979: 119).

These directive activities are a contrast to both the techniques of free association in movement and the unstructured improvisation techniques favoured by psychodynamic dance movement therapists. The Gestalt approach stresses the use of body movement via structured exercises and may involve the use of videotaping and video playback to heighten awareness and confront defences that the client may have.

Bernstein describes a young woman training as a scientist, who came to therapy suffering from migraines, and complaining of being isolated from colleagues and friends. Bernstein saw the woman in individual dance movement therapy sessions, after the woman said that she could not cope with coming to group sessions any longer. Bernstein noted that the way the woman moved gave her a sensitive, evasive, floating quality. Bernstein asked her to intensify some of her common movement phrases, as well as to associate verbally while she did so.

In one session Bernstein used the woman's fantasies to gain access to her feelings. The client said, 'I started hearing a baby crying, and I realized she was inside me, she was all locked up in the muscles in the back of my neck, right where my migraine is' (Bernstein 1979: 127). The therapist suggested to her that she move through the fantasy as though it were happening in the present. As the child, the client writhed in the floor saying, 'let me out, let me out, I want to be free'. The resulting emotional experience was talked through with the therapist and the client became aware that she had never really allowed herself any time to relax, and that coming to therapy was viewed by her as an indulgence which she had to punish herself for by giving herself migraines. After a period, she connected the fantasies with her early and rather punitive relationship to her mother, and the client was able to control her migraines once she realized her emotional source. She also began to allow herself to open up to other people in relationships.

Clearly the use of very strong and powerful emotional material through directive fantasy work including movement needs to be handled carefully, under the supervision of an experienced therapist. An example of using some of the concepts from Gestalt therapy, notably role play and metaphor, is found in an article by Linni Silberman-Diehl and Barry Komisaruk who, although not explicitly Gestalt oriented, do combine some psychoanalytic ideas with those of Gestalt role play, in addition to concepts derived from neuropsychology and neurolinguistic programming (Silberman-Diehl and Komisaruk 1985). Their type of approach illustrates the eclectic nature of the work done in DMT by practitioners who combine dance movement therapy with ideas from other therapeutic systems.

In their article entitled 'Treating psychogenic somatic disorders through body metaphor' (Silberman-Diehl and Komisaruk 1985) they discuss treating patients with psychosomatic disorders. They posit the concept of a 'body metaphor' by which patients' somatic manifestations represent specific feelings that the clients are unwilling or unable to express verbally. The manifestations often 'appear to be metaphors expressed in terms of body movement, posture, pain, or restriction of movement or feelings' (Silberman-Diehl and Komisaruk 1985: 37). For example, one of their patients had a hunched posture while she described her 'burden', the name she gave to her feelings. The word 'burden' can be viewed as the verbal metaphor and the hunched posture as the corresponding nonverbal, or body metaphor. In the same way, a verbal metaphor like feeling 'down at the mouth' describes a facial expression that illustrates sadness.

In general, in a group DMT situation with psychiatric patients, it is inadvisable to single out a particular member's nonverbal presentation to draw attention to a body metaphor; rather, general interpretations about the quality of the movement that the group is producing, or a vague statement about the quality of a movement without naming the individual, is sufficient to bring to awareness the communication the therapist has received, but about which the patient may be unaware. This issue will be considered further in clinical examples of DMT with adult outpatients.

The view of this author regarding the selective use of Gestalt therapy is in concurrence with that of Irvin Yalom, the humanistic group psychotherapist who writes that the use of structured activities such as finishing the sentence, 'Now I am feeling . . .', can often mean that patients express strong feelings without giving sufficient time to consider the ramifications of these statements, or work through these insights in the context of the individual or group therapy relationship (Yalom 1978: 449). Confrontation of psychiatric patients using structured activities based in Gestalt theory by student dance movement therapists is something to be *avoided at all costs*. A full appreciation of the humanistic and philosophical principles behind Perls' work, as well as co-work with a trained Gestalt therapist, would be the only safe way to use such techniques (Clarkson 1989). Even then, the intensity of affect they can produce would likely be counterproductive for the majority of psychiatric patients who are easily overwhelmed by the strength of their feelings, and need to learn more adaptive defences rather than having their existing ones removed by confrontation. Gestalt DMT ideas are included in this section because their work on body metaphor is of theoretical interest to therapists working in psychiatry, and because Gestalt-oriented dance movement therapists constitute a sizeable group of practitioners working with private clients.

CONCLUSION

An overview of DMT approaches from four perspectives – the psychodynamic, Jungian, ego-psychoanalytic and Gestalt – amply illustrates the diversity of methods, goals and psychological understanding of functioning which comprise DMT. It is important to remember that all the practitioners described above went on to train in verbal psychotherapy, and so carry out interpretive work in the transference in a way that would not be fitting to a DMT student. However, DMT trainings are influenced by the methods and ideas put forth by these practitioners, and as such it is important to clarify goals and methods of working that are appropriate to the level of training completed. Furthermore, it is important to look at the needs of the client in deciding how to work, as well as when considering the possibility of going on to postgraduate verbal therapy training after DMT training. This choice will be made by considering a system of thought appropriate to the therapist's views of human experience, and the relevance of a psychotherapeutic system to the patient population with which they are employed.

Comparing therapeutic aims across DMT traditions

It is useful to compare and contrast the four schools of DMT just discussed in terms of their aims and their stated goals of therapeutic change on the body level, and on the intrapsychic and interpersonal levels, and then to consider the relevance of these goals and aims to psychiatric work.

The psychodynamic approach views the patient or client in terms of a psychoanalytic model of personality development, and makes the assumption that childhood experience, and specific constellations of unconscious feelings (such as anxiety, psychosexuality, aggression, abandonment, etc.), are seen as central themes. A stated aim is 'intra-psychic reorganization through insight into meaning' (Fletcher 1979: 134). Furthermore, the use of movement to facilitate interpersonal learning is also stressed. On the body level, the aim is a physical restructuring of the body image and body ego through novel, improvised movement experiences. This is also achieved through a structured warmup, which integrates the sensori-motor, imagistic and verbal level, as conceptualized by Silberstein (Silberstein 1987). Intrapsychically, the psychodynamic dance movement therapy experience takes the form of inner sensing, where unconscious symbols arise from movement and through words, in order that unconscious ideas can be brought to awareness, and so loose their hold on the personality. Fletcher's client, for example, used the image of a 'home base' in movement to explore issues around self-reliance, and a need for others. This was also taken up on the interpersonal level, by the dance movement therapist noting the client's relationship to her in the transference (which has both verbal and movement components). This last way of working is appropriate for a practitioner like Fletcher, given her analytic training.

In contrast, movement in Jungian DMT, at least as articulated by Chodorow, is employed as a form of 'active imagination', in which a creative kinaesthetic experience is used to help integrate the conscious and the unconscious. Goals for change on a body level seem to be about allowing the unconscious (specifically in its spiritual, archetypal and healing functions) to dwell in the body, in order that wholeness of the personality, or the essential Self as Jung conceived it, may become possible.

Intrapsychic change in Jungian DMT is facilitated through allowing the patients to move, on their own, in the presence of the witness/analyst. In this, unconscious symbols are uncovered that cast a light on interpersonal relationships as well as connecting the individual to society, history and culture, giving a more complete meaning to existence. Jungian DMT goals for therapeutic change are existential, as well as interpersonal, and are rather different from trying to undo damaging symptomatic behaviour such as that seen in psychiatric patients. However, these two sets of goals may be seen as broadly related, if the sickness of one individual is seen as related to the ills of mankind as a whole. Further interpersonal goals are worked through in a manner similar to that in psychodynamic DMT, though the Jungian conceptualization of the personality means that different qualities of relating to others and to the world are emphasized, such as a struggle for balance, wholeness and integration.

Ego-psychoanalytic DMT is different again, largely due to the way in which the personality and its growth and development are considered. Ego-psychoanalytic DMT aims to resolve conflicts based in the infantile experience of the patient. This means regressing to a level of interpersonal and intrapsychic functioning at which the patient might have been stuck, or fixated. After this, the inherent connection between who the person is (intrapsychically), and who the person is in relation to others (interpersonally), is reworked in the therapeutic relationship. This is a highly specific aspect of psychoanalytic work, and is handled by Siegel in the manner of a trained verbal psychoanalyst. In DMT done by students, some regression is noticed, and there is a chance, through mirroring, to replay elements of early interaction in the hope of facilitating easier relationships to other people. These are always relationships that have become twisted and distorted through long-standing psychopathological processes in the minds of the patients, and in their communications with others. In DMT done by students, the relationship quality may not be interpreted, but the client is allowed to practise new ways of being with other people through the movement interaction, which may change as group imagery and rhythm develop and alter during the course of the DMT group.

Body level goals in ego-psychoanalytic work are broadly similar to those in Jungian and psychodynamic work, though the body *ego* is stressed, as are the use of developmental body rhythms appropriate to early stages of psychological development (Freud's oral, anal and genital stages). With disturbed patients, this bodily reconstruction in order to aid psychological reconstruction seems a major aim, and is highly relevant to work with long-term patients, as described in the clinical chapters that follow.

In ego-psychoanalytic DMT, images and bodily sensations brought out in dancing together (such as being rocked, or feeling that one's head might fall off) are explored for their intrapsychic meaning (such as recalling failures in early nurturance), and for their interpersonal source (the patient's mother who had told him she would 'lose her mind' if he kept annoying her). These are then explored within a trusting and non-punitive relationship to the analyst/dance movement therapist, who receives and tries to detoxify these fantasies and wishes, and encourages more appropriate ways of getting dependency needs met, as well as trying to undo symbolic distortions in feelings about the self and the body. Gestalt DMT, about which little has been written, and of which the work of Penny Lewis Bernstein and Silberman-Diehl are examples, aims to focus on body metaphor as a way to understand unconscious feelings that have been repressed, and are so inaccessible to awareness that they have lodged themselves in the body. The direct technical relevance of Gestalt DMT for disturbed psychiatric patients is not very great, hence the Gestalt ideas, rather than methods, have only been given brief treatment in this section.

The explication of how psychoanalytic theory is employed in DMT, as described by Fletcher, Chodorow and Siegel, is enormously rich and complex, and justice cannot be done to their work without a fuller understanding of the psychodynamic, psychoanalytic, Gestalt and depth-psychology theoretical frameworks of personality development and therapeutic processes. The sheer enormity of this material, as well as its complexity, is beyond both the author and the scope of this book, and deserves several years' study at a psychotherapeutic training institute. However, it is important to understand that within the field of DMT as a whole, there are an increasing number of verbally trained psychotherapists who are also dance movement therapists, trying to integrate movement with psychological systems. This fact offers a great future potential for therapeutic work using DMT, as well as for revisioning some aspects of psychotherapeutic understanding which seem 'disembodied' in their over-emphasis on verbal processes.

The consideration of these four major theoretical schools, including psychodynamic, ego-psychoanalytic, Jungian and Gestalt, will hopefully provide student readers with a beginning point of reference from which they can decide the direction in which they wish to explore their work in psychiatry.

The ideas and methods described by Fletcher, Siegel, Chodorow, Bernstein and Silberman-Diehl are largely developed in the context of private work with non-psychiatric clients, though Siegel describes hospitalized inpatient adolescents suffering from schizophrenia, and Fletcher's clients may have also attended outpatient clinics. Therefore, caution needs to be exercised in translating their methods (if not their theories) into work with more mentally disturbed or damaged client groups. The primary body-level goals of reintegration, and restoration of an appropriate body image and body ego are fully relevant, as will be seen later in the clinical example of a DMT group for older, long-term psychiatric inpatients.

The intrapsychic goal of bringing unconscious emotions into awareness via bodily experience and symbolization is also relevant. However, the method by which this is achieved, namely through encouraging the patient to move, with eyes closed, while the therapist, usually seated, witnesses this 'inner sensing', is probably not applicable to psychiatric patients, or at least not to schizophrenics, for a number of reasons. Primarily, such a patient actually *lacks* defences against experience of powerful unconscious emotion, and so listening to sensation, imagery and feeling might produce a massively heightened awareness of material which the patient may find terrifying or overwhelming. The group movement, the group image and the interpretation by the dance movement therapist and group members – in the context of synchronous movement done with open eyes, and in relation to others – seems a safer therapeutic container in which this process can occur.

Additionally, given the propensity of more seriously ill patients being unable to distinguish the imaginary from the real, the patient and the dance movement therapist might find that inner sensing would give rise to acting out unconscious contents, such as rage, anger, fear, and chaos, as well as feelings of explosive joy or expansiveness which, in their distorted or exaggerated form, would be difficult to integrate into everyday awareness. Therapy with schizophrenic patients takes a long time: this is usually not available in the public health sector, and nor is the specialist supervision that such work requires. Using the mover/witness model and focusing on movement as inner sensing might be possible with depressed patients, though only under careful supervision and over a period of weekly sessions lasting at least four months. Some of the ways to work, by allowing movement to generate inner sensations and imagery within the group context – which is safe for more disturbed patients – will be discussed in the clinical section describing DMT groups for high-functioning adult outpatients.

Interpersonal goals in DMT as described by Fletcher, Siegel, Chodorow and Bernstein are also highly relevant to work in psychiatry, though the method by which new learning experiences are created through the language of movement is slightly different. Rather than working individually, a group setting is usually more appropriate. Even where individual work is undertaken, the therapeutic relationship may be less intense, and transference issues might be hinted at as 'patterns of behaviour' or 'modes of relating' rather than analysed in detail, with concomitant fantasies about the dance movement therapist, and retrieval of memories from childhood about the patient's relations to parental figures. Transference phenomena do occur in movement, but they need not be analysed in such detail if the primary therapeutic aim of DMT is to liberate the patient to relate in new ways, rather than to regress, repeat, reconstruct and repair old ones.

To a certain degree, the boundary between the therapeutic work of DMT undertaken by students, and the work done by dance movement therapists who have further psychotherapy training, will always be a permeable one. The work of advanced practitioners such as those described here does influence how students are trained, though the depth, intensity and methodology of DMT differ from school to school, and from junior to senior practitioner, with or without further verbal psychotherapy training.

Because individual work with adult psychiatric patients is one area in which students should be very careful of working without advanced training, supervision and support, clinical examples of individual DMT with adults are not included in this book, the aim of which is to introduce DMT in psychiatry and its use in therapeutic group work.

The interaction of verbal psychotherapy systems (such as the Jungian, Gestalt, ego-psychoanalytic or psychodynamic, as well as object relations, humanistic, and others) with DMT is ongoing; some people in the field feel that DMT should be seen as unique in its own right, and not merely a follow-on from verbal psychotherapy work. Presumably as DMT becomes more widely used and more widely available, and when more dance movement therapists engage in theoretical and methodological interaction with verbal therapies, there will be further delineation of theory and method which is informed by psychological theory but grounded in the inherently growth-producing aspects of dance, body movement and creativity.

The next part of this chapter examines current schools of group DMT practice in psychiatry. These will be seen to be more specifically geared to the needs of psychiatric patients than the work with individuals just described, though there are parallels and intersections.

Part II: Work with groups

GROUP DMT APPROACHES

As the examples of psychodynamic, Jungian, ego-psychoanalytic and Gestalt approaches illustrate, there is a diversity of theory and technique applied to DMT with individual patients. The same diversity exists in group approaches, though the most commonly employed theories of group therapy include the humanistic, as described by Irvin Yalom, and the psychoanalytic, of which the work of W.R. Bion is an example (Bion 1961, Yalom 1970, 1983). Many DMT Master's degree trainings offer their students experience of humanistic or psychodynamic verbal group psychotherapy so that DMT students should have personal experience of both dance movement and verbal group therapy before beginning to work with groups of patients. Group DMT shares many of its aims with verbal group therapy, primarily in addressing interpersonal functioning, though DMT also pursues additional movement goals for the group. Work with long-term or chronic psychiatric patients figures highly in the literature on DMT groups, as does the use of the therapist's conscious and unconscious responses to the group as a therapeutic tool.

This part will begin with a discussion of early approaches to DMT groups, which stress the therapeutic value of dance and bodily experience. The important modes of group functioning delineated by W. R. Bion will then be summarized to enable the reader to appreciate the major contribution that Susan Sandel and David Read Johnson have made to DMT in psychiatry with their psychoanalytically informed approach – specifically with their concept of the 'nascent group'. The therapeutic factors at work in group psychotherapy will then be described and examples will be given of how these are extended into the group DMT approach. Claire Schmais's articulation of what she terms the 'healing processes' in group dance therapy will then be summarized (Schmais 1985) and the part concludes with an overview of the proposed ways of analysing what happens in group DMT, how sessions are structured, and how leadership style affects patients. It is important to consider group DMT at length here, since the theories discussed in this part underly the techniques described in the clinical chapters, and because DMT students must spend at least one year working with groups before they move on to individual work, and some students and practitioners specialize in group work during their entire careers.

DMT group techniques for movement with psychiatric patients described in the existing literature are directly influenced by the work of Marian Chace, which was described in Chapter 2. This means that groups include a warmup, a development or 'process' section, and a closure. Most groups include the use of the technique of shared leadership in which patients are asked to lead an improvised movement which the rest of the group, including the therapist, imitates or mirrors. The therapist asks the group to verbalize during the movement, and the resulting statements and imagery are discussed while the group is still moving. The final part of the group is a verbal discussion in which the participants are seated, which serves as a closure for the session.

EARLY DMT GROUPS IN PSYCHIATRY

Early DMT groups stressed the value of opening up nonverbal channels of communication to patients. This remains important, given that diagnostic criteria for schizophrenia include disturbances in verbal expression and cognitive functioning such as delusions, hallucinations, incoherence, and marked loosening of associations, as well as an inability to function in social situations (American Psychiatric Association 1987: 194). Early DMT groups did not include a verbal discussion section and instead focused on giving the patient a reintegrative movement experience using warmup exercises and free improvisation. Other aims included using movement to enable the patient to gain a sense of physical well-being. This movement-based goal is still relevant: psychiatric patients frequently remark that they have lost a sense of their bodies, that they feel numb, or have forgotten that sensations derived from physical movement can be pleasurable or energizing. A final dance-derived goal of early work was expanding the patients' expressive range of movement either through directive or non-directive movement activity (Govine 1971: 15).

Alma Hawkins' work from the late 1960s emphasized heightening sensory awareness – that is, an awareness of the inner and outer world of the patient. She attempted to provide the patients with 'an experience of interacting with one another, not in a contrived way, but at a felt level; an honest, authentic type of relating' (Hawkins 1971: 67). At the time, Hawkins worked without music because she felt it 'too often provided immediate stimuli to move without allowing the inner-directed response to grow from within the person' (Hawkins 1971: 68). Only after some time of working with patients did she capitulate to psychiatrists' suggestions to include a specific section of the group for verbal discussion of the movement experiences. Since the late 1960s dance movement therapists have been continually preoccupied with ways of integrating verbal and movement dimensions of therapy, either sequentially or simultaneously. It is the use of verbalization during movement that distinguishes DMT from pure dance, and the use of verbalization that aligns DMT with other forms of psychotherapeutically informed therapeutic work. Schmais writes that 'a patient jabbing in the air would be encouraged to verbalize who he is jabbing at and why, so that his thoughts and actions become linked. Movement alone is not enough. Insight requires a cognitive component' (Schmais 1981: 106).

PSYCHOANALYTICALLY INFORMED GROUP DMT

Before discussing the more recent work of Sandel and Johnson, a summary of some of W. R. Bion's psychoanalytic group theory on which their work is based is necessary. Bion articulated the unconscious factors that influence group behaviour. According to Bion, there are three distinct emotional states of groups derived from three 'basic assumptions': dependency, fight–flight and pairing (Grinberg 1975: 16). These assumptions represent ways in which the group members seek to defend themselves against anxiety, which Bion and the British object relations school hypothesize has its root in the primitive or infantile elements of the personality. These hypotheses were initially formulated by the child psychoanalyst and theorist Melanie Klein (Klein 1959). Basic assumption phenomena, therefore, are the group's reaction to 'anxieties reactivated by the individual's dilemma in the group and the regression this dilemma imposes on him' (Grinberg 1975: 15). These basic assumptions are 'unconscious emotional states that tend to *avoid* the frustration implied in learning from experience, when learning implies effort, pain and contact with reality' (Grinberg 1975: 15).

Bion's model of group functioning

Very common among groups of psychiatric patients, particularly chronic schizophrenics, is the dependency group. This group seeks, in fantasy at least, to obtain security through, and have its members protected by, one individual, often the leader. The group's behaviour implies that it can initiate very little, and instead, wait for instruction from the therapist. The leader is often idealized and made into a sort of superhuman parent who will take care of his or her children. The group leader or therapist may be tempted to fall into this role, and will feel invested with grandiose power with which to save or rescue the helpless group from its state of isolation and wretchedness.

However, since no ordinary mortal can possibly fulfil these fantasies, the leader inevitably arouses disappointment and hostility. One frequent manoeuvre among the group is to put forth one member as especially sick and requiring the special care of the leader. Thus, one member may be forced into the sick role, in which an emotional fragility is emphasized, when in fact this person represents for the entire group something about its underlying state. In the dependency group, members could sometimes be said to represent a group of siblings greedily demanding the care and attention of the parent/therapist (Bion 1961: 76). There is often conflict within each member between dependent tendencies and the desire to act as an independent, autonomous adult. Resentment at being dependent, as well as a wish to persist in it, is common (Rioch 1975: 25).

In contrast, the basic assumption of the fight–flight or counterdependent group is that the group must preserve itself, which can only be done by either fighting or running away from someone or something. Action is essential, whether for fight or flight, giving these groups an active character. There is often the feeling of an outside enemy which must be destroyed if the group is to survive. Both in battle and in escape, the individual may be abandoned for sake of the survival of the group. The ethos of the survival of the fittest, and the group's needs being put forward before the individual's, are those which prevail. There is no tolerance for needy or dependent members in this group, and the group is inimical to the idea of introspection. Rather, it delights in constant defensive activity, generally thought to be an avoidance of anxiety or panic, from which fight and flight are an escape (Bion 1961: 71). Bion felt that the army represented a work group that was functioning under this basic assumption (Grinberg 1975: 19). In outpatient work with psychiatric patients, there may be a shift between dependency and fight–flight or counterdependent group functioning; sometimes the group's enemy is symbolized as 'the system', which may be seen as a barrier to gaining employment, status and normality; and other times the 'enemy' from which to flee is the day hospital or unit itself, which is seen (sometimes correctly) as pulling the patient towards a regressive dependence upon psychiatric services. The most extreme example of this mode of functioning is the adolescent group, in which the need for, and rebellion against, adult or parental authority figures is of paramount concern. Scapegoating, in which all the negative feelings of the group are projected onto one member, is also an important fight–flight strategy used by such groups (Holmes and Karp 1991: 115).

A final basic assumption is pairing. Here the unconscious assumption is that the group, through the pair, can live in the hope of the creation of a new person, or a new idea, the group's 'baby', which will bring about a new life that will solve all the old problems and bring about a Utopian existence. An air of persistent hopefulness pervades this group. Feelings associated with this group are soft and agreeable. The new, as yet unborn, leader of this group will save the group from feelings of hatred, destructiveness and despair, both within itself and from others.

If a person or idea should be produced by such a group, morale would be weakened, for then there would be no idealized future to hope for (Bion 1961: 151–155).

Basic assumptions are not directed towards outward reality but towards inward fantasy, which is then impulsively and uncritically acted out (Rioch 1975: 28). The group's mental attitude and its resulting behaviour may move between these assumptions during the life of the group, with dependency and fight–flight being the most common. Dependency and fight–flight modes of behaviour are useful ways of seeing psychiatric group-as-a-whole behaviour, rather than as a number of complex and multifaceted individuals, with their own histories and symptoms, who happen to have congregated in a room. The shift to seeing the group as a whole, rather than relating to each member individually, is a difficult but important one in DMT training: experience of a wide range of groups, within and outside psychiatric clients, is helpful in comprehending group-as-a-whole behaviour.

THE CONCEPT OF THE NASCENT GROUP

Using Bion's psychoanalytic observations, Sandel and Johnson have evolved a fascinating theory of the 'nascent group', which they use to describe their work with groups of chronic schizophrenics. Sandel and Johnson recognized that ordinary outpatient group theory does not necessarily apply to such damaged patients. Indeed, the group dance movement therapist working with long-term patients is often faced with the challenge of making contact with isolated individuals for whom the notion of a group does not even exist. It is the therapist, rather than the patients, who must hold on to the mental image of the group. By acknowledging that the dance movement therapist is the container of the group identity of the nascent, or pre-group, they provide a useful framework for addressing the difficulties of work with long-term hospitalized patients, and they posit realistic therapeutic goals. They write that 'as the group develops and its defenses against relatedness diminish, the possibility increases that the patients will be able to perceive and experience the therapist's internal representation of the group which emanates from his/her behavior' (Sandel and Johnson 1983: 134).

Working with such patients over a period of time is stressful and requires that the dance movement therapist has supervision and peer support. Sandel and Johnson note that the feelings engendered in the dance movement therapist working with such patients provide a valuable clue to the unexpressed inner world of the group. Feelings include hopelessness, grandiose fantasies of rescue, and a persistent sense of chaos and fragmentation. Goals of such therapy differ from those of higher functioning groups, and so the group work can be considered

> not an intervention (i.e. a temporary action designed to eradicate 'problems' or 'disease') but rather it is a life support system which must be present in some form in order to prevent atrophy and maintain functioning.
>
> (Sandel and Johnson 1983: 134)

Nascent groups go through three stages, the first being one resembling a social façade in which the group members act in a compliant and superficially functional manner, usually to please the new therapist. In the second stage, a slow development of relatedness and intimacy occurs, usually followed by a third stage, termed dissolution, in which a more realistic picture of the internal state of the patients is seen, which may manifest itself in chaos, lack of attendance and disruptive behaviour. Without the containing function of the therapist, the group usually dissolves, but 'this stage is not characterized by any form of working through or termination as in groups of higher functioning people. The group merely comes apart, like passengers at the end of a long bus ride' (Sandel and Johnson 1983: 134). The most therapeutic part of the life of the group could be assumed to be the second stage.

It is important to note that such patients are not usually participating in any other type of therapy. Often, when dance movement therapy is being introduced into a psychiatric hospital, these are precisely the sorts of patients chosen to try DMT, which is seen as a 'novel' approach. Popular assumptions about the energizing function of movement, as well as recognition that verbal conversations may simply produce distorted speech from the patient, mean that staff are keen to try innovative therapeutic methods. Fortunately, DMT 'has been found to be especially effective in engaging patients whose capacity to participate in strictly verbal group therapy is limited' (Sandel and Johnson 1983: 134). However, it must be made clear to hospital staff that, while DMT can be effective with this group, it is also applicable, with modified goals, to higher-functioning patients.

Case example

Sandel and Johnson describe a case study in which a nascent group constructed an image of themselves as an imaginary fish stew. As the group pretended to stir the stew, the therapist asked, 'What can we do with it now?' One person said, 'Throw it away!' Others said, 'Eat it.' The therapist spontaneously responded to the first suggestion, and guided the group's movement to one end of the room where the fish stew was symbolically dumped into the rubbish bin. Several patients immediately expressed regret or surprise at this action (Sandel and Johnson 1983: 136). In retrospect, the therapist realized that she had allowed the group to reject its symbolic representation of itself. This type of group image is probably not surprising, given that patients' self-esteem is extremely low. In the experience of the present author, imagery which involves taking a creation of the group and killing, destroying, losing, forgetting, or letting it disappear are common in groups of this type.

Therapists must point out in as neutral a manner as possible the implications of such a symbolic gesture, and interpret it as a statement about the group's self image. The therapist can then try to engender a level of self-respect for the group, or at least some measure of positive regard, while not falling prey to the tendency to idealize the group. It is important to acknowledge the horrible nature of the symbol, and take it seriously, and not to brush it under the carpet, or dismiss it as 'not nice';

at the same time, it is essential to give the group the message that these feelings might become more bearable if they can be sorted out and examined within the emotionally safe environment of the group, using the modes of symbolic and movement experimentation, rather than verbal confrontation or aggressive behaviour.

Johnson and Sandel give a good example of a phenomenon that is common among long-stay or chronic patients, in which a particular member comes to embody an emotional statement which speaks for the group as a whole. For example, a disruptive patient whose actions tend to break up the group when it is engaging in synchronous movement or expressing feelings, is helping the group (and the therapist) avoid the threatening experience of the intimacy and contact that could arise from such engagement. Patients seem to monitor the degree of intimacy with flight behaviour. Such behaviour includes refusing to attend the group, or coming for the first five minutes and rushing out, returning only if tea or biscuits are offered at the end of the session. Other avoidant behaviour includes an unpredictable lack of participation in basic group structures, by either refusing to take turns at leadership, or not mirroring another patient, or possibly by becoming disorganized, and talking incessantly about topics unrelated to the group and its therapeutic tasks. All of these behaviours serve to disrupt the group's attempts at contact and cooperation, and serve as a defence against feelings that arise.

Another common phenomenon, which illustrates that chronic patients often assume Bion's basic assumption of dependency, is the fact that patients will often begin to rely on ritualized behaviour rather than fresh and spontaneous interaction each week. Patients will repeat the same turn in movement each week, and will make similar comments when asked how they are feeling. In the initial stages, ritualization seems to be important in creating a sense of relatedness among the participants by bringing a sense of familiarity, safety and structure to human contact. The ability to relate to others, even in a ritualized way, is an important therapeutic gain for patients who may assume that others are fundamentally hostile, uncaring, or threatening. However, ritualized rather than genuine interaction must not be allowed to continue indefinitely; the therapist might introduce a new prop, or warmup, or more structured format of movement in order to shift the group gently out of its ritualized monotonous harmony. Finally, the patients may concretely show their dependency needs by becoming organized and showing contentment when they are literally fed by the nurse or therapist who may arrange tea and biscuits at the end of a session with long-term or geriatric patients. For this reason, most dance movement therapists do not use the lure of tea and biscuits to get chronic patients to come to sessions unless institutional policy demands or expects it as a matter of course.

Although the difficulties in work with long-term patients have been emphasized here, the work does provide a challenging and fascinating experience for the dance movement therapist, and provides patients with a therapeutic medium that can address this largely neglected client group at a relevant level of intervention. Long-term patients in well-established groups are able to explore issues important to them, such as: feelings of hopelessness, worthlessness, loneliness or failure; anger at themselves, other patients, or staff; fears about rejoining community life; and sadness at leaving the institutions that may have been homes for many many years or even decades. Many of these issues can then fruitfully be taken up by key nursing staff, once they are revealed in the context of the DMT group (Liebowitz *et al.* 1989).

The recognition of the effect the patients' behaviour has on the therapist must be used therapeutically, in order to get in touch with what the patients are feeling. Without supervision, support, and possibly individual therapy as well, the dance movement therapist may become frustrated or exhausted in endeavouring to work with these very damaged patients. Sandel notes that 'incredible patience, optimism, and stubbornness, while in part defensive, are probably necessary qualities for the therapist, as is ability to tolerate extremes of emotion' (Sandel 1980: 30). Relatively recent research into the psychophysical effects on the dance movement therapists who work with the schizophrenic population shows that recuperative measures, such as taking time to use one's own rhythmic, integrating movement, and understanding the phenomena of countertransference, can allow the dance movement therapist to be empathetic with, rather than overwhelmed by, the feelings patients bring to the sessions (Skove 1986). These ideas are discussed further in the clinical section, which describes DMT groups with long-term patients.

HUMANISTIC GROUP DMT

In addition to DMT groups informed by psychoananalytic ideas, a second large school of group DMT is one based in theories of humanistic and existential group psychotherapy. A major practitioner and theorist in this area is Irvin D. Yalom (Yalom 1970, 1983). Humanistic group psychotherapy evolved from the 'encounter group' – a term coined by Carl Rogers in the mid 1960s for experiential groups. Yalom's work represents a synthesis and evolution from many different kinds of early group therapies including sensory awareness groups, transactional analysis groups, traditional 'T' or training in human relations groups, and psychoanalytically oriented group psychotherapy. Because they include psychodynamic ideas derived from Freud, such groups are sometimes referred to as psychodynamic, or simply dynamic therapy groups.

These verbal psychotherapy groups consist of between six and eight patients or clients as well as a therapist and co-leader who meet once a week or more for an agreed period, lasting from six months to several years. Such groups are a very common form of treatment for high-functioning psychiatric outpatients, and for 'normal neurotic' clients. Illustrations of parallels between verbal and DMT groups will be drawn before considering Claire Schmais's important theorization of what she terms the 'healing factors' specific to group DMT.

Yalom's therapeutic factors

Yalom identified crucial aspects of the process of psychological change which form a basis upon which the group therapist may base tactics and strategy. He notes that therapeutic change is an enormously complex process occurring through an intricate interplay of various guided human experiences which he termed 'therapeutic factors'. Included among the eleven therapeutic factors that Yalom identifies are a number that are also relevant to group DMT. These include: the development of socializing techniques, learning through imitation, a corrective recapitulation of the family group, group cohesiveness, catharsis and a recognition of the universal nature of many emotional experiences. These six will be considered briefly below.

The development of socializing techniques is often an explicit aim for therapy groups which prepare hospitalized patients for discharge, and for groups of adolescent patients. 'In dynamic group therapy with ground rules which encourage open feedback, patients may obtain considerable information about maladaptive social behaviour' (Yalom 1983: 17). In the course of therapy, patients learn to be helpfully responsive to others, are less judgemental, and are more capable of experiencing and expressing accurate empathy, all of which are helpful in the patients' future social interactions. Group therapy teaches the patients the kind of impact they make on others, and can improve their skills in getting along with people. In group DMT, the nonverbal elements of clear social communication are enhanced. Patients must increase their eye contact in order to follow the group process, and, by seeing their own movements mirrored by the group, obtain valuable feedback about their nonverbal self-presentation. The dance movement therapist must endeavour to facilitate the creation of an open and accepting interpersonal environment in which patients feel able to comment on the behaviour of other members of the group, and learn from others' comments about themselves.

A second therapeutic factor is that the patients learn through imitation. In group therapy it is beneficial for patients to observe the behaviour of others with a similar set of problems to their own. Even if specific imitative behaviour does not last long, it may help the patients to 'unfreeze' by experimenting with new behaviour. It is not uncommon, Yalom writes, for patients in therapy to try on, as it were, bits and pieces of other people, and then either relinquish them as ill-fitting, or integrate aspects of others into a new way of being. In dance movement therapy, in which patients are asked to mirror each other's movements, there is a rich potential for this type of imitative behaviour and learning.

A third therapeutic factor is the fact that the group provides a corrective recapitulation of the primary family group. The group resembles a family in many respects, and often groups are run with one male and one female therapist in a deliberate attempt to simulate a family dynamic. Patients will repeat patterns of interaction with the therapists and other group members which they once used with parents and siblings. Such patterns may include: helpless dependence upon the therapists/parents or blind defiance of them; attempts to split the mother/father therapists; bitter competition with other members to gain the attention of the leaders; or the formation of subgroups, searching for allies among other patients in an attempt to overthrow the rule of the therapists/parents. Being in a therapy group in which such patterns are pointed out helps the patients to understand past relationships. Creative interaction in movement in which patients may assign each other specific movement roles during group improvisation offers ample opportunity for concrete, physical examples which show the group's functioning. Interestingly, issues and group dynamics that emerge in groups do resemble strongly those that arise in DMT work with families, an example of which is given in the clinical chapters that follow.

A fourth therapeutic factor is that of the discovery of the universality of human feeling. Many patients enter therapy with the belief that they alone have certain frightening or unacceptable problems, thoughts, impulses or fantasies (Yalom 1983: 7). A patient's sense of uniqueness is often heightened by a sense of social isolation, and, because of interpersonal difficulties, opportunities for frank and candid consensual validation are not often available. As patients perceive their similarity to others, and share their deep concerns, they benefit further from the accompanying catharsis and acceptance by other group members. Yalom notes that common themes, or 'secrets' which patients do not immediately assume that others in the group might share, include a deep conviction of basic inadequacy – a feeling that if others really knew them, they would discover their incompetence and see through their bluff. A second theme is a deep sense of interpersonal alienation; individuals report that they cannot really care for or love another person. A final theme is some variety of sexual secret, often a dread of homosexual inclinations (Yalom 1983: 9). In group DMT, members share each other's movement expression and engage in cooperative formation of verbal symbols which illustrate the movement. Here, the opportunity to share an individual expression is great; patients often make more eye contact, and exhibit greater nonverbal synchrony when they repeat the movement expression of another individual with whose experience they can identify.

A fifth and related therapeutic factor is that of group cohesiveness. This is defined as the special sense of actually belonging to a group, being accepted, and approved of. The importance of belonging to childhood peer groups, adolescent cliques, a proper adult social 'in' group and one's own family cannot be overestimated. To be accepted by others brings into question the basic belief that the patient or client is essentially repugnant or unlovable (Yalom 1983: 50). The person therefore has a sense of not being alone, and belonging to a group of people who understand and accept them. Claire Schmais adds that the DMT group 'allows for controlled regression in that people can re-experience repressed and disassociated feelings that are then valued and accepted by the group' (Schmais 1985: 27). The growing sense of cohesion in DMT groups is clearly felt and illustrated in the synchrony and patterning of group movement behaviour. As groups develop, mirroring becomes more precise and members are able to sustain more rhythmic and spatial synchrony as well. In group DMT, the building of the sense of group identity and cohesiveness is a task that takes some time, but its value is illustrated by the fact that patients in an outpatient setting behave as though they regard their membership in the group as important. Often, after other aspects of their treatment have ended, they request to continue attendance at a DMT group until it finishes its planned series of meetings. In this way, the sixteen-week outpatient group often forms a useful bridge between dependence upon the day treatment unit and independent living after treatment.

A sixth and final therapeutic factor is catharsis: this is simply the ability to express feelings rather than hold them in. This includes expressing positive or negative feelings towards the leaders and other group members. Catharsis on its own is not enough; the release of intense emotions is liberating, but must be accompanied by ownership and understanding of the emotions released. In DMT there is a danger that patients will use the movement as an opportunity to give physical vent to feelings, but will not wish to reflect or verbalize their feelings later. It is of the utmost importance that the dance movement therapist does not allow the movement experience to be one of mindless release, and that he or she ensures that the physical release does not become an end in itself, but rather is understood in the context of the relationships developed in the group between members and the therapists.

Yalom takes special care to note that the operation of therapeutic factors, and the therapeutic goals derived from them, are appropriate to fairly high functioning adults, generally capable of holding down employment and perhaps maintaining family and working relationships. This is in contrast to the sorts of therapeutic goals that he views as important for hospitalized patients seen in inpatient groups, such as those seen on acute admissions wards. These goals would include: identifying problems in relating to others; alleviation of hospital-related anxiety; and giving the patients the clear message that talking helps (Yalom 1970). It is imperative for the success of therapy with psychiatric patients that the dance movement therapist sets realistic treatment goals; unrealistic ideas about 'curing' mental illness defeat the strengths of both the group and the therapist.

Further therapeutic factors for inpatient and outpatient groups not discussed at length here include: the installation of hope; imparting of information; altruism; and existential factors. Student dance movement therapists will find it of value to be familiar with both the theory and the practice of verbal group psychotherapy in order to understand their patients and clients.

SCHMAIS'S 'HEALING PROCESSES' IN GROUP DMT

Claire Schmais has articulated a number of 'healing processes' in group DMT, some of which relate directly to the work of Yalom. These include synchrony, expression, rhythm, vitalization, integration, cohesion and symbolism (Schmais 1985). Each will be described in turn, as they can provide a useful framework for examining clinical experience.

There are three different types of synchrony: rhythmic, spatial and effort synchrony. Rhythmic synchrony simply describes people who are moving in time with one another. Spatial synchrony describes people who are moving in time with others who are also making the same spatial design with body parts. Effort synchrony refers to people using the same movement quality, though this may be occurring with different body parts; that is, one person might be pressing down with a foot, and another with a hand forward into the air to the same rhythm. The term 'effort' applies to a qualitative movement analysis system developed by Rudolf Laban, which is discussed in the next chapter (Laban 1948).

Synchrony can be viewed as a recapitulation of an earlier developmental process; synchrony between mother and child allows them to engage in a shared experience. The nonverbal communications researcher Albert Scheflen viewed parallel synchronous human activity as evidence of social unification or interpersonal affiliation (Scheflen and Scheflen 1972, Scheflen 1979). Schmais notes that dance movement therapy encourages identification with the social group by structuring the activity so that people move together in time and space; in this way, synchrony promotes a sense of solidarity. This is a potentially important experience for psychiatric patients who are socially isolated. Schmais concludes that the development of synchronous activity promotes what Yalom terms 'group cohesion'. The dance movement therapist, with a trained eye, can detect members of the group who synchronize easily with one another, or those who have persistent difficulty in achieving synchrony, which might possibly indicate fear or anxiety about experiencing a loss of self in being overwhelmed by the group's synchrony (Schmais and Felber 1977: 24).

Expression, another healing factor, describes the process by which the use of movement allows internal states to be made conscious through external expression, and so appear less ominous or frightening. Schmais notes that everyday actions and emotional expressions share the same neuromuscular pathways, such that seemingly simple themes of work or play often shift into powerful emotional statements in movement. For example, the action of throwing a ball can become the plunging of a dagger into a heart; the miming of a simple task such as smoothing a tablecloth can be metamorphosized into covering a coffin, or a gesture of tender caress.

A further therapeutic factor is rhythm. Rhythms that are reminiscent of early developmental processes may create a basis for symbolic gratification of infantile demands. When the group rocks to a common pulse, it seems as if they share in a regressive fantasy that binds them together. It would be interesting to research whether dependency groups, for example, would use developmentally based body rhythms as described by Kestenberg (1975), such as rocking, which are reminiscent of those appropriate to what Freud termed the oral stage, in which psychological issues concerning nurturance and dependency figure highly. Rhythmic repetition both contains and clarifies emotional expression (Schmais 1985: 22).

A fourth healing factor is vitalization. Marian Chace wrote that

a positive quality of aliveness is present in a group of dancers which is a strong contrast to patients sitting listlessly absorbed in no activity, withdrawn from all others in loneliness. It is exciting to see one of those passively still people rise as though drawn by a magnet and move towards the living group.

(Chaiklin 1975: 203)

The very act of moving can provide the patient with a relief from anxiety, loosen physical rigidity, free the emotional and physical impulse to act, and supply the energy to do so. Schmais notes that one of the most striking aspects of DMT group sessions is to witness the energy that is liberated with the expression of angry feelings. A synergistic effect results from the stimulation of being in a group situation and from the activation within the individuals that is caused by moving, stamping, reaching, punching or slashing in unison. Moving to rhythm in a group, in the expression of a feeling, vitalizes the individual and the group, 'generating a reservoir of physical and psychic strength that can further expression, communication and competence' (Schmais 1985: 24).

Another healing factor in DMT is integration, which implies achieving a sense of unity within the individual and a sense of community between internal and external reality. The dance movement therapist strives to help the group to integrate 'body actions, facial expression and verbalization; thought and expression; feelings and words; breathing and activity; past and present; and self-image and self-presentation' (Schmais 1985: 24). She notes further that integration requires that experiences are both felt and symbolically represented; movement must be used as an experience that is then considered or reflected upon. The metaphoric dance symbol can externalize the internal state. With verbal symbols it is possible to label, classify, discuss and reflect upon this internal state (Schmais 1985: 27).

The relationship between movement and words is a complex one which dance movement therapy must consider theoretically as well as practically:

words may lead to associations and images that alter the movements and each alteration in movement evokes new verbal associations and ideas. This interaction of words and movement escalates affect and provides an associative matrix from which integrative dance symbols can arise.

(Schmais 1985: 27)

Part of what makes dance movement therapy a unique approach in psychiatry is that the therapist, by labelling affect as it appears and by reflecting the patient's movement, offers an experience that can help the patient integrate feelings, thoughts and actions in the here-and-now, present experience of the group.

Group cohesion is a further healing factor that Schmais derives from Yalom's work. She writes that 'being a part of the dance by sharing and repeating simple steps and rhythms builds a sense of community, but it is not until people actively participate in each other's symbolic statements that group cohesiveness takes root' (Schmais 1985: 29).

A final healing factor in dance movement therapy is found in the use of symbolism. Schmais hypothesizes that 'the dance symbol is threefold; in its creation, in the illumination it affords and in the actual participation in the collective product' (Schmais 1985: 31). For example, in a group of patients, the movement of walking might become heavy rhythmic stepping, which produces a verbal association of 'stamping out feelings of frustration' or 'brushing things under the carpet'. The group can recognize a feeling and acknowledge that, though they may have different sources that led them to engage in creating such a movement symbol, they can gain a sense of relatedness to others through this shared experience. Undoubtedly the most important feature of symbolism is that:

it allows for psychic distance from private preoccupations. Once it has been structurally represented, an idea or emotion can be apprehended, contemplated, analyzed, or connected to other symbolic material. The symbol can shed light on old issues, articulate current concerns and anticipate the future.

(Schmais 1985: 32)

The importance of symbolism to the dance movement therapy process will be further explored in Chapter 9, which will articulate an approach to DMT that takes the symbol as its central concern.

In conclusion, it can be seen that DMT groups share similar goals to that of group therapy; in addition to goals of improved social functioning and the reintegration of unconscious material through exploring feelings, group DMT also has movement goals of integration, release and vitalization. The achievement of a sense of the DMT group functioning as a unit, rather than as a therapist relating individually to each of a number of patients in a room, is an important one. Supervision, participation in a group, and the review of work with psychiatric patients on videotape (whether one's own or that of a colleague) can all facilitate an understanding of group process. Despite the large amount of energy required to facilitate a group with psychiatric clients or patients – particularly those who are long-term patients – the rewards are great. It is possible to see improvements in social functioning in patients quite quickly, often within a few sessions. Often the opening of the nonverbal channel of communication is a great stride forward for patients who have been isolated for a long time, and it seems to inspire them to communicate socially and verbally. The sharing of a symbolic movement and verbal therapy experience, in which patients create, explore and analyse a symbol that contains emotional meaning, can be equally exhilarating for patients and therapist.

STRUCTURAL ANALYSIS OF GROUP DMT

The arts therapies, in common with verbal psychotherapy, have little experimental verification for the assertion that their therapy is effective, or research evidence illustrating which of the elements of therapy actually contribute to its success. This section will describe some of the existing research that is relevant to DMT groups in psychiatry (Bruno 1981, Schmais and Felber 1977).

David Read Johnson and Susan Sandel have developed a systematized vocabulary for describing the events and processes specific to group DMT sessions, known as SAMS (Structural Analysis of Movement Sessions) (Johnson and Sandel 1977). This was developed from work with chronic schizophrenic and character disordered adolescent patients in group DMT and dramatherapy sessions modelled after Marian Chace's work. The basis of SAMS lies in the concept of *structure*, which is defined as the overt, agreed upon patterns or rules of organization; it describes what the group is doing.

For example, SAMS would describe the therapist's suggestion of a circle format, but would not describe the specific movement qualities that the patients provided during their turn in taking leadership. Facilitating 'a consistent and predictable group structure is one of the most important functions of the dance or drama therapist' (Johnson and Sandel 1977: 33). In their view, for the disturbed patient, being in a circle, following a designated leader and imitating movements in unison form a structure that is critical to the shared social reality within the movement sessions. Disruption in group structure 'therefore places a greater burden on the individual's capacity to manage anxiety' (Johnson and Sandel 1977: 33).

Sandel and Johnson identified three dimensions of structure including: *task structure*, that is, the observable action that the group does; *spatial structure*, which describes the physical relationship the group members have towards one another in the space, such as a circle, or line, or more irregular forms; and finally, *role structure*, the particular pattern of formal roles that the group sets up in conducting its activities, such as when each individual in turn takes over leadership at a designated signal from the rest of the group. These structures were rated for definiteness, indefiniteness during a session.

Johnson and Sandel discuss a videotaped case example of a group of schizophrenics in their early twenties. It was noted that the group had difficulty maintaining definiteness in structure at times when leadership had to be passed from one member to another. This indicated that the group was highly dependent upon the therapist and the role structure to maintain its coherence. Furthermore, the group had the most difficulty maintaining structures when there was any interruption in the music; the reliance on music as an external organizer reflected a low level of functioning in comparison with other, higher functioning groups of patients. Sandel and Johnson's work provides experimental evidence for the often quoted observation among dance movement therapists that the more disturbed the patients in a group, the more the need for structure. This might take the form of an extended warmup, the use of highly rhythmic music, or suggestions from the therapist or other patients as to what each member might offer when their turn comes to lead the group.

The relationship between the structural cohesion of a dance movement therapy session with schizophrenics and the content (or 'group process') was studied by Carol Bruno using SAMS (Bruno 1981). She noted that structure became less definite when aggressive images emerged, when the spatial configuration was disturbed, for example by a member leaving the circle unexpectedly, or when a movement task was introduced that was too difficult for patients to follow. Her work gives experimental validation to Marian Chace's views about rhythm being important for integration and structured interaction for patients. It also gives a rationale for using the Chace format in DMT in psychiatry by affirming that 'simple, definite spatial structure seems crucial for a schizophrenic group's overall functioning' (Bruno 1981: 131). Her study also showed that the use of music, and props such as balls or a long piece of Lycra stretch-cloth, increased definiteness of structure for schizophrenic groups, while they did not have this effect with control groups of character-disordered adolescents or normal subjects. She concluded that the ability to continuously create, alter and monitor group structures that best allow content or process material to emerge was a unique feature of the arts therapies. Because of this, 'participants can try out new roles and behaviours in an environment that is less restrictive than everyday life' (Bruno 1981: 133).

CONCLUSION

This chapter has shown how many different psychological models can be integrated with group and individual work in DMT, including the psychodynamic, Jungian, ego-psychoanalytic, Gestalt, humanistic and psychoanalytic theories and methods. In practice, most dance movement therapists are grounded in one tradition, though they may borrow, eclectically, from others.

It will be clear that the psychological framework used by the dance movement therapist makes a great impact to the quality and nature of the DMT being practised. For example, the movement behaviour of the patient may be read as evidence of spiritual growth (as in the case of Jungian DMT) or of psychosexual developmental fixation at oral, anal or genital stages (as it is in ego-psychoanalytic DMT) or be seen as evidence of infantile anxiety manifesting itself in group behaviour (as is the case in psychoanalytically informed group DMT). All of these levels of interpretation can exist simultaneously; it is the immediate needs of the patients and the stated goals of the group DMT that determine how movement is understood in the context of a particular theoretical framework.

In addition to being based in a psychological school of thought, DMT is based in creative movement, and the particular type of dance or movement training that the dance movement therapist has had will undoubtedly influence his or her technique. Elaine Siegel's balletic training means that she and her students would view barre exercises as an appropriate way to facilitate changes in the client's body ego. This is a direct contrast to the work of Johnson and Sandel which is influenced by dramatherapy and so employs props and encourages patients to use symbols to describe how they are feeling.

The reader who is new to DMT may be bewildered by this array of psychological and movement frameworks; generally each training institute adheres to a specific tradition or school. Also, the theory and techniques used in DMT are employed with specific reference to the needs of the patient population. A supportive group for long-term or continuing care patients may include a great deal of synchronized movement within the shared leadership format, because primary social and movement interaction is an approprite therapeutic goal. Conversely, the outpatient group, which may be aimed at exploring underlying emotional difficulties and expanding expressive movement range, might have a looser structure, including a measure of free improvisation in movement and more verbal interpretation by the dance movement therapist, because these would be most appropriate to achieving the relevant therapeutic goals.

It may be noted that the range of approaches here probably only constitute half of those currently being practised as DMT; dance movement therapists are notoriously nonverbal when it comes to articulating and formalizing what they are doing. There are a number of eclectic approaches which combine other types of dance form such as New Dance, and still further forms of DMT using other psychological theories such as those derived from Jacques Lacan, about which little has yet been published. The next few years in Britain will undoubtedly produce some interesting new ideas as American DMT techniques mix with British and European psychotherapy theories to produce further innovative forms of DMT (Higgens and McLean 1990, Payne 1992, Shenton 1990).

The next chapter will survey the ways in which movement carries meaning, by introducing the main choreographic movement analysis system used in DMT, derived from Rudolf Laban's Effort Analysis. A description of studies in movement psychopathology is provided, along with a glimpse at psychoanalytic and nonverbal communications perspectives on movement behaviour, and the chapter concludes with some ideas about body movement as a field of cultural and intellectual inquiry. Readers keen to understand the clinical application of ideas presented in this chapter could usefully read one of the clinical chapters before delving into the next chapter's survey of movement analysis systems. Although it is important to understand the technical and theoretical bases on which movement is employed in DMT, it is difficult to visualize exactly how movement is used in DMT without the aid of videotaped examples. Therefore, a glance at one of the client groups in the clinical section might put the next chapter into perspective for anyone more interested in clinical work than the technical and theoretical foundations of DMT.

Chapter 4

Movement and meaning

INTRODUCTION

The psychotherapist uses words to communicate with the patient, and takes his or her statements to be evidence of their emotional state and underlying unconscious processes. In the same way, the dance movement therapist uses movement to interact with the patient, and reads the patient's movement for its symbolic and expressive content. It is important, therefore, to consider the question: 'How does movement carry meaning?' First, it is necessary to bear in mind that the way we define the units of movement circumscribes what we can read from movement. When we say 'movement', do we mean an action, like lifting the hand vertically and diagonally at a quick pace? Or do we define movements in units of gesture, such as, for example, waving goodbye? Or is movement a kinesiological problem in which groups of muscles contract in sequence to enable a mass of flesh to move from one fixed position to the next?

Perhaps we would look only at movement in relation to speech, as in: 'The man said, "Well, I guess it's goodbye. . . " and then turned and waved.' Or would we consider the *quality* with which the man waved; was it in a silly manner, or in a somber one, exuberantly or quietly? Perhaps we would be interested to know whether the hand wave that the man performed was a type of wave specific to his culture and therefore denoted an informal, friendly wave, rather than a formal or ceremonial one. We might also speculate whether the man waved because he was in synchrony with his friend, who was also waving, so that his waving signalled the ending of their interaction.

We might make hypotheses for the underlying reasons for the man's wave. Was he happy to see the other person depart, or was he extending his hand longingly, waving it as though to stay connected to his friend for a moment longer by synchronizing his wave with that of his friend? Or was the wave perhaps a bizarre, occasional mannerism devoid of any communicational meaning, made by his arm but disconnected from his facial expression, and unrelated to anyone around him? Could the wave even have been the man illustrating how birds flap their wings to his four-year-old child standing nearby, or could he have been using the wave to illustrate the rise and fall of his shares on the stock market, such that the wave took on a symbolic meaning, and underlined his speech? This very simple example illustrates the complexity of movement and the fact that it can carry a multiplicity of meaning, depending on the units in which it is defined, the context in which it occurs, and the presuppositions of the person analysing the movement. The various ways in which we have just described the man waving show that movement can be seen anatomically, kinesiologically, communicationally, culturally, interactionally, pathologically and symbolically.

This chapter will give a very brief history of the study of movement, and then survey various levels and types of movement analysis, making some reference to their relevance to clinical work in DMT in psychiatry. Types of movement analysis that will be discussed in this chapter include: movement as evidence of psychopathology; movement as reflective of psychosexual development (Freud's oral, anal and genital stages); movement as considered by psychoanalysts in the light of theories of instinctual drives and defence mechanisms; choreographic analysis of movement such as Laban's effort–shape with its psychological correlates developed by Irmgard Bartenieff and Marion North; and finally, a brief consideration of anthropological and aesthetic writing on movement.

Historical perspectives on movement research

Our current ways of thinking about movement reflect intellectual influences from the history of its study. This history is an interesting one, beginning with Darwin's publication of *The Expression of the Emotions in Man and Animals* in 1872. Darwin formulated theories of origins and functions of nonverbal behaviour, such as the theory of 'serviceable associated habits': this argues that certain acts are performed to relieve certain states or sensations. When the state recurs, so does the action, even if it is no longer adaptive. Instances of this include the startle reflex, angry facial expressions, or scratching the head when perplexed, which occur almost automatically, or out of human habit. For example, Darwin noted that domestic animals circle and pad down the carpet before they lie down on it; this seems to be an inherited association to their wild ancestors, who would have smoothed down the grass before lying on it (Davis 1975: 11). Darwin used concepts from ethology and his evolutionary theory to try to understand the meaning of movement behaviour. Some of his ideas were taken up by researchers in the 1960s and 1970s who drew parallels between human and animal behaviour (Scheflen 1979).

In the 1920s and 1930s, experimental psychologists hoped that the study of facial expressions would provide a way of understanding the nature of emotions, how they are shown, and how they are perceived by others. Interestingly, research concluded that subjects were not very accurate at labelling emotional expressions on the faces of people in photographs. They could get the general idea, but the situational cue, or context of the facial expression, was needed to gain greater accuracy. This research showed the necessity of reading movement in its communicational context. This insight was taken up by the nonverbal communications researcher Ray Birdwhistell, who made micro analyses of movement using structural linguistics as a framework with which to understand nonverbal communicative behaviour. For Birdwhistell, the meaning of movement cannot be separated from who does it, where, when, and in which interactional sequence (Birdwhistell 1970).

From the 1930s to the present, movement research has become more specific, and can be grouped according to a number of categories: movement as reflective of personality, emotion or psychopathology, psychological interpretation of specific actions, interaction, communication, cultural comparisons and developmental patterns (Davis 1975: 12). From the 1940s onwards, the disciplines of anthropology, linguistics and social psychology took up an interest in the nonverbal dimension of the communications process. During the 1960s, nonverbal communications research emerged as a field of study in its own right, related to, but distinct from anthropology, psychology, ethology, ethnology, linguistics, psychology and aesthetics.

Given this huge spectrum of approaches to reading movement it is helpful to remember that in DMT we are concerned primarily with *how* movement happens, rather than *what* is done in movement. That is, we are not interested in the fact that the man, described above, lifted his arm from his side, to the upper right-hand space, and returned it to its original position. Instead, we are interested in whether he shot his arm up in a quick gesture of salute, or whether his hand gave a wobbly, drunken wave. The adjectives 'quick' and 'wobbly' describe the quality of the movement, from which we can make inferences about its psychological significance for the subject: this qualitative, expressive, psychological aspect of movement analysis is the one that DMT takes as its focus. The nonverbal communications researcher and psychologist Martha Davis has developed a schema, or theoretical framework, with which we can organize all of these movement analysis perspectives. She writes that, 'at any one moment, movement is simultaneously reflecting intrapsychic, interpersonal and cultural patterns' (Davis 1974: 21). For example, movement can show the intrapsychic processes of emotion, anxiety, defence mechanisms, or unconscious symbolic communication. It can illustrate the interpersonal processes of cohesiveness, relatedness, dominance, or subgrouping. Movement can also reflect cultural rituals and group interaction conventions, such as Western culture's respect for a degree of 'personal space'. Movement can reflect transitory patterns, or enduring style with repeated characteristics. The interpersonal and intrapsychic processes are subject to momentary change, while an individual's personal movement style and cultural features persist over time.

Rather than seeing movement as a mere parallel or illustration of the verbal dimension of experience, it can be argued that

> movement patterns are not simply signs of individual differences and interpersonal processes; *they are of them.*
>
> In effect, the movement dimension is a *direct access* to these processes, which

are only inferred from words, drawings, dreams, work products, or what people do.

(Davis 1974: 22)

The relation between movement and meaning, then, is an intrinsic one; there is an essential, inherent and natural connection between the movement and what it means. For example, not everyone can immediately read the sign language used by deaf people. The meanings of these specific gestures are conveyed by convention, by everyone establishing a tradition of using a particular hand movement to signify a particular word, or meaning. Movement in general, however, does carry meaning in a way that is almost universal; narrowing of facial features, contraction of the chest, and shrinking in of limbs towards the centre is highly unlikely to be a statement about something wide, expansive, or encompassing. In Darwin's terms, 'the young and the old of widely different races, both with man and animals, express the same state of mind by the same movements (Polhemus 1978: 16). Finally, it must be remembered that movement must be permitted to 'speak for itself': descriptive terms, metaphors, and criteria from other disciplines should not simply be imposed upon it (Davis 1974: 19). Given this proviso, we can now turn to specific areas of movement and meaning that are relevant to DMT in psychiatry.

MOVEMENT AND PSYCHOPATHOLOGY

The body movements characteristic of mental illness have historically been of interest to psychiatrists for their potential diagnostic value, and have engaged the popular imagination. Study in this area has continued, concurrent with advances in neurologically based theories of the aetiology of mental illness. Most current writing on the abnormal movements which characterize mental illness focuses the movement side-effects produced by antipsychotic medication. This literature will be considered further in Chapter 10.

Psychiatrists at the turn of the century delineated a series of deteriorative psychoses which Kraepelin called 'dementia praecox' and Bleuler renamed schizophrenia. For Bleuler all motor symptoms of schizophrenia were dependent on psychological factors for their origin. Hypotheses which posited a cerebral, or neurological basis for the movement abnormalities of schizophrenia conflicted with those that posited a psychological origin for such movement during the early years of modern psychiatry (Rogers 1985: 221). Movement features were used to distinguish between various types of schizophrenia, and probably played an important part in developing diagnostic subtypes of schizophrenia, such as the catatonic, hebephrenic and paranoid types. For example, catatonic schizophrenia was characterized by stupor, and varied in degree from a 'transient blocking of certain movements to an immobilization of the whole patient in a fixed posture'. Other movement features were rigidity, postural stereotypy, defined as: 'states of immobility and stereotypy in movement which covers all possibilities from simple "neurological" motor behaviour to complicated hyperkinesis of a highly symbolic character' (Mayer-Gross *et al.* 1954: 285). Most current psychiatrists, acknowledging the multifactorial aetiology of schizophrenia, would accept both a neurological and a psychological basis for movement abnormalities in their patients; however, research and training resources are directed towards the understanding of the neurological aspect of illness.

Movement was also useful in figuring out the differences in symptomatology between melancholia, mania and hysteria. The French psychiatrist Charcot used movement when he identified specific movement features that constituted the stages of the 'attacks' of his hysterical patients. Charcot employed a special medical artist, Paul Richet, to draw the patient's movements. Stages of attack included the *prodromes, tonique, épileptoïde, immobilité tonique, clownisme, contorsions, attaque démoniaque, grand attaque hystérique, violence des grandes mouvements, attitudes passionnelles, Zoopsie, l'hystérie masculine*, etc. (that is, the prodromal, tonic, epileptoid, tonic immobility, clownism, contortion, demonic attack, major hysterical attack, large violent movements, passionate attitudes or postures, animal-like movements, and masculine-type hysteria) (Simon-Dhouailly 1986).

It is interesting to note, therefore, that movement probably played a significant role in delineating diagnostic differences between epilepsy, mental handicap and mental illness in this early period of psychiatry. There was also an interesting phase in anthropological and psychiatric study called physiognomy, which sought to identify human evolutionary development and personality characteristics from the shape of facial features and various body parts (Mantegazza *c.* 1925).

The Victorians took an interest in the behavioural oddities and movements of psychiatric patients. A popular form of recreation was to stand in the observation gallery to watch 'the Lunatic's ball' in which a dance was held for 'inmates, attendants and often visitors. Charles Dickens was a visitor to one such ball at St. Luke's Hospital in London in 1851' (Showalter 1987: 39). The bizarre gestures of the then unmedicated patients inspired scientific and popular interest. Cultural and historical studies of the movement features of mental illness show how society's attitudes towards mental illness have evolved such that the abnormal movements of psychiatric patients have been assumed to be anything from possession by evil spirits to evidence of neurological impairment (Gilman 1976, 1985).

In current psychiatric literature, it is generally assumed that medication modifies the expression of the disease-based motor disorder. It is therefore an exceedingly complex, if not impossible task to separate movement which is based in the illness (with its neurological and psychological aetiology) from secondary movement disorders caused by extrapyramidal reactions to phenothiazines (Rogers 1985: 221). The divergent readings of the abnormal movements that constitute psychopathology are made more difficult because researchers in the area employ varying levels of sophistication in defining the movement parameters they are measuring. This makes comparison across research studies very difficult. For example, some studies measure voluntary movement and others involuntary; some note simply the presence or absence of 'abnormality', which is defined by varying degrees of sophistication. Few research projects attempt a qualitative as well as a quantitative description of the abnormal motor behaviour that accompanies psychopathology.

Specific descriptions of the movement patterns common in schizophrenia and depression will be discussed in Chapter 10.

PSYCHOANALYTIC PERSPECTIVES ON MOVEMENT

Psychoanalytic views of movement are diverse; some analysts see the movement as an unconscious communication, and others focus on finding manifestations of psychosexual development, or fixation in movement terms. Some writers see movement as a defence mechanism against anxiety, rather than an expression of emotion, and still others hypothesize the importance of the role of the body in psychological health. All of these perspectives are important to DMT, and can inform practice and technique.

The writings of the psychoanalyst Judith Kestenberg are very important for dance movement therapists because they combine detailed psychoanalytic observation of children with Laban's approach to movement analysis. Kestenberg's

> focus on the development of movement patterns has both reflected and given shape to important observational and psychoanalytic investigation into phase development (neonatal through parenthood), sexuality and object relations, all of which have underscored a marked concordance between psyche and soma.
>
> (Sossin 1987: 23)

Dance movement therapists, while not being fully trained in the Kestenberg Movement Profile (KMP), are able to recognize what she termed 'tension-flow' and 'shape-flow', which roughly correspond to observable variations in muscle tension and patterns of expanding and contracting in space. Recent research illustrates that the Kestenberg Movement Profile may have a high degree of inter-rater reliability (Sossin 1987).

Kestenberg hypothesizes that there are individual movement patterns present from birth. In her view, a child may have preferred rhythms that are important expressions of his or her personality, while still allowing for the fact that each child goes through stages of development where certain rhythms relate to and serve specific drive discharge. For example, she finds that a predominance of 'urethral rhythms, with growing control over starting and stopping and stress on the sagittal plane (the forward and backward dimension) are some of the motor correlates of the phase during which the child is developing time constancy concepts' (Davis 1975: 25).

Dance movement therapists observe children in the course of their training and so are aware of developmental rhythms in patients. The rhythms reflect changes in free and bound flow, and can be illustrated in any body part, or series of body parts. It is assumed that an adult patient's predominant use of such a rhythm would indicate a regression to a fixation point, or an unresolved issue in psychosexual development correlated with that rhythm. For example, the oral stage is correlated with rhythms resembling sucking or biting; the anal stage with sphincter-like twisting or straining; the urethral stage with walk-run or start-stop rhythms; the

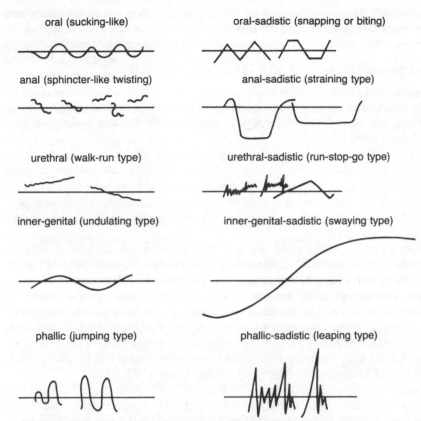

oral (sucking-like)

oral-sadistic (snapping or biting)

anal (sphincter-like twisting)

anal-sadistic (straining type)

urethral (walk-run type)

urethral-sadistic (run-stop-go type)

inner-genital (undulating type)

inner-genital-sadistic (swaying type)

phallic (jumping type)

phallic-sadistic (leaping type)

Figure 4.1. Categories of the Kestenberg Movement Profile (KMP).
Source: Sossin 1987

inner-genital stage with undulating rhythms; and the phallic with jumping or leaping type rhythms (see Figure 4.1).

In addition to Kestenberg's more recent work, some of the early psychoanalysts were interested in the psychoanalytic implications of specific postures or gestures, rather than whole body rhythmic patterns in development. For example, Felix Deutsch developed a theory which he called 'analytic posturology'. In his view, bodily sensation and movement were 'representative of relationships to objects of the past and present' (Deutsch 1952, 1962). This implies that relationships to one's parents have a kinaesthetic counterpart, and possibly accounts for reasons why families share movement patterns. Deutsch believed that 'the psychoanalytic procedure, which stirs up large quantities of psychic energy, is continually accompanied by correlated but invisible physiological adaptations and responses (Deutsch 1952: 196). He hypothesized that postural patterns appeared as 'signal and symbol during the analytical process, preceding, substituting, or accompanying verbal expressions' (Deutsch 1952: 197).

Bela Mittelmann, a psychoanalyst working with children and adults, understood movement more broadly, and felt that movement represented a drive, and was an important means of mastery, integration, and reality testing. He noted that motility 'is closely connected with nearly every other physiological and psychological striving, such as orality, genitality, evaluation of the self, aggression, dependent longings, and interpersonal relations in general' (Mittelmann 1957: 284). In his view movement represented incipient symbolic action, which represented the warding off of external and internal dangers such as fear, anxiety or guilt (Mittelmann 1957: 285).

Furthermore, he noted that movement could be evidence of psychological defence mechanisms, where an 'increase in activity may represent unconscious flight from or fight against the impulse or guilt' (Mittelmann 1957: 285). He believed that motor pathology could be the result of traumatic emotional experience. This thesis is corroborated by current work in DMT with sexually abused children (Goodill 1987).

Interestingly, Mittelmann posited the function of 'motor (imitative) identification' in which the child took on the movement characteristics of significant others with whom the child identified. The process of identification is crucial in the development of the personality, and Mittelmann's recognition that motor behaviour plays a part in identification illustrates that movement could provide useful observational data from which psychoanalytic concepts could be further understood and extended. Finally, Mittelmann, following Deutsch and Charcot, felt that there could be a motor component to memories, dreams and fantasies, and as such could be interpreted by the analyst (Mittelmann 1957: 294).

In addition to psychoanalysts who write specifically about nonverbal aspects of psychosexual development, much of the writing about mother–infant interaction is relevant to DMT. For example, Daniel Stern's work on mother–child interaction and personality development is founded on observational studies which stress the way that movement is the primary language between mother and child in their early communications. Two DMT techniques are derived from this type of research: the first is the concept of 'motor labelling' in which the dance movement therapist verbalizes the child's movement behaviour in order to facilitate a relationship with the child, and to generate an observing ego function in the child, who simultaneously experiences and thinks about his or her movement while the therapist describes its quality in words. The relations between psychoanalytic and psychological ideas on mother–infant interaction and DMT is an important area for further writing and research.

Another concept derived from this research is 'cross modal matching' (Stern 1985). This process facilitates affective (emotional) attunement and 'intersubjective sharing of affect' (Stern 1985: 141). In this, the mother responds in one sensory mode to the child's behaviour in another sensory mode. For example, the mother might respond to a communicative *noise* the child might make by using a *movement* that has the same rhythm, shape and duration. This process also works when the mother uses her voice to match the infant's movement; she can facilitate the child's emergent sense of self, and sense of agency, by responding to movement using language, or vice versa. This process of combining words and movement is a crucial one which underlies DMT, particularly in work with children, but also in work with adults. Because the child's gurgling, babbles and other pre-speech is responded to verbally and non-verbally, early communication between mother and child is facilitated. Furthermore, this process is thought to be responsible for the emergence of the child's early sense of self (Winnicott 1971). A lack of 'cross modal matching', or disturbance in this verbal and nonverbal process in deprived or disturbed mothers may result in developmental delay (Fish 1975).

Movement as a defence

The object relations psychoanalyst Esther Bick conceptualized some of the movement seen in children as a psychological defence mechanism, and she regarded a few particular qualities of children's movement behaviour as a 'second skin'. This describes a state in which a child deals with the experience of lack of integration and regression by adopting a constant pattern of continual movement which serves as a defence or protection from the experience of psychological disorganization. This perpetual state of activity functions almost literally to 'hold the child together' in a kind of partial 'muscularity', and it protects the child from the experience of catastrophic emotional disorganization in the absence of a maternal figure who can help the child reintegrate (Bick 1968: 485). The use of movement, particularly perseverant, phraseless movement as a way to avoid thinking or avoid mental pain, may play a part in what Melanie Klein termed 'manic defences' which protect the subject from experiencing the painful consequences of dependence on good loved objects (Hinshelwood 1989: 341). Dance movement therapists encountering disturbed children may describe this movement as 'endless', and 'multifocused', to convey its phraseless and spatially disorganized quality.

Body image

Another important psychoanalytic and psychiatric theorist on movement is Paul Schilder, who wrote a work of major importance to DMT entitled *The Image and Appearance of the Human Body* (Schilder 1950). He also wrote a book entitled *On Psychoses* (Schilder 1986). In the first of these books, he posited that we have a body image, a mental picture of the body that we form in our mind. Distortion of this image is evident in the illness of anorexia, in which the patient feels grossly overweight when, in fact, he or she is not overweight at all, but is often physically emaciated. Schilder thought that movement was one of the ways in which the body image could be transformed. He said that 'the phenomenon of the dance allows a loosening and changing of the body image', which is important since

> there is no question that the loosening of the body image will bring with it a particular psychic attitude: motion thus influences the body image and leads from a change in the body image to a change in the psychic attitude.
>
> (Schilder 1950: 208)

This theory underscores the psychotherapeutic value of movement in DMT.

As the works of Kestenberg, Bick, Mittelmann, Deutsch and Schilder illustrate, there is a large array of psychoanalytic concepts for which movement is held up as evidence. The most important of these include developmental stages, defences, identifications and symbolic communications. This diversity may lead a new reader to wonder whether movement is a screen onto which psychoanalysts wishfully project their desire to 'see' evidence for their hypotheses. In fact, such a diversity is probably more a function of the fact that psychoanalytic researchers have not systematized the units of movement behaviour they are examining. For example, a symbolic gesture might be momentary, whereas a developmental pattern could persist for years. This does not mean that their hypotheses are not valid, or cannot be compared, but rather that more experimental evidence is needed to support these hypotheses. Furthermore, dance movement therapists must examine carefully the clinical context and focus of their use of movement, and not attempt to read or infer too many of these categories of movement's meanings simultaneously. Videotaping DMT sessions and conferring with a qualified DMT or movement analysis supervisor can enable the dance movement therapist to bring in appropriate psychoanalytic movement research so as to enrich clinical work. It is important to maintain a clinical focus on the essential needs of the patient, whether those be to assist in movement integration (as in work with chronic patients) or to recapitulate developmental processes (as is the case in work with children), and to employ aspects of psychoanalytic movement theory in accordance with clinical aims.

CHOREOGRAPHIC MOVEMENT ANALYSIS SYSTEMS

Rudolf Laban (1879–1958) was an architect and painter turned choreographer whose artistic work flourished in Paris before the First World War. In the 1920s he went to Germany, where he founded several dance movement schools, and became a major figure in the First International Dance Congress (Davis 1978: 183). He developed several dance notations including Labanotation (also known as Kinetography Laban), and later effort analysis (Laban 1948). He was also interested in dance theory, composition and 'choreutics' or 'space harmony', which is a close parallel to music harmonic theory and describes organizations of spatial patterns in movement. He also explored what he termed 'eukinetics' or 'dynamic patterns, the piano, forte, lento, staccato, and so forth of the movement' (Davis 1978: 183). 'Eukinetics' later formed the basis for effort analysis. It is used in nonverbal communications research, and is a highly accurate notation for recording professional dance, in both its spatial composition and dynamic quality.

The effort analysis system developed by Rudolf Laban is of major importance for dance movement therapists. In addition to being a shorthand for recalling movement qualities, there is an accompanying notation which facilitates the therapist's ability to capture and record movement qualities that characterize a patient's movement profile. A single movement, when recalled by the therapist and recorded after the session, can then be examined for its psychological correlates as developed by Irmgard Bartenieff (Bartenieff 1980). Many dance movement therapists videotape their work, if patients agree to be videotaped and sign a consent form, which enables the therapist to analyse the tape after the session. There are debates among DMT practitioners and teachers as to whether it is possible to be analysing the effort qualities of a movement and its symbolic meaning in the session simultaneously. Most agree this is not possible with any degree of sophistication; recalling a mirrored movement, notating it, and thinking about it after the session is usually simpler. However, after the several hundred hours the dance movement therapist spends during training learning effort notation, observation, and analysis of movement in Laban terms, he or she will be possessed of an instinctive sense of the sorts of effort combinations being used, and will have a fairly immediate response to their meaning, both kinaesthetically and emotionally.

Laban's choice of the term 'effort' is interesting: in German, the word is *Antreib*, meaning literally 'drive towards', denoting a fundamental movement quality. 'Effort' describes the qualitative nuances of movement. There are four effort 'factors': space (direct and indirect); weight (strong and light); time (quick/sudden and slow/sustained); and flow (bound/free). Any adjective that describes movement can be translated into a combination of these seemingly simple terms. For example, 'fluttering' may be a combination of quick, light and indirect, and 'pressing' may be a combination of sustained, strong and direct. Flow refers to the element of fluency and continuity of the movement. For example, the man waving at the beginning of our chapter may have waved with quick, indirect and light effort qualities in his friendly wave, or with sustained, indirect and light efforts if his wave was a longing and extended one. The difference between the friendly and the more sombre wave is in their attitude to the effort dimension of time.

Furthermore, the effort factors have their correlates in planes and shapes. Space is correlated with the horizontal plane, weight with the vertical, time with the sagittal or diagonal. Shaping is the description of how the body fills space in movement, whether expanding or contracting in the horizontal plane, growing or shrinking in the vertical, and advancing or retreating in the sagittal plane. Shape describes the quality of sculpting through space, simultaneously creating three-dimensional forms of the body and carving space in complex ways (Davis 1987: 188). Most normal movement involves combinations and sequences of shape and effort flow; healthy movement is defined as that which is flexible, adaptive to the task or expression in movement and encompasses a wide range of effort–shape combinations. Effort–shape analysis of schizophrenia and depression will be reviewed in Chapter 10.

In her study, *Body Movement: Coping with the Environment*, Irmgard Bartenieff describes a series of psychological correlates which correspond to Laban's effort shape (Bartenieff 1980). She drew parallels between flow and emotion; space and attention; weight and intention; and time and decision. It is assumed that the reader of this book will not rely simply on movement descriptions, but will either learn about movement notation and observation in training, or, perhaps for a non-dance movement therapist, attend a dance or drama workshop that would include an

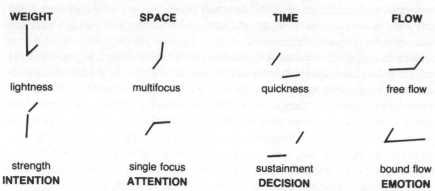

Figure 4.2. Rudolf Laban's effort–shape notation with Irmgard Bartenieff's psychological correlates (from Laban 1948 and Bartenieff 1980).

introductory demonstration and experiential use of effort–shape, a common dance notation system (Laban 1948). Figure 4.2 illustrates how each effort is represented in a notational system.

Bartenieff's effort–shape correlates

Bartenieff explains that each effort quality can be shown to answer a question. These will now be considered for each effort factor.

The element of weight answers the question, 'What is my impact, or intention?' Weight is correlated with the quality of intention, or assertion, creating a strong or light impact, sensing my weight and my self. The act of 'putting one's foot down' or 'throwing one's weight around' implies the use of the strong effort quality of weight, as in stamping, clumping, thumping or banging one's feet against the floor. Using the effort of lightness implies a sensitivity to one's impact, as when one creeps, floats or sneaks across a room with care, perhaps to avoid awakening a sleeping child. In dance movement therapy with psychiatric patients, the use of the weight effort is almost always disturbed. Patients lacking a sense of self can use neither assertiveness nor sensitivity. They are said to have a neutral attitude towards weight. Warmups, which include bouncing, bending at the knee, jumping a little, or swinging, all include the opportunity to regain a sense of one's weight in effort terms, and so become 'grounded' in the self once again.

For the second effort element, namely space, the question is: 'In what manner do I approach the space?' Space is correlated with the quality of thinking, orienting specifically (direct space) or generally (indirect space). For example, someone searching for a lost contact lens approaches space with a limited focus, or direct use of the space effort, whereas someone scanning a crowded room looking for someone approaches space with a multifocus, or indirect use of the space effort. It is important to remember here that the term 'space' refers to the *quality* of the body's movement in space, and not the arrangement of the limbs in space, or the position of the body within the room.

The element of time answers the question: 'When do I need to complete the action?' This is correlated with the quality of decision, urgency (quickness/suddenness) or non-urgency (sustainment), rushing or delaying. How do the movers exert themselves in time? Are they driven by it, as people using haste, or desperately rushing to catch a bus, or are they lingering in it, like people admiring the sea as they walk along the coast? Thinking and therefore using the time effort may require quick and decisive action, as in jumping into a train just as it is pulling out; alternatively, thinking may require the slow, easy contemplation of a problem such as choosing a pastry from the bakery counter, or mulling over a course of proposed action, which would be accompanied, in movement terms, by sustainment in the time effort.

The element of flow answers the question: 'How do I keep going?' Flow is correlated with the quality of emotion and its progression, or how to start and how to keep going, freely, or carefully. Free flow is easy, streaming out, abandoned and ready to go. In contrast, bound flow is controlling the flow, streaming inward, holding back and restrained. Free flow is the dominant element in a child's whirling in delight, or the easy bopping along of someone who has perhaps had a little to drink and is keeping time to a reggae song on the radio. Bound flow, in contrast, is shown in freezing in fear, wincing in anticipation of something coming, or restraining strong feelings. Bound flow is required (along with directness in space and lightness in weight) if one is to carry a full cup of hot coffee without spilling it.

Each effort is acquired by the child during his or her body movement development: space is dominant during the oral stage (0–1 year), weight in the anal stage (1–2 years) and time in the genital stage (3–5 years). The efforts come together in combination during the latency period, and reorganize into a more mature pattern during and after adolescence. Unresolved developmental issues in a stage might mean that the use of that effort is either used repeatedly, or possibly restricted.

It is important to remember that the efforts always occur in combination and sequence. In this section, everyday actions have been given as examples for the sake of clarity of presentation in the absence of a video or live demonstration. In therapy, we would be concerned rather with making effort–shape analysis of expressive, rather than instrumental actions. Furthermore, the combination of effort elements are important: direct space, strong weight and suddenness in time indicate a punch, whereas indirect space, light weight and sustainment in time would indicate a floating combination. There are eight basic effort combinations: floating, punching, gliding, slashing, wringing, dabbing, flicking and pressing. These are like the primary colours in a spectrum. The shades in between, and the intensity of the elements in any one combination, are what give individual character to the performance of an action. Even if two people do the same movement in nearly the same way, they each bring a slightly different degree of the effort elements, which accounts for each retaining his or her fundamental personal style within the same movement action. Quality of movement is also determined by the phrasing of the efforts in movement (with accents at the beginning, middle or end of the phrase), and by the manner of making transitions between different qualities.

Effort analysis and Bartenieff's psychological correlates can be used in a number of ways in psychiatry. It is possible to look at a characteristic phrase or piece of movement on a videotape after a session, and so get a very accurate reading of the movement, which in turn provides insight into the patient. It is also possible to recall a patient's movement when it is his or her turn to share the leadership, and then to reconstruct the movement later by remembering what it looked like, as well as actually enacting it after the session while making notes. For example, in a DMT outpatient group, a young anorexic woman took her turn in the group movement by lifting up her arms, looking to the ceiling, and then letting go, flopping over like a rag doll as she hinged from the waist. She called this 'falling over', and said she could do the movement all day, she found it so easy. The group spoke about falling, and the need for support, as well as how to be more confident or sure of oneself. Later, the dance movement therapist, with the co-worker, reconstructed the phrase, and found the efforts shown in Figure 4.3 present.

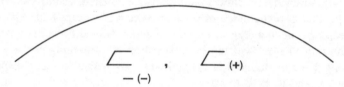

Figure 4.3 Effort–shape notation of a movement phrase from an anorexic patient (original to author)

Using Bartenieff's interpretive framework, the *quality* of the movement phrase showed a preference for spatial directness, bound flow and diminished quickness, with an absence of the weight element. The small plus and minus signs in the figure indicated relatively less quickness as her arms went up, and relatively more bound flow as she dropped forward. This indicated a state of mental alertness (in the direct space) with emotional restraint (bound flow), combined with a diminished sense of self (a lack of the weight effort). The clinical picture is one of a person who is intellectually aware, but emotionally tense, or 'holding herself together'. This described quite accurately the emotional state of this patient; she had been accepted at a prestigious university, but had been unable to fulfil her intellectual talent due to familial and emotional difficulties. The lack of the effort quality of 'weight' seemed almost ironic, given that this woman was grossly underweight in terms of body mass. She also reported to her psychiatric nurse-therapist (whom she saw for individual sessions) moments of feeling 'like a nothing, or a zero', which the movement, when analysed in this way, clearly corroborated.

Laban's original effort analysis was developed further by Warren Lamb, and by

Marion North, who was a student of Laban's, and who extended his complex theories of interpretation which are known collectively as 'Effort analysis'. North's work represents a major attempt to validate certain theories Laban formulated about the relation between individual movement dynamics and personality (Lamb and Turner 1968, North 1972).

The subtlety and complexity of effort analysis is illustrated in Marion North's work, *Personality Assessment Through Movement* (North 1972). This describes research in which she articulates theories for interpreting combinations of effort qualities. She conducted effort and other movement analyses of twelve school children during a semi-structured movement class. The movement assessments were compared with teachers' evaluations, and responses to a series of psychological tests, including IQ.

Her movement assessments included parameters such as effort patterns, balance, dexterity, symmetry, phrasing, planes, and area of space used. She made psychological interpretations based on these, such as adaptability, drive, alertness, reasoning ability, creativity, attention, attitudes toward authority, and emotional makeup. Her predictions were impressively verified over the length of the study. North's experimental work and theoretical explication of how effort may carry information about psychological dimensions illustrate the rich research potential of Laban-derived movement analysis (Davis 1975: 126).

Additionally, the dance movement therapist Penny Lewis integrates the work of Laban, Lamb, Kestenberg and North within a broadly psychodynamic framework (Lewis 1986).

NONVERBAL COMMUNICATIONS RESEARCH

In addition to a psychoanalytic understanding of developmental body movement and the psychological correlates of effort qualities in movement, DMT's understanding of movement and the rationale for its use also rests upon some nonverbal communications research (Weitz 1979). For example, nonverbal communications describes the role of movement in interaction, with concepts such as synchrony, and also sheds light on movement behaviour of individuals in a group. Nonverbal communications research relevant to DMT includes that based on the work of Albert Scheflen, Ray Birdwhistell, and Adam Kendon, Martha Davis and many others (Birdwhistell 1970, Davis 1972, 1974, 1975, 1978, 1981, 1987, 1987b, 1988, Davis and Skupien 1982, Kendon 1979, Scheflen 1979, Scheflen and Scheflen 1972). This section will briefly mention just two concepts, that of interactional synchrony and signals of relatedness in group behaviour, which are two fundamental nonverbal communications insights used in DMT.

Interactional synchrony describes the phenomenon where the movement of a listener is rhythmically coordinated with the flow of speech in the speaker. Synchrony in body position, effort elements, and gesture may occur in patterns between the listener and speaker, and constitute the way in which we can see that the two people are communicating, as opposed to being unrelated to each other.

We can conclude something of the nature of their interaction: perhaps they are highly synchronous until a point of disagreement is raised, at which time they disengage their synchrony on a number of levels, and return to different movement styles. Kendon notes that

> shared rhythmicity in movement was most conspicuous at the beginning and end of an interchange. To *move* with another is to show that one is 'with' him in one's attention and expectancies. Coordination of movement in interaction may thus be of great importance since it provides one of the ways in which two people signal that they are 'open' to one another, and not to others.
>
> (Kendon 1979: 132)

Theories about the role of synchrony in communication underpin the effectiveness of Marian Chace's technique of mirroring. Nonverbal communications research, which explores this phenomenon at its micro level, supports the view that, at the macro level, the therapist's mirroring or synchrony with the patients facilitates the patients' feelings that the therapist is empathetic and understands their communication.

The nature of synchrony and mirroring in DMT interaction is not merely 'copying' another's behaviour, but rather constitutes a system of complementary complex fluctuations in various movement elements (effort–shape, attitude, body posture, gesture, etc.); this means that the therapist is not only reflecting the patients' movements, but is actively entering into a nonverbal dialogue and interaction with them. DMT research into synchrony shows that patients perceived their therapists as more empathetic when the therapists synchronized their movements with that of the patients but allowed a brief period of time to elapse in between, such that the synchrony was *delayed* or *echoed* rather than simultaneous (Fraenkel 1983).

In DMT, the therapist mirrors some aspects of the patients' movements, while retaining elements of their own movement style. This means that patients perceive the therapists' movements as in sympathy with rather than as a mimicry of their own. Dance movement therapists are therefore taught to recognize their own effort–shape profiles, and they gain extensive experience in active mirroring of movement. They also know how to subtly disengage from interactional synchrony by withdrawing or altering some of the elements of their movement. Finally, they are able to read nonverbal signals from the patients, which indicate the patients' responses to the movement interaction.

In addition to the interpretation of the symbolic communications present in the patients' movements, which is central to DMT, the ability to have a movement 'conversation' without recourse to words allows a dance movement therapist to make contact with patients for whom verbal speech may be a distorted mode of communication. It must not be assumed that this is a magical process. Rather, DMT capitalizes on the naturally occurring phenomenon of nonverbal communication, including developmental body movement and the nonverbal synchronous dimension of ordinary conversational behaviour, by employing nonverbal communications theory and research in the support of DMT's therapeutic aims.

Albert Scheflen's work includes illustrations about how people signal relatedness in a group, or in a pair. For example, two people standing together with their backs to the rest of the group, holding eye contact, being *en face*, and being synchronized in a head-nodding movement gives everyone the clear impression that those two people are having a discussion from which they are excluding or 'blocking' the rest of the group. Standing face to face is quite an intimate act, and is qualitatively different from varying degrees of standing side by side. For this reason, in work with individual patients, the therapist generally moves beside rather than facing the patient, or may be seated while the patient engages in his or her own movement exploration, if the patient is able to manage this situation.

Affiliation of group members is achieved through synchrony in such dimensions as shared gaze, position of hands and arms, smiling, nodding and shifting gesture or posture at the same time (Scheflen and Scheflen 1972: 29). *Gesture* is defined in terms of units of movement generally involving the hands, arms or legs, which often have an expressive quality. *Posture* is a unit of movement involving initiation through the trunk or spine, such as a weight shift (when standing) or altering one's position in a chair (when sitting). A postural shift generally indicates a large shift or change of topic in conversation, whereas a gesture may function to punctuate ideas, images and sentences, or add meaning to specific words. Using the concepts of affiliative behaviour, and observing postural and gestural movement, the dance movement therapist may become aware of the phenomenon of subgrouping in group therapy before it has been verbalized or enacted behaviourally.

In conclusion, it can be seen that the same concept, that of synchrony, is used to examine both the group and the dyad. Finally, it might be noted that Scheflen makes the interesting observation that people's nonverbal behaviour often contradicts their verbal statements. An example of this is when someone says, 'I see what you mean,' while covering their eyes, or when someone tries to say cheerfully that the weekend was 'really quite all right' while they make a slumping or wilting posture, and sink into their chair, avert their eyes, and frown lightly. This contradiction corroborates the psychoanalytic view that movement may provide a symbolic communication which substitutes for, or contradicts, that provided by the verbal mode.

CULTURAL AND INTELLECTUAL PERSPECTIVES ON MOVEMENT

In addition to the array of psychoanalytic, nonverbal communications and choreographic analyses of movement, there is a wider intellectual field of inquiry to which these levels of meaning relate. Furthermore, the history of the study of movement determines paths of inquiry; ethologists, animal psychologists, and social psychologists were inspired to look at movement behaviour and its social and expressive function based on the findings of Darwin. In this section, brief mention of three fairly recent books will be provided to illustrate the breadth of intellectual inquiry surrounding movement, dance and the body.

Dance criticism illustrates shifts in assumptions about movement and meaning prevalent in intellectual and cultural circles. For example, Susan Leigh Foster has written a major study of dance which employs semiotics, or the study of signs, through which she explores the ways that dance carries meaning (Foster 1986). This work replaces a previous literary bias in which dance was assumed to tell a story. Since the intellectual development of semiotics, analysing dance as a language of its own has become possible; before this, it was expected to have characters and a narrative, in imitation of written or spoken language.

The subject of 'the body', including questions about representation, sexuality and phenomenology, is one that is periodically and currently in vogue in psycho-analytic and poststructural intellectual circles (Adams 1986, Feher et al. 1989, Suleiman 1986, Dale 1983, McDougall 1974). For example, the psychoanalyst Joyce McDougall has written extensively about psychosomatic metaphor (McDougall 1974). There are also studies of the nonverbal dimensions of the psychotherapeutic process (Mahl 1979). It would be a potentially rich source of ideas for therapists working with the body in DMT to compare their experiences with intellectual theories about the body, and bodily experience and expression.

A recent work of intellectual importance is a study by Francis Sparshott entitled, *Off the Ground: First Steps to a Philosophical Consideration of the Dance* (Sparshott 1988). This extends inquiries from the philosophy of art and aesthetics to a consideration of the dance. Sparshott sees dance and movement as being intimately related to fundamental conceptions of the self, of consciousness, and of being-in-the-world. For him,

> The dance is not an object for the dancer, who lives the dance. In fact, what dance is for the dancer and spectator alike is a modification of our way of being in the world (instrumentally, as agents) and in-the-midst-of-the-world (situatedly), temporally and spatially, in a basic human way that the reification of the body falsifies, a way explored by standard expositions of this or that variety of phenomenology.
>
> (Sparshott 1988: 363)

In other words, seeing 'The Body' as a thing does not actually reflect the dancer's experience of dancing, the experience of how creating and trying new movement inspires new ways of feeling. The physical experience of movement, Sparshott argues, provides us with insight into who and what we really are, at our essence, at the core of our being.

He also traces important historical antecedents of dance, and differentiates, for example, in Hellenic Greek terminology, *choreia* which was identified as dance in social life, and *orchesis* which described the formal properties of dance; that is, the specific movements performed and their meaning. Roman society later conflated these two words into *saltatio* to describe both of these aspects into what we now know as dance (Sparshott 1988: 390). It is important to recognize that 'dance' in dance movement therapy only focuses on expressive, creative, improvised and developmental body movement (or *orchesis*) and does not really utilize social dance forms (or *choreia*), with the possible argument that the circle formation, as used by Marian Chace, is based in ritual and folk dance. Therefore, DMT only uses a few expressive aspects of dance and movement from a potential field of many.

It is also important that dance movement therapists do not see their work in a cultural vacuum. In short, patients and staff in psychiatry will need to understand what the therapist means by 'dance and movement in therapy' in relation to their own cultural and educational understandings of what is meant by dance or movement (as well as what they understand by the term 'therapy'). Their background understanding of dance may be as diverse as having only ever witnessed dance as gyrating bodies in a disco or nightclub, to experiences of ballet training, or gymnastics in physical education classes at school. The therapist must articulate a focus on expressive, creative, improvised movement as distinct from physical exercises or social dancing, which are two of the most commonly drawn parallels to DMT by those who are unfamiliar with the arts therapies in general, and DMT in particular.

A rather different approach is taken in cultural and anthropological studies of movement, dance and social conceptions of the body. Emily Martin's feminist study, *The Woman in the Body*, explores the way in which cultural attitudes to the body in general, but especially attitudes towards menstruation, childbirth and menopause, actively influence women's views of their bodies as separate from their 'selves'. That is, they are taught to view their bodies as subject to processes of decay, waste and passive manipulation by outside forces, such as the experience of invasive hospital techniques in delivering babies, including unnecessary use of episiotomy, forceps or caesarian delivery. Furthermore, the body may give voice to feelings of rebellion against expected behaviour, but these are often dismissed as problems related to women's bodily functions, rather than considered emotional statements in their own right. Martin argues, for example, that emotions of anger and frustration are passed off as 'pre-menstrual tension', which is a cultural way of dismissing women's feelings as 'merely' part of their physiology, and therefore unconnected to the woman's real emotional life (Martin 1989). In taking a more grounded and positive attitude to women's bodies, and the processes of childbirth, menstruation and menopause, these phenomena can be removed from their culturally coded stereotypes which render them, dark, ugly, mysterious and threatening.

Cultural attitudes shape people's feelings about their bodies and about illness. For example, psychiatric patients often report feelings of disconnection from their bodies, and this may be accompanied by a sense of fear, worry and regret, although the patients may in fact be using their bodies to express an emotional statement about feeling fragmented, or emotionally numb. They further suffer by the fact that society continually provides imagery and ideas which imply that disunity between body and mind is an unhealthy state, thereby adding a sense of guilt and shame to their views about the state of their body–mind relations.

Finally, cultural historians note that the body awareness philosophies popular in the 1960s, and rekindled in current New Age interest in yoga, meditation, massage, and nutrition, persist as a societal preoccupation. Bombardment with imagery from the media has made new generations intensely aware of the visual presentation of the body, and body movement. For example, in the 1988 presidential campaign, much publicity was given the fact that George Bush employed an 'image consultant' to help him perform more 'Presidential-type' nonverbal gestures. Evidently the American viewing public was much exercised over the presentation of a President that would make him appear 'warm, but strong, decisive, in charge, tough, but not mean' (Burns and Brookoff 1988: 5). Similarly, the press in Britain noted Prime Minister Thatcher's changing image and gestural presentation style during her period in office. DMT Master's dissertations are just beginning to reflect curiosity in movement as a cultural phenomenon, as well as to consider the types of institutions and places in which DMT can be successful; hopefully this is the beginning of a wider intellectual range of reflection and analysis of body movement in general and DMT in particular.

CONCLUSION

The way movement carries meaning is derived from our historical understanding of movement and its expressive qualities. The way that we understand movement has been influenced by theories of child psychological development and psychoanalytic theory, as well as by advances in choreographic notation systems and nonverbal communications research. The cultural context of understanding the body and body movement is a further aspect that influences the theory and practice of DMT.

How are these levels of movement and meaning relevant to DMT practice with psychiatric patients? Generally, the understanding of the diversity of theories about movement and its meaning are only kept in the back of the dance movement therapist's mind while working. However, the technical tools of movement analysis, such as those by Laban, North and Bartenieff, are employed usefully with psychiatric clients or patients, as are systems based in Laban analysis such as Kestenberg's developmental rhythms, and Davis's Movement Behaviour Assessment of psychopathology in movement (which is discussed in Chapter 10). In some DMT trainings, Laban and Bartenieff movement analysis forms a crucial and major part of using and reading movement. By contrast, some trainings are not Laban based, and focus instead on the dance movement therapist's more subjective and aesthetic reading and response to movement. An example of this is Joan Chodorow's work, *Dance Therapy and Depth Psychology: The Moving Imagination* (Chodorow 1991). Kestenberg's work is very useful in DMT with children as well as with adults (Kestenberg 1975). There are many potential research avenues that could be explored in DMT from the application of movement systems to the therapy process; for example, it would be interesting to do a Kestenberg Movement Profile of a group's developmental rhythms, and to compare this with Bion's psychoanalytic conceptualizations of a group's unconscious functioning, specifically the regression to earlier, more primitive modes of psychological functioning.

Typically, dance movement therapy MA dissertations use an effort–shape analysis as a component of their research, to see how movement reflects a particular diagnostic group, such as sexually abused children or depressed patients (Noebel 1990, Biggins 1989). Furthermore, there is interest in using movement analysis systems in their choreographic and aesthetic dimensions and applying these to the therapeutic process. Claire Schmais found that the psychotherapeutic concepts of warmup, development or process and closure also had choreographic parallels (Schmais 1981).

The potential for interaction between psychotherapeutic conceptualizations of functioning and movement analysis systems appears a rewarding one: a survey of DMT writings illustrates a dizzying array of combinations of therapy and movement ideas. Hopefully, as the field continues to develop, a number of specific schools will be delineated, so that the field can begin to find its own intellectual identity and coherence. At present, it seems that Laban and Bartenieff-based movement analysis constitute a large school, and new and interesting work is continually appearing in the *Arts in Psychotherapy* and the *American Journal of Dance Therapy*. Given the complexity of movement language, and the multiplicity of psychotherapeutic schools of practice, it seems important that DMT attempts to focus on some primary ways in which movement carries meaning, and concentrate on these, rather than be tempted to see *every* dimension of meaning present in *all* movement, such that every movement can mean just about anything, depending on who is observing or describing it. Movement is an incredibly rich language; the task ahead for DMT is to clarify which voices and strands of meaning are most useful to therapeutic aims. In psychiatry, at least, systems that examine choreographic, developmental, expressive and psychopathological meanings in movement serve the dance movement therapist most rewardingly. The next chapter considers clinical examples of groups and individuals in child and adult psychiatry.

Chapter 5

Theory into practice: clinical examples and techniques

INTRODUCTION

Before considering the clinical case material, it is important to discuss the general problems that surround therapeutic intervention in the treatment of mental illness, and to consider which sorts of patients seen in adult psychiatric settings are suitable for DMT, and which are not. This will enable a general statement of realistic therapeutic goals for DMT in the psychiatric setting. There is then a brief discussion of psychodynamic perspectives on mental illness. This is not intended as a guide to clinical techniques, but will assist the reader in understanding mental illness as it might be seen from the patient's existential perspective. The chapter concludes with a look at psychodynamic aspects of schizophrenia and depression, which are the most common illnesses suffered by clients referred to dance movement therapy.

The clinical section of this book does not include an example of work with an individual adult outpatient. This type of work can only safely be attempted by qualified dance movement therapists working under close supervision, ideally while they are themselves in individual therapy, or have completed some years of individual therapy and are engaged in further training which addresses the one-to-one psychotherapeutic relationship which develops between therapist and patient. For similar reasons, work with inpatient adolescent psychiatric clients is described in general terms only, with references to literature for the student to begin reading; DMT groups with adolescents can be very challenging, both physically and mentally, and this work is probably best carried out in the latter stages of the student's training. Chapters 6, 7 and 8 will give extended clinical illustrations of DMT with adult outpatients, long-term hospitalized patients, and clients seen individually and in groups in child psychiatry settings. Each chapter outlines actual techniques, gives examples of patients' behaviour, and discusses how the material that emerged in the session was used in light of therapeutic goals.

The clinical examples are drawn from my own experience and experiments in working in psychiatry: as such the work will show my own biases in favouring a psychodynamic approach to understanding personality and group behaviour, in concentrating on movement improvisation within the shared leadership format, and in choosing to focus on the symbol, metaphor and imagery that arise in group work.

Theoretical sources and inspirations for the form and focus of this work are provided in Chapter 9, which articulates the theoretical underpinnings to my particular approach to DMT in psychiatry. Readers who already work in psychiatry will notice that in both my clinical accounts and in the accompanying theory, more interest and attention is paid to patients suffering from schizophrenia and related disorders (such as borderline personality organization) than to depressed patients. Names and details of patients have of course been changed to protect their confidentiality; and some of the material presented in the group section is an idealized composite sketch drawn from a number of groups of similar types. This means that some of the detail has been sacrificed in order to give a broader sense of the themes that arise in the life of a group over several months.

Obviously there are limitations in describing the clinical experiences of one author, and I hope that the ideas presented here will not be seen to constitute any standard or norm. Instead, it is hoped that what is written here will open up spheres for debate and comparison among dance movement therapists, other arts therapists and mental health professionals working in psychiatry. To some degree, 'the therapy is the therapist', and so every dance movement therapist chooses, consciously or unconsciously, to attend to certain aspects of experience rather than others. Readers are encouraged to compare their own experiences of groups of patients with those I have provided here, and to question how DMT group theory, which was presented in the latter half of Chapter 3, is incorporated into practice.

THERAPEUTIC APPROACHES TO THE TREATMENT OF MENTAL ILLNESS

Mental illness is an extraordinarily complex phenomenon, as is illustrated by the range of theories that attempt to understand it, and the array of pharmacological, psychotherapeutic and social approaches that exist on its treatment. It is important that dance movement therapists have a relatively clear notion of how they see their work in the overall context of psychiatric approaches to mental illness, which means that they must understand the role of psychotherapeutically informed therapeutic work in the psychiatric setting. This brief section will frame the parameters of this role and will hopefully encourage students to consider the nature of their work and read further into this area.

Anyone surveying literature on mental illness will be struck by the range and diversity of the spheres of inquiry which seek to address the subject. There are, for example, perspectives on mental illness, which are: neurological, genetic, biological, sociological, political, cultural, religious, literary, aesthetic, historical and, finally, psychological, which itself contains such dimensions as the psychiatric, anti-psychiatric, psychoanalytic, psychotherapeutic, existential and humanistic.

Some biologically oriented psychiatrists favour the view that mental illness, like physical illness, is the result of a complicated interaction of neurological, biological and physiological pathological processes. In taking this view, they concentrate efforts on trying to pinpoint genetic and neurochemical causes for illness. They believe that a pharmacological approach, using neuroleptics or anti-depressants, is the best way to tackle the symptoms of mental disease (see, for example, Trimble 1981).

In strict opposition to this view, there is an anti-psychiatry movement which argues that mental illness is not an illness at all, and that the whole concept is 'a complete fabrication – scientifically worthless and socially harmful' (Szasz 1974, Szasz cited in Warner 1987: 9). The anti-psychiatry school sees mental illness as a politically and socially constructed reality which obscures and denies the existential suffering of human beings (Laing 1975). An illness like schizophrenia, then, may be viewed as a sane response to an insane society. Feeling dissociated from reality, and from oneself, is to be expected in a society which possesses weapons of mass destruction, which divides workers from the products of their labour, and which legitimizes familial and social structures that alienate human beings from true emotional experiences of themselves and others (see, for example, Laing 1975, Laing and Esterton 1970). Anti-psychiatry approaches to treatment include long-term psychotherapy, and therapeutic communities.

Most mental health professionals take a view that is somewhere between these two extremes of either a biological or socio-political/existential explanation of mental illness. In this model, mental illness is seen as having a *multi-factorial aetiology*, in which genetics, neurology, intrapsychic and interpersonal emotional processes, and family, social and political environment *all* play a role in creating the disposition to mental illness and influence its course or outcome (Strauss and Carpenter 1981, Warner 1987).

In taking this middle position, it becomes apparent that neither medication nor therapy, on its own, will be enough to intervene in the treatment of serious mental illness. Medication may produce biochemical changes that will reduce symptoms but will not assist the mentally ill person in coping with everyday emotional, family or working life. Therapy, no matter how intense, or how long, is unlikely to reverse a predisposition to schizophrenia caused by 'mild cerebral atrophy' (Warner 1987: 27). The current practice in most community psychiatric clinics (excepting those specializing in neuropsychiatry) reflects a treatment plan that is based in this interactive, or multi-factorial model of mental illness. Patients are generally given medication, of either a short course, or continual maintenance, and they may be directed towards the generally minimal resources for individual psychotherapy. Often the patient's family is involved in treatment, and may attend one or more consultations with psychiatric staff. Most commonly, patients are offered individual meetings with a psychiatrist, psychiatric nurse, or social worker to address personal or intrapsychic issues. They are also provided with opportunities to join groups to improve interpersonal skills and social functioning (which are usually run by psychiatry registrars or interns, psychiatric nurses, social workers and occupational therapists). This general treatment plan, available in most public mental health facilities, is one which addresses itself to the biochemical, intrapsychic, familial and interpersonal dimensions of the person and his or her illness.

Within the confines of this multi-factorial approach there are further ranges of conflicts and debates surrounding the use of psychotherapeutic ideas and approaches to the treatment of mental illness. There are quite sensible arguments that contend that classical psychoanalytic intervention (which includes the uncovering of the unconscious factors in mental distress, and reconstructing the formation of symptoms from childhood experience and patterns in relating to parents) is a process that is too intensive and too frightening for those with serious mental illness to manage (Malan 1989: 221).

There are, however, a few specialized and usually private sector facilities that will undertake the modified psychotherapeutic treatment of schizophrenia; some work in tandem with psychiatric models and use medication, where others are anti-psychiatry based and may employ psychiatrists who use the minimum amount and duration of medical intervention. Some of the ideas derived from the therapeutic treatment of schizophrenia are briefly surveyed in the section on psychodynamic perspectives on mental illness on page 96.

Insofar as the patient needs to be able to function as an individual, and in family and social life, some of the concepts and techniques derived from psychoanalysis and psychotherapy can play a valuable role in understanding and assisting the patient to maintain as high a level of functioning as possible. The question is how to adapt ideas from psychotherapy to work with patients in a way that is relevant, does not overwhelm the patient, and is feasible given the meagre funding and resources available for psychotherapeutically informed therapeutic work in psychiatry.

In the view of the present author, and of a number of other dance movement therapists working in psychiatry, the arts therapies in general, and DMT in particular, may offer therapeutic intervention which fills a gap between occupational therapy and psychotherapy. Given the limited funding available for psychotherapy in the public health system, there are a vast number of patients who, while they might benefit from therapy, are unlikely ever to receive it. In addition to these patients, there are a large group whose severity of illness is such that they would probably *not* be able to make use of insight-oriented psychotherapy, but who nonetheless may benefit from some work which addresses their interpersonal and intrapsychic emotional functioning. While it could be argued that occupational therapy or social skills groups are 'therapeutic' enough in themselves, some patients can benefit from a creative arts therapies experience to safely release and grapple with at least a few of their emotional difficulties, even though they would not be deemed suitable for individual or group psychotherapy run by a verbally trained psychotherapist.

Given that some sorts of psychotherapeutic intervention confront the seriously mentally ill patient with psychological insights that could give rise to great distress, or suicidal or violent acting out, it is not surprising that many people retain suspicions about the value of *any* therapeutic work in psychiatry. Furthermore, the fact that there is such a range of therapies available (such as psychoanalytic, psychodynamic, existential, Gestalt, transactional, behavioural, insight-oriented, and supportive therapy, to name but a few), it is no wonder that psychiatric staff, when their patients are referred to groups that are termed 'therapeutic', may have difficulty in being clear about what their patients will actually be doing. This problem is exacerbated by the unwillingness or inability of a number of people using therapeutic ideas in their work with psychiatric patients to be properly articulate, or to define their adherence to specific theories, methods and goals, but who instead prefer to cloak themselves in the power and mystery of psychological jargon.

Furthermore, there is a dearth of reliable outcome studies which demonstrate the effectiveness of psychotherapeutic approaches to mental illness, though this is currently being addressed in the field of brief and focal psychotherapies (Balint *et al.* 1972, Ursano and Hales 1986, Malan 1989). A fairly recent study suggested that a short-term intensive dynamic group psychotherapy programme – which combined general systems theory (on which much family therapy is based), analytical groups, community meetings, Gestalt therapy, psychodrama, video feedback and art therapy – was able to reduce the dependence on psychiatric services for a majority of patients, and showed considerable change in self-satisfaction as assessed by an attitude test (Dick and Woof 1986). However, this study did find that there was a subgroup of 17 per cent of patients who demonstrated an increase in psychiatric service use in the post-therapy year.

It should be noted in this context that the general prognosis for those affected by psychiatric illness is variable, with patients who suffer from depression expected to fare much better than those diagnosed with schizophrenia. The duration of a major depressive episode, when untreated, may be six months or more, but 'usually there is a complete remission of symptoms, and general functioning returns to the premorbid [or pre-illness] level; but in a large proportion of some of the cases, some symptoms of the episode persist for as long as two years' (American Psychiatric Association 1987: 220). Studies of schizophrenia are less encouraging, and

> a return to premorbid functioning in this disorder is not common. Full remissions do occur, but their frequency is currently a subject of controversy. The most common course is probably one of acute exacerbations with residual impairment between episodes. . . . There is some evidence, however, that in many people with the disorder, the residual symptoms [which include social withdrawal, affective blunting or flattening and impairment of role functioning] become attenuated in the later phases of the illness.
>
> (American Psychiatric Association 1987: 191)

Research evidence suggests that, as far as schizophrenia is concerned, good prognosis is more likely in those persons who attained a high level of personal and social functioning before the onset of the illness, and for whom the onset of the illness was abrupt, occurred later in life, or developed in reaction to external life-stressors. The fact that there is a wide variety of courses or outcomes of schizophrenia, and varying degrees of impairment, supports the hypothesis that there may be different types of schizophrenia in which neurological, familial and social factors have varying degrees of influence (Ciompi 1980).

Given this information, it is clear that a great deal of psychiatric treatment is aimed not so much at 'curing' mental illness as it is at attempting to alleviate some of the more distressing symptoms and returning the person to full functioning (as in the case of depression) or in reducing the most acute symptoms and supporting the person in achieving and maintaining as high a level of individual mental and social functioning as possible (as is the case with schizophrenic patients). Until more is known about the genetic and neurological factors responsible for mental illness, and more effective medication is developed, the role of psychotherapeutically informed therapeutic work with seriously ill patients may be one that is aimed at providing support, and facilitating a manageable amount of psychological insight, rather than at eradicating symptoms as such, or attempting to prevent recurrent periods of acute illness.

So, the choice of mode of therapy, be it one aimed at insight (through revealing unconscious factors in behaviour) or support (focusing on helping the patient manage day-to-day life) depends on the needs of the particular person, and the ability of the psychiatric services to meet that need. Some insight-oriented psychotherapists feel it is utterly tragic that *all* patients are not offered individual psychotherapy. Most people with experience of psychiatric patients would agree that, for a large number of patients (particularly those who are suffering from long-term schizophrenia), a more supportive approach aimed at maintaining communication and ameliorating deterioration in interpersonal functioning is a more suitable goal. One outcome study which compared 'exploratory/insight-oriented (EIO) therapy with reality/adaptive/supportive (RAS) therapy, found that the RAS therapy decreased the patient's subsequent use of the psychiatric services, while the EIO approach improved ego-functioning. This study concluded that, for schizophrenics at least, the 'more pragmatic and less expensive' RAS was more effective (Klerman 1984). Furthermore, a Menninger Foundation outcome study found that schizophrenics benefited more from a supportive approach than from exploratory 'expressive' psychotherapy (Kernberg *et al.* 1972). In the section below, which discusses realistic therapeutic goals for DMT with psychiatric patients, it should become clear that the approach can be used in a fundamentally supportive, rather than exploratory or insight-oriented, way and as such may provide a safe and structured therapeutic intervention appropriate for outpatient treatment programmes in psychiatry.

In conclusion, this discussion of the prognosis of mental illness, and some views on the effectiveness of therapeutic approaches to it, brings us logically to a consideration of the difficult question, 'Which patients are appropriate for referral to arts therapies, specifically for a DMT group?'

SUITABLE REFERRALS TO DMT

DMT is appropriate for quite a few of the patients usually encountered in outpatient work, including those suffering from depression, schizophrenia and related disorders. Generally, DMT groups are of use to patients who:

1   would benefit from improving their interpersonal skills;
2   are felt to need some reconnection to their physical selves;
3   would be comfortable initiating any improvised, impromptu gesture or move-
    ment which the rest of the group would follow, and who would attempt to follow
    others; and
4   could manage a general discussion on the theme of feelings of anger, frustration
    or loneliness, which are typical themes that patients bring to such groups.

The usual procedure by which patients are selected for therapeutic groups offered
by an outpatient mental health centre is of course a function of the general policy
of each centre. In designing a treatment programme for a patient who arrives at an
outpatient unit, the referring psychiatrist or psychiatric nurse obviously considers
the presenting problems of the patient, and seeks to address these by combining a
number of the available treatment components offered by the unit.

It may be helpful to understand that DMT groups involve about as much physical
activity as a light exercise class, and that the group movement starts with a
therapist-led warmup, and generally takes place with the patients standing in a
circle. Then, using a structured turn-taking format, each patient leads the group in
an improvised movement. The session involves creating group movements and
images and discussing whatever has come up, either just the content itself, or what
it might express about the underlying emotional state of the group as a whole.

It is most important to recognize that the movement and the imagery that
emerges in DMT is *patient-initiated*: the patients provide the material each week
for the group, and they, along with the dance movement therapist, determine the
level of self-disclosure and level of depth of exploration of interpersonal issues. A
group that finds itself marching and stamping in unison, as though its members
were army guerrillas in the desert, might sit down at the end of the group and discuss
how distressing it was to watch the TV news footage or movies that show war
combat (as might happen in a lower functioning group of patients), or (if the group
is higher functioning) they might discuss the sources and targets of their own
personal anger and aggression, and how to manage them more effectively in their
lives within and outside the group. Both cases – in the context of the therapeutic
relationship, and the movement, along with the imagery – allow for a controlled
and contained cathartic release of anger and frustration, at least for the majority of
patients.

It is important to recognize that DMT, while it occurs within the same structured
format each week, is essentially *non-directive*. It is the patient who brings the
movement and imagery of anger. The dance movement therapist never comes in
and introduces the issue, or would never say, 'Today we are going to look at angry
feelings and how to manage them.'

In considering a referral for DMT, then, it is highly inadvisable to refer patients
who are prone to aggressive or sexual acting out, who have little or no ability to
distinguish what is imaginary from what is actual, or who are frightened by the idea

of standing around in a circle and doing marching-type movements with other people because they might fear a loss of self-control, or be terrified by other people enacting this in an imaginary way in the group.

In the experience of the present author, there are some types of patients who are *not* suitable for DMT groups. The first are floridly psychotic patients, who find that the improvisation element of the group does not help them manage or contain their emotional chaos. Until such patients are stabilized on medication, and have adjusted to the milieu of the inpatient or outpatient environment, they will be able to make little use of the creative or interpersonal learning opportunity provided by the group.

It is difficult to determine where 'free association', used in the group, may drift into 'loosening of association' (a disconnection of the logical flow of mental ideas). The creative process is linked in literature to the dissolution and fragmentation which accompanies some forms of mental illness; however, creativity is also linked with an integrative and healthy mode of mental functioning (Arieti 1976, Kubie 1958). Some hospitals do demand that therapeutic work be undertaken with acute admissions patients; this needs to be undertaken with extreme care and caution, if attempted at all, and always with full cooperation and support from ward staff. This type of work might resemble treatment with long-term patients described later in this chapter, in which movement-based goals are a primary focus. Therapeutic work with acute patients is not described in this book, as it is not really suitable for DMT students, though it has been described elsewhere in the context of DMT and verbal approaches (Payne 1992, Yalom 1983).

The second unsuitable type of patients are recently admitted anorectics. These patients must reach a safe weight before joining a DMT group, and must be admonished not to endeavour to use the warmup or movement process sections of the group as a form of exercise in order to lose weight, which is in direct opposition to treatment aims. Finally, as a cautionary note, patients with physical disabilities such as a propensity for epileptic fits or perhaps fainting must be known to the dance movement therapist and co-worker to ensure the patients' safety. On the whole, the level of physical activity in a DMT group rarely rises above that of a light exercise class, and so very few patients can be ruled out on physical grounds alone.

Generally speaking, if the patients under consideration are those who would not be suitable for art therapy and would find discussion of any emotional issues difficult or overwhelming, then they are probably not suitable for DMT. In questionable cases, the best rule of thumb might be: *if in doubt, do not refer*. Most DMT groups use a co-worker who is on the staff of the unit; that person may be the one most able to advise about the suitability of the groups for particular patients, since he or she will have actual experience of participating in DMT sessions with patients that are known.

It is difficult to predict which particular patients will actually benefit most from a DMT approach. Those with an interest in creative work, painting, films, music or literature can generally make good use of the symbolic and expressive opportunities the group provides. Patients with a limited capacity for abstract thought tend to stick to the concrete level of movement, but even these patients can benefit very much by simply being part of a group which values their membership and contribution; they can gain a great deal from movement and verbal interaction with others; and they benefit from engagement in other patients' expressive movement, even if they cannot articulate the process verbally, or engage in symbolic development of an emotional theme.

A new dance movement therapist coming to work at a unit may be able to provide a videotaped example of a DMT group which other staff can see. Some dance movement therapists choose to run one or two 'open' groups before starting the planned course of a time-limited group (typically lasting sixteen sessions), so that they, and the patients concerned, can determine who is suitable and who is likely to benefit from the group. Whether the group eventually evolves into one that is more exploratory, or one that is largely supportive in character, is dependent upon the immediate needs of the patients and the skill of the particular dance movement therapist.

Verbal psychotherapists have been known to recoil in horror at the thought of DMT groups that use bodily experience and movement activities combined with free association to create imagery that is then used to address the affective life of the group. Many imagine that a great deal of touch is involved (when in fact it is actively discouraged), or that massage must be included (which it never is), or that DMT must be gratifying the patient's propensity for the release of sexual and aggressive impulses. Obviously, any group of people standing in a circle moving synchronously in a style of their own choosing could become sexualized (in the manner of disco dancing) or aggressive (in the style of a tribal dance). It is the responsibility of the dance movement therapist to slow down, alter, or stop the group if this type of movement gets out of hand, or becomes therapeutically counterproductive.

The therapist can alter the group's movement behaviour by providing a prop, such as a stretchy Lycra cloth, or foam ball, or large plastic physiotherapy ball, or can direct the group to alter the movement choreographically by changing its phrasing, its shape, or possibly exaggerate some element of the movement such that it becomes a caricature-type illustration of the feeling, rather than a direct expression of it.

Usually, the patients themselves use the shared leadership format to stop and change the movement if it becomes uncomfortable: they merely say 'pass' and the person next to them in the circle introduces a movement, which may either counteract or extend the movement quality currently being used. The therapist can also alter the quality of movement by the use of verbal or nonverbal interventions, by articulating the group's discomfort, or by expressing concern that the movement is being used mindlessly, or gratuitously. The fact that much of the movement takes place accompanied by imagery of things or places (being 'like' soldiers or 'like' swimming in treacle or 'like' climbing up a mountain) is also a containing factor: there is usually a sense that the movement has the status or quality of exploration, or play. If the movement is sexualized or aggressive, it is not a raw and direct expression of those feelings towards other persons in the group; it usually has an 'as if' quality which prevents it from becoming too much to handle.

There is no question that movement is a powerful tool, one that could be potentially damaging as well as helpful. The containing structures of the shared leadership format, the use of imagery, and the therapeutic relationship between the clients and the dance movement therapist are the things that assure that movement is used in a manner appropriate to therapeutic goals. It is important that staff of psychiatric facilities be fully aware of what they are recommending for their patients, and that the dance movement therapist and staff have good working relationships to ensure the psychological safety and well-being of their clients. Given the flexibility of the creative arts approach, and its patient-directed material, it can be used in ways that vary with patient needs. The next section discusses some of the different ways in which DMT can be employed.

Insight-oriented and supportive groups

It will be seen in the clinical examples that follow that group behaviour in DMT varies depending on the particular client group with which it is being used. Outpatient groups tend to be somewhat higher functioning, and can use the movement and the verbal imagery and associations to explore unconscious material. Inpatient or chronic groups tend to be more supportive in nature, and the primary benefits are probably found in the warmup phase of the group, and in the interpersonal gains made in the highly structured turn-taking format of the group. Some externalization of unavowed feelings can occur via the use of movement and imagery, but this is less evident than in higher functioning groups.

The distinction between these two types of groups can be usefully thought of as one between 'glue' and 'solvent' (Dulicai 1988). For the high-functioning outpatient group members, the DMT group sometimes acts as a solvent; it helps dissolve unhelpful patterns of relating, it opens the patient up to new experiences, and helps reach through to the emotional difficulties that are preventing the patient from being sufficiently in touch with his or her problems in order to think about how to do something towards managing them more effectively.

In contrast, for the long-term patients, who may be continually aware of distorted or frightening feelings, and who do not have adequate defences to deal with them, the DMT group can function as a sort of 'glue', which holds each patient together. The extended warmup is aimed at awareness and integration of body movement, which produces changes in the patients' states of mind: they become more alert, more active, and more coordinated and organized in their appearance. Secondly, they can recognize, in synchronous group movement and shared imagery, that they can connect to others. Isolation can be alleviated, and the structured group movement provides a sort of supportive social connection or 'glue' for patients. Furthermore, by the concrete and physical enactment or expression of feelings (for example, generated by stamping, or being gently rocked while holding a Lycra cloth to which the whole group is connected), a patient's emotional life becomes somehow more basic, and slightly more manageable than the fragmented and confused morass of memory, imagery and voices which seem to be a feature of some long-term patients' affective lives.

The higher functioning patient has the ego strengths, and the defences, or common sense to be able to withdraw from a particular movement if it feels too threatening. In contrast, the long-term patient needs validation from the group and the assistance of the therapist to be able to gauge how much expression and exploration of emotion is possible.

With lower functioning groups, the dance movement therapist rarely makes direct comments on an individual member's movement behaviour, or interaction with another patient. Instead, *whole-group* comments and interpretations are offered, which, while less intensive, are less threatening than comments directed at individuals, which might be deemed to be appropriate for a higher functioning group (Kahn 1984, O'Brien 1975). This idea has its parallels with the concept of the nascent group as defined by Johnson and Sandel in Chapter 3, and will be discussed further in the section on groups with long-term patients, on page 143.

Another useful distinction in considering the function of DMT with different sorts of psychiatric patients is that between a 'top down' and a 'bottom up' approach, as described by Krueger and Schofield in their combined DMT and psychotherapy work with anorectics (Krueger and Schofield 1986). This metaphor describes the idea that for some (generally higher functioning) patients, the aim of therapy is to get down to the historical point in their lives where psychological conflicts that are presumed responsible for their dysfunction may lie. Once this traumatic memory or mode of relating to others can be found, the patient and therapist can begin to rework the patient's traumatic experience, or try new patterns of relating to others in a manner that is more adaptive, and causes the person less emotional pain (Balint 1968).

In contrast, the 'bottom up' approach sees the patient's difficulties as essentially ones of deficit, or lack. Usually this is a lack of early maternal psychological care, or possibly an area of development which was missed out (such as the achievement of a separate identity from that of the mother during infancy, or the establishment of autonomy in adolescence). Once the deficit or difficulty has been recognized, the therapist and patient can go about the task of working on whatever emotions or modes of relating the patient needs to develop. Usually this can be done in a modified form – the patient does not literally regress to infancy or adolescence; instead, memories, dreams, drawings and movements can be used within the therapeutic relationship to build up the area of missing development.

The 'glue and solvent', the 'top down' and the 'bottom up' approaches are mentioned here to underscore the need for students to make every attempt to be clear about their understanding of psychotherapeutic models of behaviour, personality, symptom formation and therapeutic goals, and to have a realistic grasp of what is possible and appropriate for the various levels at which psychiatric patients function, and at which level of working their training will permit. Dance movement therapists who, after completing a Master's level training, go on to have supervision or further training at a psychotherapy institute may work at deeper levels, perhaps using the transference or therapeutic relationship quite intensively.

In conclusion, DMT is a potentially beneficial and exciting form of psychotherapeutically informed therapeutic work which can be used within the spectrum of treatment interventions to mental illness, alongside occupational therapy, psychology, psychotherapy, nursing and psychiatric approaches. It is *not* suitable for all patients, and careful planning and monitoring of the role of DMT on a patient's treatment plan must be considered. DMT must not be used as a last resort, as a substitute for exercise or physical recreation, or as a simple diversion from verbal work. DMT has a role to play in psychiatry as one of the arts therapies, potentially filling a gap between occupational therapy and psychotherapy, and always used as an adjunct to or alongside the many other components of effective mental health treatment.

THERAPEUTIC GOALS FOR DMT IN PSYCHIATRY

In order to support the contention that DMT can provide a safe form of therapeutic work with psychiatric patients which fills a gap between occupational therapy and psychotherapy, an attempt will be made here to extrapolate three primary therapeutic goals that are specifically appropriate to work in psychiatry. The formulation of these goals has been achieved by combining reflections on five years of the author's experiences in running DMT groups with the concepts of group therapy which inform DMT as it is currently taught and practised. These three goals are based on four group therapy theories, which were described in detail in the latter half of Chapter 3. These four theories are: Irvin Yalom's existential/humanistic approach; Johnson and Sandel's psychoanalytically informed work (which owes a debt to W. R. Bion); Claire Schmais's 'healing processes' in DMT (which are themselves dance and movement-level goals related to Yalom's therapeutic factors); and, finally, Marian Chace's 'shared leadership' group DMT format, which, like Yalom's work, owes a debt to the interpersonal and psychodynamic tradition of Harry Stack-Sullivan (Bion 1961, Chaiklin and Schmais 1979, Johnson and Sandel 1977, Rioch 1975, Sandel 1980, Sandel and Johnson 1983, Schmais 1981, 1985, 1986, Sullivan 1932, 1940, 1956).

It is important that students enter work with psychiatric clients or patients understanding that they cannot 'cure' or 'fix' patients, and that 'helping' really cannot mean offering superficial cheer or assistance to patients suffering such degrees of mental distress and disorganization. Students familiar with psychoanalytic literature should not be tempted to use the patient's personal reaction to them – that is, the powerful tool of the transference – to rework the patient's personality until they have had experience of personal therapy and have undergone some verbal psychoanalytic or psychotherapeutic training. This level of working, which combines movement and psychoanalysis, is carried out by senior dance movement therapists who have also trained as psychoanalysts (see, for example, Chodorow 1991, Dosamantes-Alperson 1987, Fletcher 1979, Siegel 1984).

If the dance movement therapist attempts to hold in mind such diverse goals as alleviation of symptoms, behaviour modification, understanding of family and childhood problems, life history, fantasy life and dream material, as well as movement psychopathology indicators or choreographic qualities, he or she will undoubtedly feel flooded with a massive amount of information from the patient which is virtually impossible to organize, let alone endeavour to work with. If, instead, the dance movement therapist is intellectually fairly familiar with one or two theories of behaviour, personality and models of psychopathology (such as Jungian, Freudian, or psychodynamic), and is committed to facilitating a safe, creative movement experience for the patient, he or she will be well on the road to being of some therapeutic use to the majority of patients referred for DMT groups.

Three fundamental goals

With these things in mind, three fundamental goals for DMT in psychiatry can be stated. These are:

1 body-level reintegration
2 facilitation or maintenance or improvement in interpersonal functioning
3 provision of a safe, contained forum to address emotional issues by using group movement, imagery, symbol and metaphor.

Each of these will now be defined in some detail, as they are applied to adult and child psychiatric patients. Readers may wish to refer the clinical material, described later in this book, back to these stated goals.

Movement-derived goals

First and foremost, DMT offers the patient an opportunity for body-level reintegration. This includes goals such as vitalization, integration, activation and motivation of the patient using both directive movement warmups, and non-directive improvised movement (Schmais 1985).

Although experimental validation is intangible, many authors stress that with new body movements, a new body image and body-ego (or sense of bodily/affective self) can be formed (Boas 1952, Chace 1953, Christrup 1978: 302, Delaney 1973, Dosamantes-Alperson 1984, Gilroy *et al.* 1989, Higgens 1989, Kluft *et al.* 1986, Krueger and Schofield 1986, Poteat 1981, Robbins 1980, Schilder 1950: 208, Shenton 1988, 1990, Siegel 1974, 1984). It has been suggested that movement experience for schizophrenic patients can increase levels of self-synchrony, or organization in movement (Lawler 1979, Lefko 1974, Lipshutz 1978, Silberstein 1987).

Further important movement-level goals in DMT with psychiatric patients include expanding the patient's expressive movement range, and opening up new, primary, or 'authentic' ways of interacting with others on a nonverbal level (Hawkins 1971). Simply getting the patients to feel a sense of their own impact (or weight) as their feet touch the ground in walking, stamping or hopping often gives them the appearance of being more grounded, and more connected to their surroundings. By contrast, in work with child psychiatric patients, movement-based goals include tension discharge, gaining impulse control, and replaying parent– child interaction on a nonverbal level. With abused children, DMT aims to help build a more adaptive movement profile, decrease sexualized behaviour, and assist the child in forming an age-appropriate sense of their bodily experience. This last goal might be understood as an attempt to normalize the nonverbal dimension of their 'psychosexuality', a term defined by Freud (Freud 1905, Goodill 1987, Goodill and Leatherbee 1986, Leatherbee and Wood 1984, Weltman 1986).

Interpersonal goals

The second major goal consists of using the DMT group to provide the patients with a group interactive movement experience which allows them to maintain or increase their level of interpersonal functioning. By initiating their own expressive movement in a group, in effect 'leading' others, the patients are able to develop a preliminary sense of personal effectiveness and autonomy. By following the movement of other clients, they can develop nonverbal empathy with others. Furthermore, group members actively cooperate to achieve movement tasks, such as pulling a stretch cloth for a tug-o'-war, or bouncing a ball on top of a cloth. They collaborate in the creation of movement sequences (which employ verbal and nonverbal free association) and these are accompanied by their own created images, such as climbing together up a mountain, or swaying in unison to a rocking rhythm. The DMT group offers the nonverbal dimension as a mode in which to develop socializing techniques (exemplified by turn-taking), to learn via imitation (through mirroring), to participate in group cohesiveness (through synchronous, rhythmic, or complementary movement) (Schmais 1985, Yalom 1970). With child psychiatric patients, movement – whether structured in a game or improvised – provides a channel through which relationships can be formed or repaired with peers and adults, thus often decreasing isolation and chaotic behaviour.

Emotional release and externalization

The third primary therapeutic goal for DMT groups with psychiatric patients is to offer a safe and contained forum in which to address emotional issues. This does not mean an in-depth exploration of the unconscious or infantile roots of their difficulties, but rather some quite elementary interpersonal and intrapsychic experiences in the context of improvised group movement. Each patient's move-ment is reflected or mirrored, and thereby accepted by the group and the dance movement therapist, in much the same way as a verbal statement might be reflected back to a patient during counselling or therapy sessions.

The arts therapies all offer a no-fail experience for the patient: virtually whatever the patient does, however minimal (provided it is not too frighteningly bizarre or disturbing or aggressive towards others), is enough and is valued and appreciated by the group, such that some confidence is developed, and each patient engages in trying to do more ordinary or interesting and difficult things next time his or her turn comes around, or the next time he or she is asked to speak.

The therapist facilitates a turn-taking or other structure in which the patient's movement can allow for controlled cathartic release of feelings such as anger or frustration. Doing a movement that the group labels 'strong' is a way to externalize feelings so that they are amenable to management, and not stored up and waiting to be acted out within the patient's usual social environment. Patients often report that they feel good to be 'doing something' about their feelings, rather than 'just talking' about them.

Perhaps, most importantly, movement is not simply done for the sake of 'dancing'; movement statements are connected to verbal statements in order that some insight is gained into the impulses or feelings that may have led to that movement. Sharing a group movement which resembles falling, and being able to discuss scary feelings of 'losing control' or 'falling forever' or 'falling apart', allows the patient to externalize the feeling, recognize it as common to other people as well, and therefore (hopefully) conclude that such feelings may not be over-whelming, but may offer a point of connection and understanding with others. Using movement and word symbols gives 'psychic distance from private preoccupations' (Schmais 1985: 32).

In work with abused children, DMT capitalizes on the children's ability to use movement language to clarify feelings, replay parent–child patterns of interaction, and address directly the body-level sensations and memories of sexual abuse. DMT uses the kinaesthetic component of the child's emotional life in order to promote the exploration of worries, fantasies, or traumatic memories. Children have an immense love of movement and expression of feeling, and they desire to share and validate each other's experiences in movement and verbal symbolic play. Thera-peutic work with children using DMT capitalizes on the child's natural inclination to mental health through an integration of body and mind, fantasy and reality, memory and present experience.

DMT as an arts therapy

These broad goals of body-level reintegration, improvement in interpersonal functioning, and the provision of a safe, contained forum to address emotional issues by using movement, imagery, symbol and metaphor are generally in keeping with other writing about the therapeutic role of the arts therapies (Karasu 1984,

Zwerling 1989). The existing literature stresses that 'the nonverbal media employed by creative arts therapists more directly tap emotional rather than cognitive processes in patients' (Zwerling 1989: 23). Furthermore, the intrinsic social or reality-based character of the arts therapies is held up as a benefit, in that there

> is a visible or audible or tangible link to society in a session involving a creative arts therapist and a patient, and it has a qualitatively more immediate, more real presence than does the person or thing that a patient may talk about.
>
> (Zwerling 1989: 25)

Most importantly, the use of drawing, painting, dance movement, music and drama offer the patient an exit from self-preoccupation, offer a different, hopefully less distorted channel of emotional expression than verbal discussion, and serve to orient the patient towards reality and towards the people in his or her immediate environment (Zwerling 1989).

In addition to employing psychological theories, DMT is also based in the arts and as such can address the patient's relationship to culture as a whole. Culture and the arts, understood broadly, are concerned with the struggle to create meaning out of the general chaos of modern existence. The arts offer the opportunity to use symbolism to express difficult issues in the life of one person and the life of society; for example, themes of birth, death, separation, loneliness, relationships, despair and hope. Creativity taps the ability of the client or patient to draw upon creative resources in thought, action and expression.

These goals may seem a little removed from outpatient psychiatric groups, but in fact they are integral to the use of the arts in therapy. For example, adolescents who bring their own music to DMT sessions can address psychological developmental issues such as attaining a measure of emotional autonomy from their families, but may also deal with broader personal and sociocultural issues. For example, the verbal and nonverbal material that they bring to sessions is concerned with themes such as being conformist or nonconformist, making a transition from wildly idealized romantic love to a realistic search for a partner, worries about drugs, violence and nuclear threat, concerns for the local and global environment, and hopes for the future, for themselves in particular and for the world in general.

While it may be tempting to make grand claims for the role of the arts therapies, overstating their potential effect is hazardous, insofar as the distinctions between the role of the arts in therapy, and in education, religion or culture become blurred. 'Art' is different from the arts therapies in that catharsis and symbolic exploration (which are two of the main arts elements used in DMT) are used by the artist as only a small part of the means by which an artistic product is created. The aim of DMT is not to awaken the latent artist inside the patient, but to use the therapeutic potential inherent in the creative process to aid the patient towards better emotional and social functioning, and possibly point the way towards psychological growth.

Client's views on DMT

There are as yet no full-length outcome studies on the arts therapies, though journals like *The Arts in Psychotherapy* do feature studies of their effectiveness in particular contexts (Callaghan 1991, Johnson 1987). Anecdotal evidence from patients suggests that they find DMT a useful part of their treatment programmes. In an informal survey carried out by a co-worker of the present author, employed by a community voluntary agency mental health organization (MIND), the following comments were made by psychiatric clients about DMT. One particularly articulate person wrote:

I found the dance movement group helpful in many ways. The actual physical movement with others, the revelation of a sense of union of emotions and physical feelings grew the more I attended the group.

A further statement was:

I found the dance movement therapy helpful in releasing pent-up emotion and frustration which really prevented me from moving forward. I had a great deal of anger in me; this therapy helped me to release some of this, and held out hope for the future, which to a large extent I had lost.

Another patient said:

As a person who was unemployed when I attended the group, and feeling that unemployment and states of depression/anxiety are often connected, I feel that movement dance therapy can be very important in alleviating feelings of emptiness/depression, and giving people an idea that they are 'involved' in a dynamic process.

A group of long-term patients, who attended a DMT group while making the transition from hospital-based to community care, said things like: 'We enjoy it very much. It's good. We do different things every week. You can be yourself. Nobody laughs at you' (Higgens and McLean 1990: 11). One long-term patient, upon leaving the eighteen-month long DMT group described later in this clinical section, was asked if he had got anything of benefit from his time in the group. He gave a smile and a knowing look, and said something to the effect of, 'Well . . . it's alright I suppose . . . good to move about, you know, do something with your-self . . . get yourself going. . . . And . . . well, it's sort of something different, innit?' [isn't it].

PSYCHODYNAMIC PERSPECTIVES ON MENTAL ILLNESS

What distinguishes a mentally ill person from someone who is not ill? A few mutant genes, or their dopamine transmission rate? Or their distorted ideas, such as paranoia, delusions, or anxiety attacks? Perhaps they have bizarre ways of getting attention, or withdraw from contact with others? Mental illness, as defined in psychiatric terms, comprises: biochemical changes; intrapsychic states (a person's sense that he or she is troubled, tormented, or in some form of mental pain); interpersonal relations (feel cut-off, or isolated, or unable to maintain satisfactory relationships with family, friends and colleagues); and social role functioning (can't, even if desirable, fulfil duties at work, or function as mother or father, wife or husband, sister or brother). But what is it like for the mentally ill person? Existentially, there are probably as many responses to being mentally ill as there are people who suffer the illness. However, there are certain features that clinicians from psychodynamic and existential perspectives have identified as common to those suffering from mental illness.

It is helpful to consider some of this literature in the light of the therapeutic goals of DMT, specifically in improving interpersonal functioning and helping to manage emotions. Some dance movement therapy students, keen to get onto the job, may not see the relevance of reading Freud or large tomes on existentialist theories of emotion. However, the understanding that comes from such reading forms the dance movement therapists as individuals, and it is those individuals who employ themselves and their responses as therapeutic tools in their encounters with patients. DMT students often worry, and ask, 'What should I *do* when I meet the patients?' It might be most useful to take the view that one should initially do nothing but listen, accept, try to understand and try to connect.

Once work starts, one can use one's human response and psychological understanding to make the patients' lives more bearable, first, by helping them maintain contact with others, perhaps through feeling valued by a group, and, secondly, assisting them in externalizing, expressing and managing their feelings, perhaps employing symbolic communication in the context of the DMT group. Simply being able to survive the patients' emotions, to witness their struggle away from illness and towards health is an important endeavour.

For example, a woman in an outpatient DMT group, who was withdrawing from tranquillizers, said that she was glad that she was not treated as a leper or a freak by the group, as someone whose panic was something to run away from; instead, she later explained that because her symptoms were not repugnant to everyone, she began to think that she herself might survive them, and go on to return to day-to-day life once again. This section will briefly examine a few ideas of psychodynamic thinkers on schizophrenia and depression. These are not intended as a guide to clinical practice, but merely as a starting point for reading about mental illness and considering things from the patient's point of view.

Schizophrenia

Early treatments of schizophrenia included 'moral treatment' advocated by Philippe Pinel (1745–1826) at the Bicêtre in Paris, and Samuel Tuke in England. This approach eliminated cruelty and physical punishment and restraint. Instead, they emphasized treating patients as human beings, giving them attention, living as normal a life as their conditions and the institution permitted, and attempting to restore them to a normal place in society. Productive work and interesting activities were encouraged (Karon and Vandenbos 1981: 9–17). Economic constraints and a lack of training of professionals to provide a second generation of moral treatment, as well as advances in descriptive psychiatry around the turn of the century, saw the decline of moral treatment. After this, some of the early psycho-analysts took some interest in psychoses, but they had many theoretical and practical differences among themselves. Freud initially took a pessimistic view of the treatment of psychosis, when he hypothesized that the libido was invested in the self, and therefore not available for a transference relationship. Many believed that this might be a technical obstacle around which someone might find a way, and the early analysts, including some following Melanie Klein's theories, had a degree of success in such treatment (Karon and Vandenbos 1981: 19).

Two later influential figures in the modified psychoanalytic treatment of schizo-phrenia were Harry Stack Sullivan and Frieda Fromm-Reichmann, who worked in the USA from the 1930s to the 1950s. Their work still exerts an influence on psychodynamically oriented mental health professionals. In contrast to many writers in that period who argued that disturbance arose largely as a result of intrapsychic dysfunction, Sullivan argued that personality should be conceived of as

the hypothetical entity which manifests itself in interpersonal relations, the latter including interactions with other people, real or fancied, primarily or mediately integrated into dynamic complexes; and with traditions, customs, inventions and institutions produced by man.

(Sullivan 1932: 302)

He believed that the symptoms of mental illness could be realized when their interpersonal context was known; by understanding the patients' relationships to themselves as a reflection of their relationships with others, including those with their families. The theory that schizophrenic disorder is exacerbated by irreconcil-able contradictory messages from the family has been developed further in both anti-psychiatry and empirical psychology studies (Laing and Esterton 1970).

At the Shepherd and Enoch Pratt Hospital in Maryland, Sullivan trained special psychiatric nurses to facilitate the creation of a warm, caring, trusting environment on the psychiatric ward. He stressed the opportunity for work and activity, because he felt that the lack of meaningful work or relationships could generate or make worse existing psychotic symptoms. It was at this hospital that Marian Chace conducted some of her pioneering work with dance movement therapy groups for psychiatric patients, where she was undoubtedly influenced by the working culture of innovative treatment approaches (Greenberg 1974, Green 1964).

The psychodynamic treatment of schizophrenia consists essentially of getting the patient to build a relationship with the therapist and then to use the therapist as a bridge to the external world. Sullivan and Fromm-Reichmann tried to understand the complexities of interpersonal relations and the preverbal experience of the infant in order to understand the details of the states and symptoms of the schizophrenic individual. In their view, the primitive affect of the preverbal child resembles the psychotic experience, such that theories about the birth of the psyche and the monumental chaos, joy and distress of the infant can be applied (with modification) to comprehend the raw emotional experiences of psychosis. Their treatment stressed repairing the person through relationships, particularly with persons of the same gender, in the manner of friends or allies, rather than parental relationships, or relationships with partners or spouses. In Sullivan's view, building peer relations was crucial for the schizophrenic, who, unlike the neurotic patient, was generally lacking in any sort of contact with others.

In terms of intrapsychic problems, the psychodynamic approach to schizophrenia contends that problems with anger and isolation are more prominent than those concerning sexuality, which might be more prevalent among neurotic clients. The importance of loneliness and the fear of closeness are primary issues to be addressed (Fromm-Reichmann 1954).

In their clinical writing, both Fromm-Reichmann and Sullivan emphasized the extraordinary patience and kindness necessary in developing an interpersonal relationship with the schizophrenic person. They see the schizophrenic patients as people who are frightened, and do not fully understand what is happening; who are afraid to communicate clearly because they fear it may be used against them; who are typically angry because they have been hurt so badly in the past, although they remain afraid to express anger directly towards the instigator, if indeed they are aware of who the instigator is. A schizophrenic person inexplicably shifts attitudes and behaviour during any single hour, as well as over days or weeks, and will typically create puzzlement and confusion in the therapist, and be difficult to contact (Karon and Vandenbos 1981: 152). Other psychoanalytic writers believe that

> because schizophrenics find needs painful and sometimes terrifying, they also experience the process of living in a similar fashion. They live in a transitional space, but they are developmentally paralyzed, not able to move into the outer world because they feel totally vulnerable, helpless, and completely out of control.
>
> (Giovaccini 1986: 265–266)

Sullivan was adamant that clear, simple communication was the best approach, and that getting into the patient's delusions, or trying to use one's own imagination to enter the schizophrenic's state, was too difficult and unreliable for most clinicians (Sullivan 1956: 364–368). He added that a schizophrenic person has 'never achieved the degree of self-esteem and certainty of ability to get along with other people that makes some major field of interaction safe' (Sullivan 1956: 364). This is echoed in contemporary psychotherapeutic work by, for example, Silvano Arieti, who notes that the therapist

> must at first become an exception for the patient – not a person to be mistrusted like others, but a person who is willing to share whatever anxiety and fears the

patient has, and finally a person who nourishes (psychologically speaking), who interprets things in a different way, and most of all who relieves anxiety and inspires a hopeful expectation for the future.

(Arieti 1979: 107)

In making contact with very ill patients, Sullivan felt that the problem was 'to find a way to relate to what is communicative in the patient's productions'. Both he and Fromm-Reichmann, and their contemporary revisionists such as the psychologists Bertram Karon and Gary Vandenbos, attempt to make psychotic phenomena meaningful to patients, as reactions to life phenomena, without accepting psychotic distortions. For example, one patient hallucinated that he could speak to the dead; instead of dismissing this, the therapist offered the suggestion that this patient was in fact missing an incompletely mourned family member who had recently died (Karon and Vandenbos 1981: 182). While this did not rid the patient of hallucinations, it did open up issues about loss and longing, fear of death, and a wish to be accepted and loved by members of the family.

Importantly, most psychodynamic clinicians argue that interpretations of unconscious processes or wishes, typically used with neurotic patients, should be *avoided* for schizophrenic patients, on the assumption that their conscious life is already dominated by unconscious material that floods them with primitive affect that threatens to overwhelm them (Karon and Vandenbos 1981: 143). Fromm-Reichmann believed that a psychotic patient's statements could make sense if they were analysed in a manner similar to dreams; the same processes are at work in the two phenomena: allusion, distortion, condensation, conflation, displacement, and symbol formation (Freud 1900: 381–628). These processes are primitive or primary, in psychic terms, and belong to the earliest or most archaic period of development of mental and emotional functioning.

Karon and Vandenbos hypothesize that the

> distortions of schizophrenic individuals are attempts to deal with their problems symbolically. The essence of the symbol is that the contents of the unconscious are expressed, and yet the individual is preserved from the awareness of what he is expressing. The schizophrenic person is constantly trying to solve his problems, but he is too frightened of them to deal with them directly; he represses the real problems and deals with the symbols.
>
> (Karon and Vandenbos 1981: 143)

For example, they suggest that the voices some patients hear may take the place of relationships for a lonely patient, and that superego or parental figures may be represented. In Sullivan's view, the 'schizophrenic distortion is one that comes from the very time when the more primitive type of mental process was the natural and only prevailing type of mental process or symbol operation' (Sullivan 1956: 363).

Clinically this means that schizophrenic individuals may fear that their aggressive impulses will lead to the damage or destruction of whoever they are involved with, and that they fear being overwhelmed, or being dissolved into another person through contact; both of these fears lead to longstanding withdrawal (Kahn 1984). In trying to enter the world of schizophrenic individuals to deal with their angry behaviour, clinicians contend that the patients functioning on the primitive level can only perceive others as they perceive themselves. So, if patients are threatening or violent, the therapist might say, 'It's alright, I won't allow anyone to hurt you, you are safe here.' This sometimes successful intervention is based in the notion that the reason that patients wish to hit someone is partly to do with the fact that they fear that people want to hit them first, or that they wish to be safeguarded from their own feelings of murderous rage or anger. If patients feel angry towards staff but cannot cope with this, and so believe that staff are angry with them, they may either withdraw or threaten violence in self-defence.

Because of these distortions in emotional functioning and communication, psychodynamic approaches focus on the need for clear, structured, and open communication from therapist to patient, and the encouragement of mature behaviour. As patients are treated with positive regard by the therapist, their own self-image can become more positive. Karon and Vandenbos write that,

> in talking with the schizophrenic patient, we often refer to 'giving', and the word 'giving' is not chosen at random. It really is a question of giving and taking, of dynamics going back to the early mother–child relationship. The typical schizophrenic patient has felt deprived all his life. It is important that the therapist do whatever possible to be perceived as a giver and not a taker, and to be perceived as a nonpunisher and nonpoisoner.
>
> (Karon and Vandenbos 1981: 165)

In conclusion, it is important to appreciate that communication from the seriously ill person to the therapist may be distorted, and that the patient's view of interpersonal interaction is one that is fraught with danger and difficulty. Furthermore, it is important not to enter into the patient's convoluted intrapsychic material, but rather to simplify it to a most basic emotional or interpersonal communication, and gently guide the patient back to the here-and-now interaction of the group. For schizophrenic patients, an important psychodynamically derived DMT goal is the alleviation of isolation through participation in the emotionally nurturant interpersonal environment of the group. A further goal is the concrete and physical externalization of primitive affect through movement and symbol. This latter goal is secondary to the improvement of interpersonal functioning.

Depression

As is the case with schizophrenia, there are a multiplicity of theories that try to account for the aetiology, outcome and the existential experience of depression. There are biological, cognitive, intrapsychic, interpersonal, familial and sociological perspectives on depression. Some theorists are most concerned with biological and chemical factors, while others stress the cognitive component, or set of beliefs which function to reinforce the depressed person's symptoms (Akiskal and McKinney 1975, Beck 1976, Gelman *et al.* 1987). Feminist and psychodynamic writers note that almost twice as many women as men are diagnosed as suffering from depression, suggesting a psychosocial factor in the incidence of the illness (Brown and Harris 1978).

Recently, family therapists and systems theorists have posited features of family functioning which may predispose or exacerbate depressive illness (Keitner and Miller 1990). An early study by Cohen and associates emphasized the patterning of interpersonal relationships rather than intrapsychic functioning as a factor in the development of depression. They noted that a depressed person might be characterized by a high level of dependency, concern about expectations from authority figures and hypersensitivity to signs of disapproval (Cohen *et al.* 1954). Similarly, Arieti and Bemporad's work postulated that the depressive person has had a childhood characterized by extreme receptivity to others with a tendency to rely less than the average person on autonomous resources, by basing self-esteem on rewards from others (Arieti and Bemporad 1980).

Psychoanalytic theory postulated that the loss of a significant attachment figure, or a loved object (such as the mother), whether actual or imagined, might give rise to depressive symptoms (Bowlby 1988, Freud 1915/1917, Spitz 1942). Additionally, Freud noted that the depressed person's self-reproaches might in fact represent feelings of hatred towards an ambivalently loved object, which were then turned back upon the self. Indeed, 'this mixture of love and hate for the same person is one of the deepest and most painful conflicts that human beings suffer from, and depressive patients will do everything in their power to avoid it' (Malan 1989: 130). However, the primacy of Freud's view, that depression is the result of anger or aggression that should be directed towards another person but is redirected onto the self, has been questioned by clinicians (Malan 1989). Instead, a constellation of problems around miscarried grief, ambivalent feelings towards others, guilt, hostility, self-punishment, fear of retribution, and a desire for reparation are often features of the depressed person's emotional life (Malan 1979: 124).

Cognitive approaches to depression conclude that depressed persons have a belief system (originating in childhood) which offers a distorted view of themselves and others. When those people lose a significant other person, or lose a goal or role in life, they may feel themselves devoid of meaning, or unworthy, and helpless. Aaron Beck, one of the leading cognitive theorists, posits that the depressed person's initial reaction to a loss (real or imagined) may be reactivated by the breakup of a relationship, loss of a job, or failure to attain an important goal or high expectation. The individual may exaggerate this loss, and see it as being due to some self-deficiency, or as evidence for a negative view of the self (Beck 1976). Beck's summary of typical cognitive distortions in depression includes negative view of the self, negative expectations of the environment, and negative expectations for the future (Beck 1976). These are conceptualized in therapeutic terms as a set of beliefs that are causative of depression and include: (1) a devout belief in one's personal inadequacy; (2) a 'horror' of not having what one needs; and (3) a view of the 'awfulness' of the way things are (Walen *et al*. 1980: 93). Furthermore, the pessimism becomes absolute, the current defeat is perceived as continuing indefinitely, there is no future, just an extended present of pain (Noebel 1990). Beck adds that these 'depressogenic cognitive structures generally related to interpersonal conduct and evaluation' (Kovacs and Beck 1978).

Research into the interpersonal dimensions of depression shows that the person may possess high levels of interpersonal sensitivity, showing hypersensitivity to perceived self-deficiencies in relation to others. This includes sensitivity to rejection and criticism and a sense of inadequacy and inferiority (Davidson *et al*. 1989). The psychologist Dorothy Rowe notes that the interpersonal context of depression is one in which the person feels cut off from others, and, to a certain degree, has chosen to do so. She adds that

> the structure by which a person organizes his world originates in the baby's interaction not just with his physical environment but, more importantly, in his interaction with other people. The structure develops and changes, transforms through continued interaction with others.
>
> (Rowe 1978: 29)

In terms of interaction in therapeutic work, specifically in groups, Yalom writes that the therapist cannot treat depression *per se*, because the interpersonal dimension of the illness is heterogeneous, or differs from one person to the next. He adds that

> it is necessary, first, to translate depression into interpersonal terms and then to treat the underlying interpersonal pathology. Thus the therapist translates 'depression' into its interpersonal issues – for example, passive dependency, isolation, obsequiousness, inability to express anger, hypersensitivity to separation – and then addresses those interpersonal issues in therapy.
>
> (Yalom 1970: 22)

In the DMT group, patients who are beginning to make a recovery from a major depressive episode can make important interpersonal gains, some of which can be related to the existential and psychodynamic perspectives on depression described above. If the group initiates a stamping rhythm, a depressed person who had appeared quite slow, or immobile, may often use the movement to express disavowed feelings of anger, and later report, 'I didn't know I had it in me.' Furthermore, depressive self-reproaches may be somewhat lessened in their intensity by the expression of positive regard for the depressed person by other members of the group. Additionally, ambivalence is expressed clearly by many depressed patients in that they often say that they do and do not want to come to the group; they may say that they do not need the group, or that it consists of patients who are more disturbed than themselves (i.e. schizophrenic patients); however, after completing a group, it usually emerges that they initially felt themselves to be inadequate, rather than inappropriate for a group. Clients or patients coming out of a period of depression often constitute the highest functioning members of outpatient DMT groups.

In conclusion, these brief introductions to the theories that seek to understand the development of mental illness, and attempt to describe and address the intra-psychic and interpersonal experience of mental illness, offer the dance movement therapist a few fundamental concepts on which to base further reading and understanding, which can inform their therapeutic work in both inpatient and outpatient psychiatric settings.

Chapter 6

DMT with adult outpatients

PRACTICAL CONSIDERATIONS

This chapter gives a full account of the practice of using DMT in an adult psychiatric day centre or hospital. Many dance movement therapists work in this setting as a primary focus in their careers; therefore this chapter is of an extended length. Furthermore, clinical experience with this client group raises many interesting theoretical and practical issues about technique. With this in mind, the structure of a typical DMT session is described at length, with examples of material from the opening discussion, warmup, movement and process section and closing discussion. The therapist's use of a co-worker, the shared leadership format, the use of props as projective tools, as well as whole-group comments and interpretation are considered. Also, the concepts of psychomotor free association, movement symbols, and the psychodynamic reading of group themes such as falling, going on a journey, repressed anger and separation and ending are described with clinical illustrations.

It may be argued that the training of dance movement therapists and their own preconceptions and expectations shape and form the experience of DMT for their clients. The illustrations given here from clinical work undertaken by the author under supervision from British dance movement therapists, with a background in the English object relations tradition, mean that the work described is of a particular bias and character. Readers may wish to refer to other literature such as the Jungian or ego-psychoanalytic by way of contrast, and keep in mind that clinical objectivity is probably an impossibility; what emerges in a DMT group with adult outpatients reflects the unique character of each member of the group and his or her particular struggle, and the ability of the dance movement therapist to attend to the member's experience and shape it into something meaningful.

Before describing clinical examples, the context in which the dance movement therapist works should be considered. This initial section will describe how most dance movement therapists work on a sessional basis, how they decide which patients are suitable for a group, the use of time-limited groups, the qualities necessary for a co-worker, relations with other staff, and suitable rooms and equipment. This section will be most relevant to DMT students beginning work at a new job or placement in adult psychiatry.

Workload

Most dance movement therapists work on a sessional basis for outpatient day hospitals or day centres, which means that a typical day might consist of two three-hour 'sessions' in which, during a single session, a 90-minute group can be run. Then the remaining 90 minutes can be used for note-making, debriefing of the co-worker, and attending meetings with the rest of the treatment team in order to feed back insights about patients gained from the DMT groups. A generally agreed workload among arts therapists is to run either two groups per day or to run one group and see two individual patients or to see four individual patients over the course of two three-hour paid sessions. Some dance movement therapists are employed on a private sessional rate, and others on a salary scale comparable to their colleagues in art, music and dramatherapy, which is in turn linked to that of occupational therapy, under current British public health service or National Health Service (NHS) guidelines. Setting up the group by meeting patients, speaking to staff about patients beforehand, and delivering information afterwards, as well as making notes for later supervision or for patient records, and collaborating with the co-worker, all take a considerable amount of time.

Familiarizing staff with the DMT approach

A further point regarding the relationship of the dance movement therapist to the institution must be made: the dance movement therapist will quickly find that a rather large portion of his or her work consists of explaining, succinctly and clearly, to other staff members and patients what exactly dance movement therapy *is* and how it works. It is therefore useful to give an in-service presentation to as many staff as possible before beginning work in a psychiatric treatment facility. This may include a video illustration of a DMT group, providing the consent of the patients has been obtained, as well as providing written literature or articles for anyone not attending the presentation. Positive regard for therapy by staff members is one of the keys to the group's success (Yalom 1983: 9). An example of an information sheet on DMT for staff is given in Appendix 1.

Feedback

In addition to the direct treatment benefit to the patient, communicating therapeutic insights to the rest of staff forms an important part of the dance movement therapist's contribution to the mental health team. This feedback must be given without betraying the patient's confidence, by making general, abstract remarks, rather than particular personal examples from the patient's movement or verbal material.

It is often useful to prepare a paragraph-long statement after the fourth, eighth, twelfth, and sixteenth group, to be included in the patient's case notes. Some community mental health centres will require instead that the dance movement therapists enter their observations in general nursing notes, or in a file describing the therapeutic progress of patients. It is important that the dance movement therapist follow the centre's guidelines, as appropriate. Additionally, the dance movement therapist must make time for supervision. The group must be warned one or two weeks ahead if the student's supervisor is to attend the group. The importance of live or videotaped supervision cannot be stressed highly enough: without it, the dance movement therapist can become lost in a complex group process, or countertransferential muddle, and thereby knowingly or unknowingly inhibit the development of the group (Sandel 1980, Skove 1986). If the group is to be videotaped, each member's written consent must be obtained, after permission is given by the psychiatrist. Videotapes must be erased after use in supervision, or after they have been played back to the group. Strict efforts must be made to ensure the patients' confidentiality. The dance movement therapist must confer with the supervisor and make informed judgements about videotaping: some patients find the camera anxiety provoking, or even persecutory. Some dance movement therapists feel that this effect is mitigated by having a camera operator, others feel that this makes the situation more uncomfortable. Clearly, therapeutic considerations cannot be overridden for the sake of having a videotape of the group; if the clients are disorganized, or the group is wobbly or unstable in membership or behaviour, it is wise to delay the making of a videotape, or to give more time for the group to prepare itself for the taping. At all times the dance movement therapist must seek guidance from mental health centre staff regarding videotaping of patient groups.

Group composition

The decision as to whether to see a particular patient in a group or individual session is usually dictated by the economic constraints of the day centre, and the clinical decisions of the referring agent, commonly the intake psychiatrist or psychiatric nurse key-worker, who usually designs a treatment package or programme for the patient. In general, a group is most useful for patients who have difficulties in interpersonal functioning. Those with very high anxiety or panic attacks, or who have suffered recent trauma such as bereavement, or who perhaps have made recent disclosures of sexual abuse, may be too fragile to participate in a group, and may require individual counselling or therapy by a member of day centre staff, or one-to-one dance movement therapy, before possibly considering entering a time-limited group. It is helpful if patients are within a broadly similar age range, and are a mixture of recent arrivals or admissions to the centre and those who are reducing their attendance on the centre; this allows lower functioning patients to have behavioural models in the higher functioning patients, and allows the latter to make gains by helping others, and by realizing how far they themselves have progressed since initially attending the centre.

DMT groups function in the context of particular psychiatric day treatment units, and as such reflect a selection from whatever identified groups of patients are attending the centre. Some facilities run specialized groups, such as those for women only, or those open to long-term patients living in the community, or therapeutic activities aimed at mentally ill mothers and children, or after school groups for teenagers who may have stayed for a short time in a psychiatric inpatient unit. Some facilities run groups based on specific diagnoses, such as groups for sexually abused adults, and others organize pre-discharge groups for patients leaving the day centre. In general, DMT can be modified to suit most of these types of groups, and, like verbal group therapy, probably works best with a reasonable mixture of patients of both genders, a reasonable age range, and varying degrees of illness and health.

As discussed in a previous section describing suitable referrals to DMT, there are only a few types of patients who are not appropriate for DMT groups. These are: floridly or acutely psychotic patients before they are somewhat stabilized, and dangerously underweight anorectic patients who may attempt to use the movement component of the group as a way to burn calories and lose weight. The dance movement therapist must be made aware of any patient's physical disabilities (propensity for epileptic fits, fainting, etc.) to ensure safety of the group members.

Medication effects

In beginning groups, it is often necessary to take referrals who may have only been attending the mental health centre for a few weeks. It is a good idea to say openly that such members need only partake in as much activity as they can manage. This means that some depressed patients may show severe psychomotor retardation, and schizophrenic patients may show akinesia, or sluggish movement, at least for a few weeks, and so may be permitted to partake in only as much activity as they can manage.

The patient who doesn't move

There are different theories among dance movement therapists as to whether some group members can remain seated during a session if they say they don't want to move, or are too tired. If letting people sit down means that a large number of the group will decide to take the opportunity to flop down into a comfy chair and doze off, then it probably isn't a good idea. However, if it is recognized that the patients would participate if and when their physical state would permit, it is a good idea to allow them to be seated, provided the other group members don't feel uncomfortable about being observed by that person. Making references to the seated person for their comments, or ideas, or asking them to describe in words a movement idea that others can follow, helps keep them 'in' the group rather than outside it. Referring to the seated person as 'the fly on the wall' (as appropriate) can often help group members metaphorically stand back, and imagine what they might look like to an observer, which can be a useful development in their ability to think about their behaviour.

Patients may evidence some side-effects of medication which will initially inhibit their free movement in a group: these include, for anti-depressant drugs, drowsiness, dry mouth and possibly some dizziness or blurred vision; and for anti-psychotic drugs, minor side-effects include drowsiness, apathy, dry mouth, constipation and nausea. These side-effects do not usually persist much after two months, but they must be taken into consideration when assessing whether the patient is genuinely disabled by unpleasant physical sensations, or is using medication effects to evade getting on with work in the DMT group. Dance movement therapists should *always* consult the co-worker in these matters before making any assumptions about movement and medication. On the whole it is best to avoid lengthy discussions in the group about medication; referring the client to the key-worker, nurse, or psychiatrist is best if the concerns are fairly specific. Only if the general issue of medication concerns the whole group is it useful to facilitate a discussion on this issue in either the initial or closure section of the group.

Medication effects need not inhibit or disqualify a patient from participation in a group. In one instance, a woman who was withdrawing from tranquillizer use and was suffering physical symptoms of dizziness, tremor and sensations of tingling, numbness and weakness, was helped by the group to stay grounded in reality. While the group admitted their anguish at not being able to help her, it did allow for a free discussion about the benefits and costs involved in taking medication.

Time-limited groups

It is difficult to predict which particular patients are best suited for the DMT approach; it is helpful if patients themselves express an interest in coming, and if they are given a choice by their key-worker as to whether or not they want to participate in the group once they have understood (either through speaking to the dance movement therapist, or attending one or two sessions) what the group is about. Average length of patient contact with a day treatment centre varies between two and six months, with attendance on one day or several days per week. Groups optimally consist of no more than eight patients and no less than five, plus the dance movement therapist and co-worker. It is probably most practical, as well as economically sensible, to run groups for a time-limited period, such as sixteen sessions over a period of approximately four months. The fixed time frame may allow more disturbed patients to master their anxiety about joining a group because they know it has a limited life span (Ryle 1990). Time-limited groups, in contrast to open-ended ones, help keep therapists and patients focused on the therapeutic tasks of group cohesion, trying out new interpersonal behaviour, and dealing with issues of loss and separation when the group concludes (Yalom 1970).

In some instances, when patients' other therapeutic activities at the day centre are winding down, the completion of a time-limited DMT group may be one of the last elements in their programme to finish. This means that the group can provide a transitional space between dependence on treatment and a return to post-treatment living. Depending on the referral procedure used by the day unit for arts therapies, some dance movement therapists run two 'open' DMT groups during which the patients and therapist can assess suitability for the group. One can expect a drop out rate of approximately 30 per cent, and so from a group of ten patients, a core of seven or eight can be formed for the sixteen-week group (Yalom 1970: 284).

Groups have a 'stable' rather than 'closed' membership, and it is generally agreed with the patients at the beginning of the group that, should the membership drop below five, new members may be introduced, providing no more than eight of the sixteen sessions have elapsed. Some other settings, such as community centres or voluntary mental health organizations, may require a more flexible membership policy in accordance with aims of long-term emotional support, rather than an aim to provide an experience of interpersonal learning and facilitating behavioural change.

Co-workers

It is best to have a co-worker who may be either a psychiatric nurse, occupational therapist, psychiatrist, or other mental health team member. This enables a full-time member of staff to experience, and then to understand, what DMT groups can offer patients, and so make further appropriate referrals to new groups. Also, the co-worker can provide the dance movement therapist with updated information on patients' behaviour, and can also feed back to the rest of the team observations from the DMT group at other meetings during the week, when the dance movement therapist may not be working at the centre.

The co-worker must be able to participate in the group, and not use the session for personal therapy. The co-worker must also be able to restrain his or her own emotional process. He or she can aid the dance movement therapist in observing patients' behaviour, and comparing it to behaviour seen outside the sessions in the patients' attendance at other activities at the centre. It is helpful but not necessary for co-workers to be experienced in group therapy; a neutral and open manner, good communication with patients, as well as willingness to try movement and encourage the patients' exploration of new behaviour are the most important qualities. It is crucial that the co-worker be able to attend all of the sixteen sessions in a time-limited group, so that therapeutic consistency is maintained. It is useful to meet the co-worker once or twice outside the group time, to get to know one another a little, give information, or have a detailed discussion of the life of the group a couple of weeks before it is ending.

The room, props and music

Groups must be run at the same time each week, in the same room, and begin and end on time. The physical setting of the room is important. It must contain enough chairs for everyone, which can be pushed back to make enough space for the group to stand in a circle and allow a fair degree of free movement without fear of bumping into the next person. The dance movement therapist must ensure that the room allows privacy; curtains must prevent outsiders looking in, and a sign on the door to prevent people walking through the room is helpful. Nothing is less conducive to creating a safe atmosphere for exploring feelings than the threat of intrusion or interruption. The dance movement therapist must begin and end the session on time; stability in boundaries of the session allows for a sense of emotional containment, and differentiates the special time and space of the session from activities during the rest of the day. Patients must be warned, at least a week or two in advance, of a visit by the dance movement therapist's supervisor, and several weeks in advance of bank holiday breaks. Patients should be encouraged to forewarn the group if they themselves intend to be absent for a session. Many changes in staff and sporadic absences by patients which go unexplained are not helpful; the idea is to keep all elements of the group as stable as possible to allow for a sense of an interpersonal learning laboratory to be conveyed to clients and staff.

The dance movement therapist provides about eight tape cassettes of music for the group to choose from, and may bring a portable tape-cassette player to sessions. It is a good idea to bring a mixture of popular, classical, ethnic and possibly jazz or experimental music; it is not a great idea for dance movement therapists to bring their own personal favourite music, or to express a clear preference for anything in particular, since patients themselves are the ones who should have most say in what music is used. Once the group gets started it is helpful to encourage patients to bring music that they would consider suitable, or to get tapes of what patients request, perhaps from the local library, because generally patients do not have the money to purchase many music cassettes for themselves.

Props such as Lycra stretch cloths, measuring at least two metres by two metres, or of varying square or rectangular shapes, are useful tools with which to focus a group. Lycra is the stretchy material that swimming suits and cycling shorts are made from, and is available from fabric shops. Quality Lycra that has a vertical and horizontal stretch is essential: cheaper versions that only stretch one way can shred if the group, standing in a circle, decide to have a tug-of-war!

CASE ILLUSTRATION

The following are a series of composite sketches from clinical work with groups of adult outpatients. Some of the material from these groups was presented (in much abbreviated form) in Helen Payne's *Dance Movement Therapy: Theory and Practice* (Payne 1992). This section will describe clinical material from each component of a typical group, including the initial discussion, the movement warmup, a 'process' section in which the main emotional work of the group occurs, and the closing discussion in which the events of the process section are considered or interpreted by the group with the help of the dance movement therapist and the co-worker. What follows here is not an actual clinical transcription of a single session, but a series of 'snapshots' over the four months of the life of a group of psychiatric outpatients.

The first meeting

The very first group meeting is one in which the dance movement therapist provides the patients with an introduction and orientation of the DMT group. This first session may be an 'open' or trial group held for approximately eight or nine patients, before patients enter a verbal agreement or contract to attend a fixed number of weekly sessions (typically between twelve and sixteen). One can expect one or two members to drop out, or to be unsuitable or unwilling to contract for the remaining sessions. It is important to state that regular attendance is expected. If a regular member is absent for one session, an empty chair should be left in the group circle, as a concrete reminder that someone is missing.

Clients or patients will want to know what the group is for and what they will be doing every week. A very simple statement about the use of movement to get activated and motivated, and to use the group as a safe place to share and examine feelings, is a good place to begin. It might be helpful to mention that the group work isn't just a poor substitute for individual therapy or counselling sessions, but that good learning opportunities are offered by a group in which we can learn how to relate to others, and learn how other people see us, which will hopefully help everyone in the group to have more clear and satisfying relations with family, work colleagues and groups of friends.

One can continue by saying that the group can be seen as a special instance of learning ways of relating to people, and where it is acceptable to make comments about feelings, to try new things, to be creative, and to get and give support, to listen to others and to learn, and share problems. It is sometimes useful to mention that the group is not a forced confessional, but that as people get to know each other, they may wish to share more about how they are feeling, from week to week. It is a good idea to say that some people will feel more comfortable sharing more about themselves than others, but that each person must find what is comfortable for him or her, and not feel pressured.

It alleviates clients' initial anxieties to know that everyone has some difficulties in common, both in relating to others and in handling feelings, despite how very different each person's problems might seem. It is important to mention that expressing honestly one's positive or negative feelings about others, and the leaders of the group, and the group's shared activity, is one of the main unique features of group therapeutic work. While society often frowns on an open expression of feeling, the group embraces it (Yalom 1970).

The fact that the structure is the same every week (with initial discussion, warmup, taking turns at leading the group movement, and closing discussion) deserves mention. The idea that any sort of movement is fine should be stressed, as well as the point that the aim is not to move beautifully, or perform gracefully, but to use the movement to get feelings out, maybe have a bit of fun, be a little creative, have a go at something different, as a way of being together as a group.

Sometimes new members ask how they have been selected for DMT, and so some comment about how the other community mental health team members felt that they might benefit from what the group has to offer can help patients understand the rationale behind group DMT, and what they are expected to gain. The idea of openly sharing the aims of therapy with the patients is one that is derived from brief, or short-term therapy (Balint *et al.* 1972, Ryle 1990: 17).

It is also a good idea to mention briefly the fact that there may be stumbling blocks at the beginning: for example, that it is hard to see how coming to the group can help with personal problems, and to articulate how nervous or funny or peculiar people will feel both moving and talking together until they know each other a bit more and get used to each other. At some stage in the early meetings the dance movement therapist could mention how people may feel annoyed with the dance movement therapist and co-worker for not having all the answers, but that the aim of the group is to try to express and deal with feelings more clearly and effectively, and to get along better with other people. After this initial meeting, or meetings, it is a good idea to give the remaining group members a calendar with group dates clearly marked, including public bank holiday breaks. Expressing positive regard and hope for the ability of the group to engage in the task at hand can alleviate some of the initial anxiety clients may have about their ability to manage in the group. Lastly, group members should be told that if they really do find it too difficult or too uncomfortable or too much for them they can speak to their day centre key-worker in private (rather than having to address the group as a whole) about dropping out at either the initial or middle stages of the group.

Phases in the life of the group

After the introductory meetings, the group work can begin in earnest. Although it need not be stated to the group members, the dance movement therapist expects certain phases and events in the life of the time-limited group. Irvin Yalom writes that there are three stages to groups: the 'in or out, the top and bottom, and the near and far' which illustrate issues about acceptance, inclusion and exclusion, followed by issues around competitiveness, conflict, and rebellion and a final stage in which the group grapples with issues of closeness, cohesion and separation (Yalom 1970: 301–310). In Claire Schmais's view, the group's task, both within each session and throughout the life of the whole group over time, is to orient itself to the situation, and then, once the patients are used to the group, to begin a process of differentiation (taking on distinct roles, and allowing for self-related and interactional exploration) and finally concluding the group with the task of separation (Schmais 1981). In her view,

> there tends to be a sequential order in the group's uncovering emotions. Behind the depression we find anger. When the anger is experienced with full intensity,

people are ready to acknowledge their dependency needs and their yearning for closeness.

(Schmais 1981: 104)

This sequence, which includes: a period of getting used to the other people and the structure of the meetings; followed by a period of growing exploration and revelation of feelings; seeing the value of others in the group; and concluding working through the feelings evoked by ending or losing the security of the group, are tasks with which each group grapples over the sixteen sessions in which they work together. However, the group members do not need to have any of this explicitly stated; it is important for the dance movement therapist to be ready for any signs of shifts in group functioning, and to reflect upon them generally in the light of group therapy theory, as well as to be open to surprises.

Initial discussion

Every week the group begins with some sort of initial verbal discussion, lasting about 15 or 20 minutes if the session runs for 90 minutes, or 10 minutes if the session is an hour long. It may be useful to establish a routine of asking the patients, in turn, to say how their week has been, to list one positive and one negative thing that has happened to them, or that they have done or felt, and then to ask them to rate their week on a scale of 1 to 10, with 10 being a really great week and 0 being a dreadful week. This allows people to begin to reflect on their experiences from week to week, and to compare their experiences with those of others.

Interestingly, some people report very positive events in the week, and then rate themselves a 3 out of 10 because they 'felt low and miserable'. The numbering format is not necessarily vital to the conversation, but it may help the dance movement therapist and co-worker to accurately sum up the state of the group once each patient has gone around in the circle, and said something about his or her present state of mind (Kahn 1984: 51).

The co-worker and dance movement therapist also take a turn, though they ought to be careful to gauge the degree of their self-disclosure at a little lower level than that of the patients: patients need to have some confidence that the leaders of the group are generally able to manage their own feelings, such that the patients do not need to worry about the emotional fragility of the leaders, or how they are coping with their lives. The DMT group is for the benefit of the clients or patients, and not for the staff. Staff support groups and supervision are ideally part of the community mental health team facility, and can help prevent group workers surreptitiously using therapy groups for their own emotional benefit, either by bringing their own problems to the group, or by expecting the patients to perform wonderfully, and thereby validate the leaders' good feelings about themselves through their work.

The main aim of the initial discussion is for everyone to get a sense of the feeling tone of the group as a whole on that day. The dance movement therapist should try to set the tone of the group by being sympathetic but neutral, expressing positive regard for the group, without exaggerated cheerfulness or expectation. The aim is to get the group to feel that the atmosphere is one that is conducive to a creative experience, to be comfortable enough to 'see what happens' to a degree, or at least be open to structured exploration. As the weeks go by it is a good idea to feel ready and open for new ideas and movement, and to project a feeling of confidence that the group will be able to come up with some material to work with. Surprisingly enough, the confidence of the co-worker and the dance movement therapist, in themselves and their group, very much affects how the group will progress.

Group profile

The material for the initial discussion varies directly with the composition of each particular group. The group from which the clinical material for this section was drawn was composed of five clients, plus a male student psychiatric nurse co-worker, and a dance movement therapist (the present author). It was held in a large sitting room of the psychiatric day centre. This was a fairly young group, aged between 25 and 35. There had been a sixth member, another female client who had attended the first meeting but was unable to become involved in the group's movement, which she found somewhat overwhelming. Another patient had been selected in her place, but had difficulty getting to the group at its stated time, due to another weekly appointment, and so the group began with one or two members less than might be optimal.

Two of the patients, John and Joan, had been diagnosed as schizophrenic, but had been relatively stable for some time. John's repetitive psychotic episodes, which occurred about two or three times per year, effectively prevented him from working. His grandfather had also suffered from schizophrenia, which was something he found quite upsetting. Joan had had a child eight years before, but had been unable to care for the child, who was subsequently placed with foster parents when the child was two years old. She was also unemployed. Each of the patients was being followed-up monthly by a psychiatrist.

Paul, the youngest member of the group, was referred for anxiety attacks and some obsessional behaviour (such as needing to check and replace things, or count several times before leaving a room, or straighten several objects in his room before leaving it). He received behavioural management sessions with an occupational therapist who endeavoured to help him extinguish the behaviours, and trace their sources to a certain degree. During the group he was involved in doing voluntary work with the elderly, in the hope of being accepted to a job training scheme. In the end he was not accepted for this, and we all harboured suspicions that his honesty with the employment officer about his mental health record was a factor in this. However, a month or so after the group ended, he did get a permanent job doing clerical work in a warehouse.

Luke, aged 25, was coming out of a second major depressive episode, which had featured some psychotic ideation. It was unclear whether he might be showing early signs of schizophrenia, but he had not been formally diagnosed as such. He had been unable to regain his motivation, and found it difficult to think of getting a job. Since leaving school at 18, he had been sporadically employed doing manual and farm labour. Eileen, who was in her mid-30s, had suffered recurrent major depressive episodes, some general anxiety, and reluctance to leave the house at times, and also had a number of unspecified physical complaints that were thought to be related to her mental problems. She had been divorced two years before she joined the group and, though unemployed at the time, hoped one day to go back to clerical work. Both Luke and Eileen had weekly meetings with their nurse key-workers. Finally, there was Gary, the student psychiatric nurse, who acted as co-worker; he was an outgoing, athletic person, interested in learning about various therapeutic approaches.

Example of an initial discussion

The group ran from the end of November to the end of March. A typical initial discussion, which occurred about two weeks after Christmas, went something like this: Paul said he had just had an interview on a job restart scheme, that it had been all right, and that he had decided that he would tell the interviewer that he had been unemployed due to having attended the community mental health centre for counselling. He said he felt better being honest about this, because he had struggled about whether or not to mention his psychiatric history. He had also been out that week with one of his sisters, and had been playing video game machines at one of the arcades. He said he was glad the holidays were over, because he had been getting bored, and feeling cramped in the bedsit where he lived. He gave his week a 7, for the sheer relief of having survived his interview and because he had felt quite good that morning.

John reported that he had made a great effort to enjoy his Christmas, and that it had worked. He mentioned that he had a hard time getting to the group that day, because he hadn't felt very well since the doctor had cut down his medication, and he didn't like having to take capsules each day instead of having weekly injections. Most of the group made sympathetic murmurings and noddings, and so the dance movement therapist commented that it seemed that people could empathize with how John felt about his difficulties. Luke said he could relate to this issue, whereupon Paul began to look nervous, because he'd never had medication, and had once said that he didn't want any.

It is generally advisable to avoid detailed discussions about patients' medication; any factual information they really need is only available from their nurse or psychiatrist. However, some patients do wish to speak about their anxieties and ambivalence about medication. Many feel grateful for the symptomatic relief, but fear prolonged dependence, side-effects, or blunting of the feelings that led them to seek treatment. In this context it is important to maintain neutrality, and not to undermine the patients' drug treatment by suggesting that they might be better off without their medication. If patients want to reduce their medication they must do so under medical supervision, or they risk harmful withdrawal symptoms; if they later need or decide to return to having medication, they may feel that you will look upon them as 'weak' for requiring it, should they believe you disapprove of their taking medication in any way. Discuss specific issues with other staff, and always refer the patients' concerns to their key-worker or the psychiatrist. John continued that at least he was in a better state this year than he was last year when he'd been 'on a slippy slope' as he described a phase of an acute psychotic episode for which he'd been hospitalized at that time. He rated his week a 3 or a 5 maybe, and made a vague gesture with his hands.

Joan said she'd spent Christmas with her cousins, and eaten too much. She added that she was still settling in to her new council flat, and bought terribly expensive curtains when out with her aunt that morning, and it was all taking some getting used to. She said that she rated her week a 7 out of 10, which the dance movement therapist said was an improvement on last week's 2 or 3 out of 10.

Eileen reported that she'd cooked a meal for some of the residents of her group home, and otherwise hadn't done much, and was generally all right, she supposed. She mentioned that she had been really 'low' over Christmas, but had managed not to call the Samaritans at the last minute, and she felt good that she'd managed on her own. She said she'd been watering her plants, which were coming along nicely. She rated her week a 6 out of 10. This was all delivered in a flat tone, and the therapist, making a mental note that a number of Eileen's examples were mostly to do with concrete events rather than about how she was feeling, asked: 'And how have you been, *in yourself*?' Eileen looked directly at the therapist and shrugged, making the upper part of her body heavy and limp, saying, 'not too bad, really'. The dance movement therapist, noting the contradiction between her words and her speech, said, 'Really?' in a fairly neutral way, to which Eileen responded, 'Well, I've been feeling a bit out on my own – you know. . .'. This finally seemed the most honest explication of her feelings, and so the next person in the circle, Gary, the co-worker, took his turn. He said he'd had an okay holiday, though he'd been ill with 'flu, and there had been no heating in the nurses' residence. He said that this actual week he rated a 6 out of 10, because he'd worked an extra shift, and then stayed out late, and he smiled when he said he was very tired, even too tired to dream. There were giggles and speculation by the male members of the group as to the source and content of Gary's wild weekends, which he often reported, since the group ran early in the week. Some discussion about dreams followed. Paul mentioned nightmares, and Joan said she didn't dream at all; John said he dreamed but they disappeared quickly.

This discussion of dreams, though interesting in a way, seemed somewhat tangential to the 'checking in' function of the conversation, which was dragging on longer than usual, and the therapist signalled that it was Luke's turn. The dance movement therapist's role in this initial discussion phase of the group is to guide the social interaction somewhat, curbing talkative patients, drawing out the reluctant ones, and possibly trying to model verbal and nonverbal ways in which to listen and attend to others, such as not allowing subgroups to chat while someone else is speaking. Luke said he'd stayed home and watched TV most of the week and he rated the week 4 out of 10. He said he had eaten too much over Christmas, and was glad to be back to ordinary life. He added that he had been told by his mother that he should sell his motor bike, since it seemed likely that with the medication he was taking, he'd never get a proper job anyway, and there was no point in his bike sitting in the shed, gathering dust. He seemed quite detached from this, and the co-worker said he wondered if the bike had to be sold so soon. Luke perked up and said that it was his mother's idea, which she'd got after speaking to the psychiatrist. He looked questioningly at the dance movement therapist and co-worker, as though for reassurance. The co-worker said that he at least ought to wait a while, to see how things went along; not everyone who took medication became unable to drive. Luke seemed momentarily pleased, but then went back to staring at the floor. It seemed important not to offer false reassurances, and so, after sympathetic looks were exchanged among many group members about Luke's plight, the dance movement therapist, who came next in the circle, took her turn. She said that her week had been busy, and slightly rushed, since relatives had come to stay. She mentioned some mischief that her new cat had got up to over Christmas, by climbing into the tree; this elicited a predictable smile and nod of recognition from the group who were probably a bit fed up with the continuing saga of her cat. She rated her week a 7 out of 10.

She commented that the group was a mixture today, with John and Luke and maybe Eileen feeling somewhat low, while Paul and Joan seemed more energetic than in previous weeks. She added that it sounded like people had coped better with Christmas than they had expected, but that there had been some sadness associated with the holiday for some members of the group. She commented that people generally found holiday periods stressful because they were a break from the usual routine. It is a good idea to try to summarize the state of the group as a whole at the end of the discussion, to give the group a sense of feeling themselves as a unit, rather than isolated individuals. In this instance, the mixture of feelings was mentioned, and the feeling that some people seemed to want to start things off slowly, and others (Joan and Paul in particular) wanted to rush back into the work of the group, and day-to-day life after the holiday break.

Choice of music

The dance movement therapist then produced a box of tape cassettes, and asked the group to choose some music. One should always stress that the music is only for background, and not for dancing. It is important that the music provides a comfortable backdrop, but that it not be so rhythmic or overpowering that it determines the quality of the movement. Patients should be encouraged to bring music from which the group can choose – usually a mixture, such as pop or light rock, folk, possibly some classical music or guitar, African or other ethnic music – to allow for a range of moods. Jazz, meditation tapes, or experimental music that has little internal structure are not advisable since they tend to encourage attending to oneself in movement, and is not music which facilitates interaction. What and how the group chooses can be a valuable indication of the mood of the group, and can prefigure the way the patients relate to each other. Do the patients follow a strong member, or does the therapist need to institute a vote if the group is highly dependent, such that nobody will express a clear preference? These issues are often a very early indication of the sort of group process that is to follow in the central section of the group, the improvised movement process. In this case, the group was divided: Joan wanted to have African drum music and Eileen said she didn't mind, but she'd prefer some orchestral music. Paul and John said they weren't bothered, but weren't keen on African, they might prefer the Beatles. Eventually, Paul got John and Gary to agree that it was a Paul Simon tape, 'Graceland' that would be the best compromise between African music and the Beatles. Paul was often the member of the group who smoothed over conflicts of interest.

Movement warmup

The group got up slowly, and shifted their chairs out of the circle, leaning them against the wall. The therapist started the usual warmup, which runs in a sequence designed to activate and motivate, to facilitate whole-body integrated movement, and to provide an initial introduction to some new components of an extended movement vocabulary. It is helpful if the warmup contains all the movement qualities from Laban's effort–shape choreographic elements, and so does not too much reflect the personal movement preferences or profile of the therapist. The warmup used qualities of weight (strong and light), space (indirect and direct), time (sustained and quick) and flow (bound and free), which were done with their shaping components (rising, sinking, growing, shrinking, widening and narrowing) as described in Chapter 4 (see Figure 2).

Typically, the warmup began by bending at the knees, and then shifting weight from one side to the other, firmly pressing into the ground, gradually involving not only the legs but the trunk and arms as well. Images to help get these qualities are provided, such as when the dance movement therapist asked the patients to feel the ground underfoot in an attempt to get the weight effort mobilized. This was followed by reaching up high, down low, side to side, and through the diagonals. This purposeful working through all the planes of movement (vertical, horizontal, sagittal) is to increase the kinesphere, or sphere of movement. Some facial self-massage was included to counteract the tendency of some clients to move every part of their bodies, but leave out expressive facial movement. In addition, as the weeks went by, some more interesting and novel movements were added, some of which sought to address specific effort–shape deficits which members of the group showed. Paul, for example, could not use free flow with indirectness, and so the therapist introduced this combination. The warmup usually ended with some form of rocking, swaying or swinging which involved the whole body moving in a grounded or weighted fashion. The warmup was not exactly the same each week – it should never be too programmed; if people don't seem ready to move, one can add more warmup, especially if people seem a bit disoriented or flat. If people seem highly strung and ready to fly off into the movement session without hesitation, doing some sustained movement and grounding them can prevent a flurry of movement activity being used in a defensive way.

The movement warmup can be added to, and the style of the group and the dance movement therapist can be taken into account. In general, one must aim for a progression from single to whole body parts in the warmup, and for an increase in the choreographic richness of the movement in shapes, planes and dynamic colour. Doing a circle or rolling motion with the neck is best avoided; it isn't very good for the vertebrae, and can exacerbate the dizziness or nausea some patients may have due to medication, or lack of eating breakfast or lunch before coming to the group. Doing a twist at the waist helps mobilize what is often a stiffly held body area, and reaching through the space using the arms in a sequence which runs through the diagonals of up, down, side to side, forward, backward, in the horizontal, vertical and diagonal planes (in the manner of a star or a tetrahedron) is a good way to increase the kinesphere or spatial scope of the clients' movements.

Process section

Following the warmup, the group retains its circle formation, and begins the process section. The term 'process' refers to the idea that this part of the group focuses on the interaction of the members, the new emotional learning experience which occurs during the movement section of the group (Yalom 1970: 137). It is this central section of the session in which the group plays out or works on whatever material, conscious or unconscious, is of concern to the individuals and the group. In this section, each person in turn is asked to do any movement, small or large, whether a little gesture using just hands, or a whole body action such as a jump. The dance movement therapist tells the patients not to plan what they'll do, but to do anything at all, 'off the cuff, and then we'll all do it together', indicating that the rest of the group will try to follow that person. One can give examples, like walking forward into the circle, or making a gesture of throwing something to the front, or reaching into the middle of the circle as if to take something out. This first given example is narrated by the dance movement therapist, 'So if I reach like this, what could I be doing?' Someone usually says the movement is like swimming (if the dance movement therapist has used indirect space, free flow, and sustained time effort elements). And the therapist might ask, 'So where are we swimming? In a warm pool maybe, or in an ocean full of sharks, or whatever? So then we might talk about scary stuff like sharks, or even scary feelings, or how nice it might be to swim in a pool.' He or she might add that 'When we've done that for a while, just say "Pass" and the person next to you in the circle will take a turn leading the group.'

The dance movement therapist quite deliberately introduces the technique of using movement to gain a free association in words. Significantly, the words then affect the movement; one swims in a much less relaxed way if there are sharks around; this further change in the movement (which might be termed movement or psychomotor free association) can go on to produce still more verbal associations

(Boas 1952, 1989, Schmais 1981). This process, which moves from movement to image to interpretation, is one that is given or taught to the patients in much the same way that in art therapy one might be introduced to the technique of how to draw without planning or censoring the subject matter (Stanton 1988, 1991, Stanton and Stanton 1989).

It is very important to stress that the aim of using movement in the group is not to perform, or dance, or exercise. Instead, the dance movement therapist must try to facilitate a creative and supportive atmosphere for movement exploration in which it is the expressive aspect of the movement that is valued. The idea of movement as dance or performance is disclaimed by the fact that the group almost always moves while formed in a circle, rather than in two straight lines facing each other, or in an audience/performer format. The circle is a communal space, which allows people

> to move and to feel in harmony with themselves and with others. This structure is democratic: patients and therapists are on the same footing, standing side by side: no one is higher or lower, nor is status protected by the barrier of a desk. By removing people from the spatial conventions of interpersonal discourse, the circle offers the choice of making eye contact or of turning away.
> . . . The circle is a malleable entity, expanding to accept newcomers, shrinking to a solid mass or expanding into the far corners of the room. People can dance as part of it, inside or outside it. People can easily enter the circle or escape. The circle can be highly active, turning faster and faster like a wheel or it can be still, forming a barrier to shield those within its boundaries.
>
> (Schmais 1981: 106)

In addition to these benefits contained within the spatial structure of the circle, the shared leadership role structure also has the fundamental benefit of offering group members the opportunity to gain a sense of personal success and autonomy by leading the group in a created movement. At the end of the group some members remark that they thought they wouldn't be able to think of anything to do, but are pleased to have managed to fill their turns, using their own, simple or complex, created movement sequences and verbal associations.

Shared leadership

The following are a number of examples of the sorts of things that members of the circle did when it was their turn to initiate or lead an impromptu movement over the course of several months. It is interesting to note how these movement turns persisted over time, how they were elaborated, and how they became a common vocabulary among the group.

In the third session, the group had begun with a continuation of its discussion about difficulties and frustrations in finding employment. Paul in particular felt the pain of feeling unacceptable, and not gaining much encouragement from either employment agencies or prospective employers. Luke was deemed unsuitable for a voluntary job, which upset him, though he tried to make out that he didn't want the job anyway. Joan had a period of being a bit more disturbed in the third to seventh sessions, and was somewhat paranoid and unpredictable at times. John seemed very out on a limb, and lonely, or at least isolated for a few weeks following the reduction of his medication. Eileen was well, and trying to go out more with friends from her group home.

In this session, Paul began his turn with a movement of stepping forward on one leg, and bending at the knee, while looking down, so that the overall effect was like bowing down. He said he might be picking up something. By eliciting various people's associations, variations on this nearly identically shaped movement (but using different choreographic qualities and phrasing accents) allowed it to become: bowing down on bended knee, being knighted, arriving at a royal court, doing a courtly dance, surfing, balancing, and eventually, walking on a tightrope. This simple motion of bowing, of balancing one's weight on the front leg while leaning forward, gained extended meanings by repetition week after week.

The dance movement therapist, upon seeing any patient's movement turn, says something like, 'Okay, let's all do that again.' Or, 'Let's do that together.' The movement took on various meanings in interaction with others: we all bowed solemnly together, and did a 'hmmmmm' noise one day when John suggested it was like paying respects to something or other. We added a rhythm to it, and synchronized, becoming tribal dancers; and later, in making it the first move of an unplanned sequence (using sustainment and lightness efforts), it became the opening for a minuet of robots. This particular movement, like many others given within the shared leadership format, generated these meanings from the group by the continual process of the dance movement therapist asking for associations by saying: 'What could this be like? What quality does this have? How could we put a picture to this? What could we be doing? What is this about?' etc. In the early stages, it feels like one is forcing associations, but later this becomes easier, at least for some members of the group.

Psychomotor free association

Even the simplest movements can elicit associations, once the technique is familiar to the group members. In some senses it resembles the process in charades, where people have to guess what the gesture is meant to signify, but in DMT, the movement can hold many meanings. For example, simply walking forward into the circle and back out again could be 'putting your best foot forward', 'taking one step forward and one step back', 'stepping out', 'sneaking up on someone', 'going back and forth and not getting anywhere', or any number of things, depending on the emotional tone of the group and the movement quality with which the person walked.

Also, the movement can change its meaning week after week with little or no modification. Paul's bowing became a stage type introduction, like Al Jolson arriving on stage, or like Charlie Chaplin saying a silent hello. Associations elicited for this were, 'Tah Dah! I'm here!', and later, 'Like it or lump it!', followed by an interesting discussion of acting, and television, and social façades. The dance movement therapist asked what sorts of image people wanted to give out, in a job interview, or at home in private, to which the group added the necessity of 'putting a brave face on it' or 'putting on a happy face' even when feeling quite depressed.

When the tightrope image came up, a number of members of the group began to experiment with their own ways of walking on a tightrope (using different qualities, but all appearing more 'involved' in the movement, because more full effort–shape combinations were being used); this signalled to the dance movement therapist that this image and symbol were ones which the group were highly engaged in and also could share. The therapist suggested that people take a moment to 'make the movement their own' or walk on their own tightropes, and play with that for a bit, to see how it felt. Eileen said it was scary, and Gary wondered if there was support underneath. Luke bravely said that he didn't need a safety net, and John, who was rather emotionally unstable at this point, took extreme care (using bound flow, appearing tense and cautious) while doing this movement, suggesting that, for him, entering into the tightrope symbol might have been a way of trying to keep on the narrow line between health and illness, or survive a dangerous balancing act. Joan couldn't take it seriously because she found that the movement quality it required was too focused and bound for her free, easy-going movement style. But she did acknowledge that she wouldn't push someone off a tightrope if they came near her.

Movement and imagery

It is important to realize that *not all movements contain an accompanying image.* Perhaps half or less of the movements led by the clients yield associative symbols, imagery or metaphor. However, some movements are rich in association, and take the group's imagination, and allow them to enter a shared symbolic experience (rather like children who join together to play the same imaginary scenario in their groups in the playground). Sometimes if a movement does not yield imagery, or a shared symbolic experience, but none the less seems to capture the group's nonverbal attention, it can be useful, if the group can stand the slight lifting of the turn-taking structure, to let people stay with the movement for a moment, and follow it, or indulge in it for themselves, or with others, to see where it will go. Should this become anxiety provoking, this slightly looser structure can be stopped at any moment simply by asking whose turn it was next.

Many, or even the majority of movements do not yield imagery because they are too concrete, or obvious, or are actions in themselves (like a golf swing, or a goodbye wave), or are obscure, or perhaps have a symbolic value to that person alone, of which they may or may not be conscious. At any rate, doing a movement with the group, without an image, has value in itself; the rhythmic synchrony and shared movement are of value in getting the group to cohere, and in learning to imitate, empathize and identify with others by taking on their quality of motion.

In this group, Paul's bowing gave way to Luke, who did reaching. The group reached to the side, as he did, first doing it separately, and then all together, as though grabbing. When the dance movement therapist asked what this might be, he said it was pulling a boat out of the water. The group did not connect with this symbol, so it was left as it was, as a shared movement. It was John's turn, and he did a motion of walking, accenting the vertical plane (like a soldier marching on the spot, lightly) using only the lower half of his body. The dance movement therapist asked after a moment if he could maybe use his arms in it as well, and he did, making it appear to Eileen that he was climbing up a rope. The group suggested it might be a ladder, and John added he'd been watching a video of Harrison Ford in *Indiana Jones and the Temple of Doom*. The male group members laughed at the notion of themselves as this tough, rather macho hero. This theme returned a few times over the sixteen weeks, and the dance movement therapist wondered later whether this might have been a compensatory image for their feelings of being outside the usual social order by virtue of their unemployed status (which was largely due to their mental illness) and lack of wives or girlfriends (which may also have been caused by their periodic illness, and the social isolation that can accompany it). Joan took up the image of Harrison Ford for her turn, but changed the arms, and continued walking, saying we were in a jungle. Paul mentioned the law of the jungle, and when Joan quickly said, 'Pass', Paul made a sweeping motion with his arms, which he said was like clearing the reeds in a swamp. In the experience of this dance movement therapist, imagery using animals is quite common (Bender and Boas 1941). Whether this has been introduced largely as a result of her suggestion is a possibility. However, groups do pick up on this and use it spontaneously afterwards. It may have some correlation with the primitive or primary self, the instinctual self who has basic drives including hunger, aggression, or sexuality. In some instances these 'animal instincts' were presented as healthy, and in other cases destructive or perhaps childish, but in most cases they were interesting enough to engage the group in playing alive, vital and energized characters when they used this imagery.

Movement and image dyssynchrony

Once, when the group returned to jungle imagery, Joan sat down, when it was her turn, and spun round on her bottom, in a somewhat autistic phrasing; without clear initiation or conclusion. Eileen asked (without thinking) what animal she might be doing, and she said, 'a polar bear!'. This struck most of the group as very funny, because it was so far removed from 'where they were at' symbolically. Because the group had been chatting about animal behaviour, while moving, the dance movement therapist asked what sort of things polar bears did, to which Joan coquettishly said, 'hunting', 'hunting humans, no . . . fish'. In addition to this thinly veiled annoyance with the dance movement therapist, it expressed Joan's position in the group. The dyssynchronous image of the polar animal versus the jungle ones, accompanied by a shape, rhythm, and level-change in movement, was to prefigure other times where Joan was not in synchrony or even in relation to the group. For example, if someone did a vertical scissoring movement with their arms, and the group as a whole did this simultaneously, she might suddenly use her arms in the horizontal plane, or if someone did stepping forward, she would step backwards. Perhaps, for Joan, she needed to maintain separateness from the group, and not feel engulfed by it. These image, rhythmic, shape, and other dyssynchronies did serve to put her on the edge of the group often, and now and then threatened to make her the easy target or scapegoat for criticism by a subgroup.

In the circle, it was the dance movement therapist's turn next. She got up off the floor and made a forward-reaching movement, which went from side to side and from shoulder height to knee height, using a long phrase and lightness, in the manner of a scythe cutting through grass. This seemed the best way to portray a composite picture of the movements of the three people who had come before (John's marching, Paul's clearing and Joan's spinning). It is generally a good idea for the dance movement therapist not to use his or her own improvisation style, at least not completely, but to try to make an effort–shape composite of the group's movement, or to return to a similar movement to the one that most interested the group, which in this instance might have been John's marching. This time the associations produced were to walking along, and cutting through the grass, or to clearing a path through the jungle (a theme Paul continued), to get to a clear place. The group, moving together, has a tendency to synchronize, especially in the early weeks of the group, and so this scything movement turned into pulling, and then pulling away, and then throwing something behind one's back. Sometimes, if the group seems too synchronous, or stuck together in rhythm, encouraging people to attend to the movement on their own for half a minute can help refocus them on themselves, reintegrate them back into themselves, rather than feeling swayed by the group mentality if this is not desirable. In this instance, the scything did change after a while into people throwing something behind their backs and then resting. Then the dance movement therapist said, 'Pass'.

The use of physically demanding movement

The next person in the circle was Gary, the co-worker, who sat down and did a stretch like runners do before a race, touching his toes. Some group members found this difficult, but there none the less followed another entire set of leadership turns around the circle in which nearly everyone did some athletic-type movement. It is important to realize that sometimes movement can be a defence against feeling (indeed this is what one might expect from a non-psychiatric member of a group), and that doing these concrete athletic actions, which provoked no associations and which furthermore usually concern the self rather than interactional movement, can also work as a defence against interacting. In this instance, the dance movement therapist tried to push or force an interpretation onto this movement, in which she saw the group as wanting 'to push themselves to do more', 'to get fit again', 'fighting fit perhaps'. The dance movement therapist then expressed some exasperation to give voice to feelings that Eileen was having in not being able to keep up with Gary, physically. She wondered aloud why the group were pushing themselves so much that day. Sometimes this type of movement gave one the feeling that the men, in competing in some way, were showing the women that they could be physically strong, or perhaps attractive to them. This competitiveness was mainly focused in the central weeks of the sixteen sessions.

In response to the therapist's somewhat forced associations and comments, Luke said, 'Well if you do the hard things first, the rest is much easier. Otherwise, you build up and then it's all over.' The therapist capitalized on this remark to ask how the group as a whole dealt with difficulty, whether stressing oneself and trying hard things quickly, or building oneself up slowly to a challenge. This gave rise to John saying that he wanted things to go well and be perfect immediately, and Eileen saying she liked that, but it never worked that way, really. In the end, Gary said that his life seemed like the Olympics, like a real struggle. In this instance the discussion sparked by the movements was not a symbolic interpretation of them, but rather a tangential association that had some value in allowing the group to interact, and share an ordinary, unplanned, conscious discussion, which is also important in developing confidence in social situations.

It was important here for the dance movement therapist to support the two members of the group who could not keep up with some of the exercise-type movements. Initially she requested that the leader at that time do 'something else for those of us who can't manage press-ups', to which Paul, who had been lounging on the floor observing, immediately took offence, and pushed himself into doing press-ups. It is a good idea to appreciate that if some people are not doing the movements it is not necessarily because they can't do them, but rather because they may not wish to do them, or even to try. A comment to a patient who is doing something that is physically beyond the skills of the group (or at least a sizeable subgroup) might be, 'Can you do a movement that everyone can do?' In this instance the dance movement therapist chose to keep mirroring the lower-level movements of the two members not following along in the more difficult move-ment, while the co-worker went with the high-energy movement.

If a client does a movement that is difficult, and persists in it despite requests for modification, this is sometimes worthy of comment. A patient in another group, who had once been a fashion model, persisted in doing cossack-style jumps, despite protests from the group. In the end, someone said to him, 'We know you're better than us. Does it really matter?', which prompted a discussion, and the realization for him that, because he looked as he did, many people assumed that he had an inner confidence to match his outer air of diffidence, which meant that he felt that the demands made upon him were far in excess of his capabilities. At other times, doing a movement that is very different in size, rhythm, scale, or quality from everyone else's can be a way of gaining attention, or appreciation, or being separate from everyone else, all of which tells something about that person's relations with other people.

Movement symbols

An interesting theoretical point can be made here regarding movement symbols. They can simultaneously represent an immediate interpersonal and intrapsychic statement, as well as provoke a memory, or pattern of relating to others. As an example, a patient in a community group for long-term patients, run by another dance movement therapist, decided to come off his chair to join the group on the floor, something he had not done in the four months he had attended the group. He said he wanted to 'hear people better', so he'd 'better come down on their level'. The group was pleasantly surprised by this move. Later on in the group he spoke about his being upset recently when a female friend had criticized him for looking down his nose at her. Furthermore, he mentioned, in the opening discussion phase of the group, that he had been feeling very distanced from people. Then, during someone else's movement turn, which involved pushing something down from high to low, he suddenly had the childhood memory of when he was stuck indoors, looking down from the second storey window, wishing to join his friends, but not being allowed to by the will of what he now saw as snobbish parents who deemed the street children unsuitable.

The movement symbol of changing levels was about altering his style of unsatisfying interpersonal relationships (looking down on people), and it was also saying something about his intrapsychic state, in feeling distanced from others; furthermore, it was connected to a childhood experience. Therapeutically, one can choose the dimension on which to enter the image or metaphor. In this instance, the dance movement therapist chose the interpersonal level, and she commented on how this man's coming down to other people's level meant that he could now see them more equally than he had in the past, and that this made the other group members feel more accepted by him and accepting of him (Higgens 1990).

A further occurrence in DMT groups is the extension of symbol or metaphor into an idiomatic reference to body parts. For example, being 'stiffnecked' means being inflexible, 'keeping your head together' stands for keeping mental balance, while 'keeping your head above water' signals you are coping. Furthermore, 'putting your back into it' means using a lot of energy while 'getting your back up' implies getting annoyed or upset, and 'putting your best foot forward' means making your best effort. Idiomatic references to body parts seem a natural progression in using movement symbolically.

The use of a stretch cloth

In the first weeks, the group moved along comfortably, exploring and repeating movement within the shared leadership framework. Alliances were forming between Paul and the dance movement therapist, and between Gary and Luke and

John, while Joan was out on her own, and Eileen appealed to the dance movement therapist for validation. In the fourth week, the usual room was unexpectedly unavailable due to repair work to the telephones, so the group was moved. Paul had had a lousy morning, having been refused a job, whereas John was feeling better for having increased his medication. Eileen did not want to participate, and sat down instead. The group did not seem able to come into much significant synchrony at all, did not enter into each other's imagery, and were quite ungrounded, and drifting, rather than being anchored in the circle.

At this point the therapist introduced a Lycra stretch cloth, which is useful, as is any prop if the group feels as though it is fragmenting, or losing focus. Everyone stood somewhat closer, with one or two hands holding the large table-cloth sized stretchy blue fabric. No instructions were given, initially, though it was stated that anyone who had an idea could suggest it, or it can be requested that each member in turn suggest something the group can do with the cloth. Paul started pulling the cloth, making big waves through it. For him, this became a storm, and then a hurricane, which then became calm again. This brought comment from Joan about the hurricane of 1987 and surviving storms. The dance movement therapist said, 'How *do* we survive storms; how do we cope with surprise weather like that?' There was some chat about this, and the therapist added that the change in the room that day, at last-minute notice, was a bit unsettling, and she reminded the group of Joan's comments about her recent move of house, and how it was taking time to adjust. Paul asked how to keep one part of himself still while all the rest was changing; this seemed a comment related to both the movement and his somewhat obsessional need for routine and checking, but it was left as an unsaid thought, as it would have been far too threatening for him to be confronted with it. John went next, deciding we would all hold the cloth up as high as we could, which he or someone else labelled as being like a blue sky. Luke said something about reaching for the sky, and Eileen said she wished there was a blue sky. The therapist noted that John had said he'd been trying to look on the bright side of things, in saying he was doing better than he was last year at this time when he'd become ill.

The theme of falling

Gary introduced the idea of parachuting, by bending at the knee, putting the cloth on the floor, and then moving right up to holding it as high as possible, and then letting the cloth float down, while lightly holding it with one hand. This evolved into a repeated rhythmic sequence in which the group held the cloth, and simultaneously pulled themselves away from it while they lifted, swooped, and then caught themselves, in a near crouching position, holding the cloth with one hand for balance. This was a whole-body integrated movement, involving level shifts, from tiptoe to near-kneeling on the floor. Some of the group, namely John, Luke and Joan, became disorganized a little in movement when they got near the floor, whereas Eileen, Gary and the dance movement therapist remained more stiff, or closed in, as they knelt down at the end of the phrase. The movement prompted imagery and discussion of falling, with Gary beginning to say that he was going to try parachuting in a week or two. The therapist wondered aloud how it felt to fall, or how people imagined it might feel, and Joan, who was a bit paranoid at times, said, 'Well, I suppose it would be alright as long as you're not pushed.' Luke said he hated falling, and hated the idea of anything like that; Paul said he'd hate to hit the ground, and speculated on landing on concrete, or whether anyone really ever got rescued by those firemen who offered nets to people jumping out of fires in high-rise buildings. The extended movement synchrony of the group (who were moving while talking) and the ensuing discussion alerted the dance movement therapist to the fact that this discussion might be about feelings and how to manage them. She said that maybe some feelings were like falling, where they didn't feel in one's control, whereas at other times one could jump into a feeling. John mentioned 'falling in love', and Gary said he 'fell for a girl with red hair once', and Eileen mentioned that women were said to 'fall' pregnant. As some of this was going on, the dance movement therapist noted a change in the phrasing of the movement such that people were using the cloth to support themselves, and keep more upright as they fell; she pointed this out, and the group agreed. She added that maybe, in some instances, having other people around made it seem like there was something to hold one together when falling, and that one didn't have to fall, like in falling apart, if there was something to hold on to, or some way to get support.

The stretch cloth provides an object onto which people can project feelings and imagery, and may serve the function of what Winnicott has termed the 'transitional object' (Winnicott 1953). The prop also organizes and structures movement activity, concretely connecting the members to one another, and allowing them to adopt a similar rhythm, or to carry on with their own, but feel the rhythm of others through holding on to the cloth.

This particular session ended with the dance movement therapist mentioning it was nearly time to finish, and asking the group to come up with a movement to conclude the process section. Nobody wanted to be responsible for ending the group, so the dance movement therapist, who noted that Paul was swaying slightly, began to sway herself, side to side, and pull the cloth gently in this way. Soon, the group was gently standing and rocking, using the cloth in a smooth, undulating 'oral' rhythm (Kestenberg 1975). This calmed and refocused most members of the group, perhaps allowing for the symbolic gratification of infantile needs or, at least in this case, a somewhat more adult way to be rocked, calmed and gently held. Here, the use of the prop (the stretch cloth) and the falling image served to unite and contain the group, whose capacity to manage change had been pushed to the limit by the change of room, and by the events emerging in their lives, as well as by the unconscious emotional processes that were present in the group as a whole.

At the end of the session that day, in the closure discussion, the group decided that the falling image and the work with the cloth was the most rewarding part of the movement because it was fun, a bit scary, and allowed for a big whole-body stretch, as one went from ceiling to floor level. John was able to articulate his fears about falling to pieces a year ago, and how he felt that the 'slippy slope' of becoming ill was a lot like sliding and falling. The closing discussion that day was subdued, with Paul reporting he had felt anxious about the falling, but better at the end during the side-to-side swaying.

Joan told Gary that she didn't really try to fall in the movement because, since he had been across from her, she couldn't be sure that he would hold on to his side of the cloth to balance her weight. We did not push this issue specifically with Joan, and instead spoke generally about 'people needing trust and support from others'.

Whole-group interpretation

Direct interpretations of people's statements should be avoided, as should direct comments about a single person's movement: leaving comments at the level of *the group as a whole*, especially if there are psychotic members, is generally safer (Horowitz and Weisberg 1966). In the view of this author, almost all statements to the group about its behaviour, even when one wants to address a particular person, are best left at a general level, and should always be open-ended in nature. Prefaced with 'maybe' or 'perhaps' or 'possibly', the dance movement therapist's comments on the group become suggestions about how to think about their experience, rather than definitive statements about the group's underlying unconscious process. Instead of saying, 'Are *you* afraid of falling?', it is better to say, 'What is it that *people* find is scary about falling, do you reckon?', or even 'I wonder why we find falling a frightening idea?' This whole-group perspective also has an important parallel in movement terms:

> the anxiety level experienced by virtue of confronting a new group situation is substantially reduced because individuals don't present themselves singly; they move together. Moreover, movement itself discharges tension, further reducing anxiety.

> (Schmais 1981: 104)

Here, the use of the prop (the stretch cloth) and the falling image served to unite and contain the group, whose capacity to manage change had been pushed to the limit by the change of room, and by the events emerging in their lives, as well as by the unconscious emotional processes which were present in the group as a whole.

The theme of the journey

In the eighth session, a theme was introduced which was important for this group, and is a quite common one; the group, while doing a walking movement, decided they were going on an adventure, a journey or a voyage, or a holiday. This may represent a desire to change, or change one's surroundings at any rate. In this instance, the specific example was that of a mountain-climbing adventure. The group, while moving, assigned roles to different members of the expedition. This role assignment may bear resemblance to Yalom's view that groups offer a chance at a recapitulation of roles from family dynamics. In this case, Joan was assigned to be the brave person who would go ahead and check out what the terrain looked like, Gary would protect us against intruders or aggressors, John would try to navigate or orientate us, and the dance movement therapist was requested to bring along the lunch, a sort of concrete expression of the group's hope that she might feed them or psychologically nurture them, while Gary would take on the role of father/protector. Marching and miming climbing movements and making the circle larger and forming subgroups, making it an irregular shape, changed the feeling of the session from one of leaders alternating turns in a circle to one that was more loose, and free. If the group initiates a change in the structure in this way, it is safe to follow, but it would not be possible to force a very new group to try to adopt this looser spatial and role structure. This is in keeping with the differentiation and competition themes that are appropriate to the middle phase of a group.

The band-of-travellers image offers a sense of group cohesion, of being a selected person taking part in a special event, doing something together, and being valued for oneself and one's skills. In this instance, John said he didn't feel that he was anybody worth following, and Eileen protested that he seemed always to know where he was going, or he looked much more confident than she did, at any rate. Eileen said she wouldn't be able to come on any mountain climbing expeditions due to her fear of heights, and her preference for holidays close to home. This encapsulated her fear of the unknown, and her fear of changes. The closure discussion at the end of this session allowed a lot of open exchange about the group members' desires to change, to explore new things, and to work together to 'get somewhere'. Eileen was quite quiet during this discussion. The therapist pointed out how doing stuff together made them a working unit, rather than a bunch of isolated strangers. At the end of the sixteen weeks, groups are often amazed at how much they have become part of a project, or adventure, and the dance movement therapist can usefully point out that the ability to start off not knowing anyone, and come out appreciating each person and belonging to the group, is a skill that can be generalized to other, new situations, and meeting new people and new challenges.

Repressed anger and frustration

In the ninth session, a crucial theme emerged: that of repressed anger, or frustration. It began when Luke did a digging movement, and Joan said it might uncover worms or something awful. John said it might be a mine, like one he read about in the papers, which had been left over from World War II, but had been buried for many years in a farmer's field near the London Orbital motorway. The therapist gave a playful expression of surprise, and asked, 'What would we do with a mine, or a bomb in here?' The group's movement changed and became more tentative, and they circled the bomb. The buried explosive seemed an obvious metaphor for buried or underground feelings of anger, aggression, or frustration.

While the shape of each person's individual movement was somewhat different, the overall pattern of circling, and the light indirect sustained quality suggestive of suspicion, were common to all. Claire Schmais comments that 'whereas the moment to moment content of the dance reflects individual expressions, the sequencing of themes is determined by the group's needs, moods and fantasies' (Schmais 1981: 104). Initially Luke said that it was Gary's responsibility to be the bomb disposal expert, and deal with it. John later said he wondered if the dance movement therapist would get blown up by it if she touched it, or if she could handle it gently enough. This paralleled his general fears about getting out of control at times when upset, and throwing things around in his room at the hostel, and also was expressed by his worries about hurting the therapist if he threw a ball too hard, or pulled too much in a tug-of-war with the stretch cloth. While there was some genuine concern because he was physically stronger, the repeated mention of the issue suggested an emotional component. In subsequent groups his ability (along with those of other members) to use very strong and aggressive stamping movements, and to have these accepted and acknowledged and shared in the rhythmic synchrony of the group, allowed him to feel that his angry periods might be survived by other people, rather than be overwhelming of them.

The process continued, and the therapist asked whether she and Gary would be expected to deal with the bomb, or whether they might get some help. Joan clapped her hands, and was told off by Paul, who didn't want her to provoke any damage if it did go off. In the end, the group used a stretch cloth, and put the imaginary bomb into the corner of the room, using a great deal of care and cooperation to move across the space. Despite Gary's suggestion about defusing it, the group decided that his efforts were in vain; he thought he could make it inactive using imaginary foam, but the group brought it to life again, refusing to bury the issue, or the imaginary bomb. There was audible and visible relief once the task of leaving the bomb fairly contained in the corner was accomplished. Eileen said that if this had been a few months ago she guessed that she wouldn't have minded taking it, since it didn't matter to her at the time if she'd died. She said she wasn't so sure now. The therapist commented on Eileen's being willing to sacrifice herself for the group, and added that even if she felt bad, there was no way she should put her life at risk. She added that Eileen was a useful group member, and was necessary for their adventures. Paul suggested leaving a flag near the bomb, so we would remember where it was buried, so we didn't step on it the next week. We did this, but Luke said we should all jump and yell and pretend it exploded, and then put it away. After obtaining most people's agreement, we all took a massive leap backwards from the circle, opening our arms and trying to make a big thud. This degenerated into seeing whose shoes could make the loudest 'thwack!' on the floor, which seemed purely unsymbolic catharsis, but was perhaps necessary to release the anger and built-up tension for the group.

Containing anger in the closing discussion

In the closure section, the dance movement therapist asked what people thought the image of the bomb might mean, if anything, and all agreed it was about explosive feelings, or tension. The therapist commented on how dealing with the bomb might be like dealing with feelings; one could hope that other people on whom one could lean (the leaders) could take them away. The therapist also suggested that the group had acknowledged that everyone had some similar feelings, and that in setting about putting the bomb somewhere safe, they could cooperate in understanding and defusing the feelings lying underneath. This idea of the leaders managing and taking care of the group's emotion is consistent with Bion's concept of the dependency group.

The group was then able to have a discussion about ways of getting anger out without hurting people – specifically by being aware when it started, getting complaints off one's chest and not storing them up, and also realizing that anger didn't always have to be terrible when it did explode. John gained a lot from the discussion. He said he wondered if his angry spells drove people away from him, or if his moods pushed them away. He seemed to be asking if a show of the full extent of his feelings would overwhelm people, particularly when he was in an acute phase and, generally, even when he was quite stable. When in hospital the year before he had in fact hit out at a member of the nursing staff, and had suffered enormous guilt over the incident. Eileen said she had buried her anger towards her husband who had left her, and that it came back with a vengeance a few months later when she saw him in the town.

That angry feelings are a feature of many outpatient groups is supported by Harry Stack Sullivan's observation that anger as well as loneliness are important issues for psychiatric clients (Sullivan 1932, 1940, 1956). The feelings may take many forms, either in pure movement expression or in images and symbols. On a movement level, angry feelings may be expressed by or may emerge during jumping, pulling, stamping, punching in the air, karate chopping, mock jump-kicking, leaping, heaving imaginary heavy objects, flailing arms in a helicopter-motion, etc. Imagery for such feelings is endless and in the experience of this author includes things like explosives, ferocious animals, tribal stamping rituals or rain dances, hunting down terrorists, monsters, bubbling acid, hurricanes, etc. Characters from films and videos are also invoked, in particular, horrific half-humans like those featured in the film *Nightmare on Elm Street*, and absolute non-humans such as *Aliens*, who attack unsuspecting people at random, as well as *Robocop*, the robot-policeman full of unrelenting violence. While the imagery does not take away the anger, or provide an answer about how to manage it, the symbolic movement and the images provide a way of externalizing and manipulating amorphous feelings and open up discussion in which the issues can be addressed and shared. In this way the patient's concerns about unmanageable emotions can be dissipated somewhat. The safe use of such movements allows the group to work with anger in a cathartic, constructive and active way, and not merely to embark on a general abstract or theoretical discussion of difficult emotions.

Movement as a defence

It is important not to allow the group to get into a mindless or unthinking physical catharsis of angry feelings without connecting them to the present tense, or to real life, in general terms at least, during the process section and in the discussion afterwards. As work of Claire Schmais suggests, and the psychodynamic work of Diane Fletcher illustrated in Chapter 3, 'movement alone is not enough, insight requires a cognitive component' (Schmais 1981: 106). Movement release of strong feelings needs to be connected to how the patient is actually dealing with these themes and issues, or managing these emotions. It is essential to keep the group as safe and relaxed as possible when exploring or discussing such emotions, and discussing the conduct of individual members is not a good idea; instead, one must make very general statements, preferably while still in the image or metaphor or movement, and make only general connections to everyday life or events. For example, it was important not to address John directly in the group, but to say things like, 'What makes *people* afraid of buried things?' as opposed to 'What makes *you* afraid of what might be under the ground?' The removal from the individual of responsibility for the creation or ownership of direct feelings related to the image allows for less threatening exploration of the imagery and the emotional issues underlying them.

That the theme of anger emerged at this point in the group is also consistent with Schmais's view that depression or dependency can give way to anger. This session was a turning point for the group, one where they felt progress had been made, and which they recalled animatedly in our 'memory lane' of the life of the group in the very last session. Most remembered the release of energy, and all remembered feeling good about managing a dangerous situation, even if it was an imaginary one.

Props as projective tools

It is important to recognize that a group's movement can progress without much symbolic elaboration. Sometimes only a few people can use the free-associative, or movement-to-image process; or maybe some subgroups will, while for other patients even the most expressive movement can only ever be 'waggling and waving your arms about'. In other groups there are symbols, but they are not shared, or are only relevant to one or two people. If feelings cannot be externalized into expressive movement or into an image, they can at least be projected onto props. On one particularly low day in February, the group was sullen, silent and unable to speak very much. A large hollow plastic physiotherapy ball about 60 centimetres in diameter was taken from its box, along with a very long stretch cloth about 5 metres long and 1 metre wide. The group laughed when the ball kept rolling around on the uneven floor. Luke said it had a mind of its own, and Paul said it wanted to play. For a while it was the naughty child, the 'id' aspect of the group; it became Gary's bank manager and was bashed around the room, it was rolled about, and then 'became seasick' when lolled about in the stretch cloth, hammock-style. Objects become symbols for the group, and as such must not be used outside the group room, or be damaged or disparaged too much: one person's 'old rubbish' or old rag may be another person's 'favourite blanket'. One day, when the group was particulary distant and apathetic, the dance movement therapist found herself cradling one of the stretch cloths in her lap!

In one session the group was like an orchestra, as Joan said, having conducted a sort of obstacle course for the ball, in which it was bounced and caught by them in a big cloth, then deposited or bounced over for someone else to catch. This was directed initially at Luke and the dance movement therapist, but then shifted around to different members. Sounds accompanied the rise and fall in tension as the ball perilously balanced at the edge of the cloth; people were applauded if they managed to get the ball back on track; the group made annoyed or sad noises if the ball fell off too quickly. This was linked by the dance movement therapist to the difficulty of 'staying on the straight and narrow', and was picked up as a theme during the closure discussion, about how the group could help one another and be supportive in the difficult tasks that faced them, practically and psychologically. The dance movement therapist suggested the group try to switch roles, which they did.

When the ball threatened to become used unimaginatively, as a football (which was boring for Eileen who couldn't keep up, and a bit anxiety provoking for the dance movement therapist who was worried about it knocking over the potted plants or hitting the windows), some restrictions were suggested to elaborate the movements being used: 'Okay, so could you play football on a video in slow motion, or in fast forward?', 'Could you only use your left foot or one hand/elbow to move the ball?' etc. We experimented with the group, adding suggestions about how to pass the ball to each other – for example, by rolling, slamming, pressing, whispering, shuffling, shovelling, or passing it 'like a wimp, or a wally, or like Gazza', the English football player. Softer qualities made the ball 'like a baby' and prompted Luke to say 'Shhhhh', changing the mood of the group, and Paul to say it was like a little dog who needed a rest, which said something about the group's infantile dependency needs for safety and a containing space in which to rest.

At this point, Gary, somewhat unthinkingly, put the ball up to his chest, and leaned towards Paul, so that the two could walk with it together. This appeared to provoke anxiety in the female members of the group and in poor Paul, who blushed. The dance movement therapist said that permission ought to be asked if one was going to lean against someone, even with the big ball in between. Joan said she didn't want to get dusty, and the game was dropped. Even this remote touch was not easy for the group to manage: on the whole, as discussed in Chapter 3, touch ought to be avoided or quietly discouraged: it is too powerful (positively or negatively) and does not generally constitute ordinary adult social behaviour. At the end of this session, the ball was wrapped up in a stretch cloth and 'put to bed'. This might be read as a veiled sexual wish, or an expression of the group's infantile needs, not necessarily through a verbal symbol, but through the mediating projective screen of the props or objects. Paul added that the ball 'was like the feelings and junk that we bring to the group and only bring out here, and sort of leave here as well'. John said it was probably 'sea sick and worn out' after its adventures.

Props promote good whole-body integrative movements, and flexibility in response (the effort of quickness in time can be induced in even the most psycho-motorically slowed or slurred client when a flying physiotherapy ball comes near them!), and offer a concrete way to use movement interaction to promote shared-focus, team-work, cooperation, creativity and cohesiveness in a group. Props can, by their unpredictable nature, energize the group and get people out of ritualized or familiar patterns of interacting among a subgroup. A tug of war with a stretch cloth can provide a release of energy, and it can then be used to make a peaceful breeze, so that the group can share both the building up of tension and the calm cooling down after the exertion of physical and emotional energy.

It is important to use the closure discussion at the end to look over the experiences of the group, as a simple recall exercise if not as an exploration of what the movements or images might say about the life of the group. Remembering what x felt when y did something, or laughing about funny moments, or commenting about the ebb and flow of energy and ideas in the session are all valuable ways to assist in getting clients to monitor their interactive behaviour, learn about other people's responses to their spontaneous (nonverbal) behaviour, gain confidence in unplanned actions and acts, and feel valued as part of the group. As long as interaction rather than skill are the focus, props are a good way to initiate interaction and to reclaim the more playful and creative parts of the personalities of the group: as Winnicott wrote:

> playing facilitates growth and therefore health; playing leads into group rela-tionships; playing can be a form of communication in psychotherapy; and lastly, psychoanalysis has been developed as a highly specialized form of playing in the service of communication with oneself and others.
>
> (Winnicott 1971b: 48)

Perhaps this middle section of the overall life of the group – around sessions nine to thirteen – which was more concrete and used more props, was more about competition and individuating, or cohering as a group. Instead of 'oral' rocking rhythms, there were more 'phallic' jumping rhythms; which developmentally are associated with autonomy and separation (Kestenberg 1975). This developmental shift might also correlate with a slow edging out of the dependency mode and into counterdependency (Bion 1961). In later sessions, when themes of anger re-emerged, members felt more desire to work out their own strategies to tame the ravenous monsters, rather than expect to be rescued from these personifications by the leaders. There was also less rhythmic synchrony, and more attention to spatial configurations which were complex, and went outside the circle.

Loosening the leadership and role structures

In the latter sessions, sometimes the co-worker and the dance movement therapist lost track of whose turn it was in the circle because they became disorganized or were tired. Other times they lost track because the movement sequences of: initiated movement, followed by an association, followed by altered movement, and affected by an interpretation to give yet more movement, and new associations got very long (lasting 10 minutes or more) and complex. Certainly 'as people move together, the energy level rises, movement phrases become longer and more complex. They take more space, use more of themselves, and reach out to others' (Schmais 1981: 194).

Only a professional training in DMT can enable the dance movement therapist to judge when to facilitate a change in the structure of the DMT session. As Carol Bruno's research into DMT session structure suggested, the ability to continuously create, alter and monitor group structures which best allow process material to emerge is a unique feature of the arts therapies (Bruno 1981). The crucial factor in deciding whether to shape a change in the structure (via a verbal or nonverbal intervention) is the ability of the patients to manage the anxiety that the shift to a more free structure will provoke, and whether they can make use of the self-directed and interactive therapeutic opportunities that the new structure will provide.

For example, once a shared leadership format in a high-functioning group has been extended to the point where each person's turn lasts several minutes and members may only get one turn at shared leadership per group – and the spatial shapes made by the group within those turns means that they often end up back in a circle in a different order such that it is often hard to remember who comes next – then the group is probably ready for a new structure. One such structure involves the dance movement therapist or another person initiating a movement which others agree to mirror. There may be no words for several minutes, and the therapist does not elicit associations. There is a pressure on the group to synchronize in some dimensions – which in the experience of the present author is usually the rhythm or effort (movement quality) dimensions of the movement rather than the shape.

Once this synchrony has been achieved, a subtle interaction of the qualities of each movement takes hold, and the group creates a shared movement interaction in which they can keep their own qualities and enter those of the group at the same time. Movements overlap, interact, conflict, and are reshaped in this extended nonverbal interaction. Often the movement will come to a crescendo, and subside. There is often a sense of satisfaction after such a sequence, of something well expressed. In this, the role of the dance movement therapist is crucial. He or she is trained to pull out the choreographic and symbolic or expressive elements of the theme and to contain these within his or her own movement, embodying and signifying rather than simply mirroring the qualities of the group. The group, who are probably under some social influence to conform, may follow the dance movement therapist's lead, but the dance movement therapist is in fact reflecting a composite of the group's movement! In the end, a strong rhythm, or sound, or even image could emerge from this process. While the process does not probably owe as much to any sort of 'mysticism' as to unconscious group pressure, it does resemble speaking without words, and as such often does not require words for its completion. The group may discuss the process and how they felt at certain times, being in or away from the group, synchronizing and withdrawing. Perhaps it can be considered a totally unverbal version of DMT, to which verbal content is added later. It resembles the mover/witness model of the Jungian individual approach, which stresses listening to inner impulses to move, but it is interactional in content. Of the utmost importance is the dance movement therapist's ability to judge whether the group will be able to manage the anxiety involved in taking responsibility for themselves in what appears to be leaderless movement, and whether their own mental processes are coherent enough so that moving, or 'dancing' silently with others, does not unnerve them.

On the whole, this shared movement (without a 'leader') is only possible in the later stages of a high-functioning group. For the most part, the shared leadership structure is easier to maintain, and, once the group masters it, it can be used at a high level by having each member's movement turn last as long as 10 minutes, so that each person only gets one turn per group, but the safety of the role structure of the shared leadership is preserved. Some movements will yield longer interactions and others will not. In this instance, the group speaks while moving and 'the synergistic effect generated by group membership and physical activity creates the emotional intensity which can cut through defenses and promote new behaviours. The energy created is transformed into symbolic dance gestures' (Schmais 1981: 105).

This particular group entered into just such an extended sequence about two thirds of the way through the sixteen sessions in which everyone took on the manner of a robot, and passed a ball around using this style. This prompted discussion of being 'on automatic pilot' and having 'metal around yourself' and was an interesting insight into the members' perceptions of the way they held themselves together emotionally. Some members shuffled and dropped the ball or walked past each other, which was quite humorous for everyone. Further discussions included how people can get into a rut, and remain rigid about things, until they feel safe to loosen up (in movement and feelings) and ready to try new things.

Separation

If this sort of extended shared leadership format is in operation, the group is working well, and can then go on in the last four sessions to address a final issue: separation. The group is reminded of the end of its meetings at each session. Sometimes a symbolic 'death' or mourning is enacted, possibly involving a prop. One needs to take this seriously and ask what it can represent, and point towards issues of loss, as appropriate. In groups where a dead body may be represented, or where some old thing is dug up out of the ground, like an archaeological discovery, or something from TV or films is introduced (like the bog monster, or the spirit of a long-dead relative or figure from the past), this image may be an important communication about the ending of the group, which is something of a death, or perhaps the feared death of relatedness. It is important to stay with the discomfort this provokes, and simply say something like, 'some people look a bit sad, or shocked'. Not everyone will enter the image in the same way, and this needs to be respected and articulated by the dance movement therapist. One can say, for example, about a blob on the floor, made of a ball and stretch cloths, over which people are standing, quietly mourning: 'for Luke it's like a body, but for Eileen it's not' – or mention other people's ideas also, while keeping with the sober or sombre mood that usually befits an ending or a departure, or even a sort of death. This group created a sand castle image, and invoked the story of the man who told the sea to turn back, which seemed a way of trying to keep back the inevitable time of separation, and expressed the end or dissolution of the house or 'mansion in the mind' in which the group had lived in our minds for four months (Williams and Waddell 1991).

Often at this stage issues of need or dependency do arise. This can be expressed in symbols around food. The creation of an enormous imaginary picnic gripped this group. It began with Eileen making a smoothing gesture, which Paul said was like laying out a table cloth. Luke said he fancied lunch, and said a picnic would be nice. Gary initiated a stirring type movement, and John decided he could be stirring cream for a strawberries and cream tea. Movements became larger and more grandiose, and soon there was an imaginary cake that filled the room. Joan said that there might be poison in it, or at least too much salt, one didn't know, comments were made about 'too many cooks spoiling the broth' and the questions were raised about the therapist's culinary abilities, or ability to provide for the group. Paul mentioned that eating too much could make you sick, and Eileen said one could store things up for later, by taking stuff into our pockets, which we pretended to do. Gary said we could hoard food like animals in winter. In the closure discussion, we discussed this image, and the sort of hunger it represented. The dance movement therapist suggested that food expressed other emotional needs. John said he'd feel a bit empty of things to do on the morning that the group ran once it had ended. Joan agreed that even she needed food and shelter. Paul said he'd got a lot from the group and that he would miss it. We spoke about food in general, and how people and ideas could also be nourishing or even 'food for thought'. The loss of the fantasy of the therapist providing for all of the group members' needs is one that sometimes affects the mood of final sessions (Wolff 1977).

Closure discussion

The issue of food led into a discussion about the end of the group itself, and how it was important to say good-bye properly, though this was sad, because the group had been valuable and people had been 'fed' by it. They had gained an ability to express themselves, and had come to know each other. The dance movement therapist hoped that the group members would be able to take away some of the gains they had made, in being able to approach others with slightly less trepidation, and in seeing the value of expressing feelings.

Schmais writes that

the final task of every session [or group] is to deal in some measure with the issue of separation and the feeling of loss. People often regress, becoming listless, bored, inactive. Some cling while others withdraw prematurely. A closing ritual prepares the group for separation and at the same time symbolizes the continuity of the event, reminding people of the session before and the sessions to come.

(Schmais 1981: 105)

Each weekly group session may also have a group movement ending, which takes place before going back to being seated and having a discussion about the day's events. This is achieved either by the group creating a shared movement for closure, or with the therapist leading a 'warm down' exercise involving centring or breathing and perhaps slow synchronous movement designed to bring members back to themselves, and into a reflective mood to do the closing discussion.

In the closing discussion each week it is best to describe the images and movements that emerged, rather than to engage in a lot of interpretation or speculation about them; it is important to try to make sense of what the group has done, but this is always most effective if the members can endeavour, with assistance, to do this for themselves. The dance movement therapist might start by asking, 'Why do people think we got into that type of movement, and does it say anything about how the group is feeling today?' 'What might all that stamping have been about?' 'It was interesting that nearly everyone really got "into" the thing about falling which someone just mentioned, does that say anything about what's on our minds?' This leaves the group open to choose to discuss issues or not, and leaves it open for the dance movement therapist to leave things at the level of symbol, or to try to connect it to some general statement about emotional functioning. It is not a good idea to get into making connections to specific people's life events, unless they do so themselves; they may be making connections between imagery of falling and feeling 'let down' but may not be comfortable sharing those connections with the group; they may wish to take this to their key-worker, or to a friend or family member.

Endings

Often people don't come for the last sessions, or come late, or come but repeat or regress to what they did near the beginning of the group, in response to some of the stress of losing a useful point of contact with other people who are generally positive in their regard for the person.

At the last few meetings, it is useful to stress the generally ambivalent feelings the group may have about leaving; perhaps they are glad to finish part of their treatment, or to leave the day unit, but are afraid of the stress of coping on their own. It is important to say that though people may see each other in passing, a proper good-bye must be said, because though members may see each other, the intimacy and regularity of the group will be lost, and it will be different. Sometimes groups that have been functioning intensively do go through endings in a way that, it is said, mourning occurs: there are stages of denial, grief, anger, sadness, and then sometimes a coming to terms with the fact that the experience was both negative and positive, both bad and good.

Last movement sessions may recapitulate some of the typical movements and imagery, and the therapist may give a few highlights to the group members about what they have done, and how things have progressed. It is hoped that members will have gained some strengths in relating to others, and have felt supported, and possibly gained a renewed sense of themselves, particularly in connecting physical sensation and mental activity, and hopefully even a glimmer of hope or a belief in their potential for change.

Feedback and notemaking

After the patients have left the session, the co-worker and the dance movement therapist should take about half an hour to discuss and recall the events of the group. Examples of things that can be addressed are making notes about changes in people's behaviour, and comparing their state to the previous weeks. Sometimes the two can puzzle over symbols or behaviour in such a way as to be prepared for what might come next, or entertain hypotheses about what behaviour might have meant in the group that day. They might agree to mirror a member more actively if he or she is out of touch with the group. In this group, the dance movement therapist tried to empathize more with Joan, in movement and action, though this was difficult and often simply meant staying seated or kneeling if Joan was sitting on the floor, rather than standing with other group members. This was an attempt to keep her in the perimeters of the group, rather than lose her altogether. Gary noted that John had been making odd pushing movements with his tongue, and he wondered if John might have been trying to reduce his own anticholinergic medication, without supervision from the psychiatrist. Gary felt nervous about the verbal anger that came to him from Joan. The dance movement therapist shared Joan's concerns that John was physically much stronger, and wondering how to allow for a release of aggression towards a more general target, rather than engaging in tug-of-war.

Gary agreed to feed back some of the information to the daily staff meeting – notably Joan's being a bit out of sorts, and John's tongue pushing – and to give some positive feedback about Paul's contribution, and his being less shy and awkward than in previous weeks.

CONCLUSION

The members of the group described above took a lot of energy to manage, but progressed well in using the movement and props to try new ways of relating to each other, and were very successful at using imagery to express and explore a few of the many emotional issues that were problematic for them. The level of verbal disclosure about details of their lives was not very high, but the level of nonverbal participation and interaction, initiated in increasing degrees of spontaneity between members, was enormous progress for all of them. It is hoped that this interpersonal learning generalized itself to the clients' everyday living situations.

The simple expression of anger, physically, through the use of stamping or imagery was something that was positive for all the members, and one that took some courage and mastering of anxiety on all their parts. The fact of expressing strong feelings and still having good relations with people was probably a novelty for some, and allowed them to question whether their own emotions were so powerful or distorted that they could not be shared, and instead ought to be locked away or denied. The occupational therapist working with Paul reported that he valued the group since he found physical expression and activity quite problematic. John and his key-worker both said independently that John seemed more relaxed than he had been at other low periods, and they each said this could have something to do with having a place to 'let off steam' each week.

Students should not be disappointed if their groups do not appear as highly tuned as this one: the moments described here were few among sixteen hours of sometimes quite random or concrete movement and interaction, and so they represent highlights rather than the continual mode of ordinary functioning. The energy and creative spark among several of the members made this group challenging and interesting; not all patients come to work in DMT groups with the same level of interest or commitment. The policy of allowing members to choose whether they want to continue a group after a few trial sessions probably contributed to this sense of high motivation.

Despite the large amount of physical and emotional energy needed to sustain a group like this through its low and dull times, this does pay off when the group surprises itself and invents ideas and stories (like the orchestra with the stretch cloth, or the journey, or the unexploded bomb scenario), which tell something about their emotional lives. While not reaching the deeper levels of insight or disclosure possible with higher-functioning outpatients, or in DMT with non-psychiatric clients, the group does provide a useful creative forum for group members which they and other staff felt provided something unique and creative, and which balanced the primarily verbal groups in the overall treatment programmes offered by the mental health day centre.

Chapter 7

DMT with long-term patients

INTRODUCTION

One of the most exciting contributions DMT can make in the psychiatric setting is in addressing the needs of long-term or chronic patients. This is becoming increasingly important as mental health professionals struggle to cope with the rehabilitation of long-term patients, and encourage many to return to community life in programmes of deinstitutionalization. Although DMT groups with long-term patients may appear very similar to those with adult outpatients in both form and structure, there are important differences in goals, in the therapist's role, and in the common issues which emerge in DMT groups of this type. This chapter gives an example of a DMT group with patients in hospital who were being prepared to move into the community, and makes reference to some existing literature in this area.

The role of DMT in psychiatric services for long-term patients

Long-term patients are those whose conditions are generally expected to be chronic, with periods of remission and exacerbation, and who can attain variable degrees of functioning, from near self-sufficiency to almost complete dependence upon psychiatric, social work, nursing and other support services. The majority of such patients are schizophrenic, or have personality disorders, or some other long-term neurotic or reactive illness which prevents their recovery or a return to the standard of everyday living and functioning they attained before becoming ill (Higgens and McLean 1990).

DMT groups for long-term patients may take place as part of rehabilitation and resettlement into the community, or as part of hospital-based occupational therapy or psychiatric assessment and preparation of the patient's readiness to enter community life (Liebowitz *et al.* 1989, Payne 1992). The DMT group for long-term patients, which usually runs for at least a year, may also be a very useful part of their support programme once patients have left hospital and are living in the community (Higgens and McLean 1990). Although there is not very much literature describing or evaluating group approaches for long-term patients relative to the amount concerning higher functioning outpatient groups, the research suggests that supportive verbal group psychotherapy for schizophrenic patients 'improves medication compliance, reduces rehospitalization rate, and may improve social and occupational function' (Kahn 1984: 150). DMT may also offer a few similar benefits to those offered by verbal psychotherapy, given that such patients 'require long-term psychotherapeutic support to enable them to function to the limit of their capacities' (Kahn 1984: 149).

Dance movement therapists who have worked in this area believe that there are a number of benefits to patients, including, 'improved sense of self and self esteem, improvements in independence and initiative, a feeling of being accepted and valued by others, a growing ability to "play" and engage in spontaneous enjoyable interaction with peers, and a facility in self expression through movement' (Higgens and McLean 1990: 11). A recent survey concluded that, relative to the whole spectrum of treatment which long-term patients received, 'dance movement therapy stands out as being a particularly positive experience for the patients' (MacDonald and Ochera 1990).

It is important to recognize that long-term patients in hospital, or those in the community, may be receiving varying amounts of contact with different types of mental health professionals. For example, a long-term patient may be seen monthly by a psychiatrist to review medication and to discuss the patient's general state of mental health. He or she may have a psychiatric nurse key-worker who lives in the ward, or a community psychiatric nurse who may live in the hostel or community home, or who may visit the patient at agreed periods of anything from bi-weekly, weekly, monthly, as the patient's condition and the community psychiatric nurse's schedule dictate. Patients in hospital may attend hospital-based occupational therapy sessions, or may participate in ward-based activities. Long-term patients in the community may attend psychiatric day centres, or drop-in centres run by social services or community organizations, or facilities run by voluntary organizations, all of which offer varying levels of input to help the patients to live in the community. The patients who come to DMT may have been referred by a community psychiatric nurse, psychiatrist, or occupational therapist who is aware that DMT is available in the hospital or in the community.

Appropriate therapeutic goals

It is important to set realistic goals for work with long-term patients, and to note that these goals may be quite different to those with higher functioning psychiatric client groups. Initial movement-level goals include activating and motivating the patient, not in an intrusive or cajoling or directive way but through the use of movement warmup and the Chaceian shared leadership format. The patient-led movement encourages autonomy and allows a small forum for the patient to explore ways of breaking out of passive institutionalized behaviour, or what may be a dependent mode of functioning.

In the middle phase of the life of a long-term group, the highly structured sessions – which include the initial discussion, warmup, shared leadership and closing discussion – perform the function of giving the group a reliable space in which they can learn how to interact, and a stable and reliable framework in which to form or consolidate their inner, mental representation of the group and their role within it. In the final stages of the group, the members may be able to go beyond their own ritualized or repetitive modes of interacting, and make a small step towards spontaneous, self-directed interaction with other group members. Over the long term, each member gains something, existentially, by being connected to other people and by participating in a creative shared experience.

The DMT literature on long-term groups, specifically Johnson and Sandel's concept of the 'nascent group', was described in detail in the latter half of Chapter 3. Essentially, they understand the goals of work with very long-term patients as more of a life-support system than a therapeutic intervention, and one that seeks to make contact with socially isolated patients, and to ameliorate the further deterioration in their interpersonal functioning which is a key feature of long-term mental illness (Sandel and Johnson 1983). In their view, realistic goals are necessary for such work in order to diminish the frequently encountered negative attitude towards group work with this client population. Many people take the attitude that there is 'nothing that can be done for them', and use this as a rationale for a policy of non-intervention or even neglect of the therapeutic needs of this hard-to-reach spectrum of psychiatric patients.

In a fundamental sense, the end-point or goal of therapeutic group work with long-term patients is to get the group to *feel like a group*. In work of this kind, 'the group therapist is often faced with the challenge of making contact with isolated individuals for whom the notion of a group does not even exist' (Sandel and Johnson 1983: 131). In this instance, it is the therapist who must work very hard to establish the group's identity in the initial stages, such that the patients eventually internalize this idea themselves, and can later come to regard themselves as belonging to the group, as opposed to being in a world of their own, cut off from the others around them. Sandel and Johnson note that

> to be a 'member' psychologically is to establish an internal representation of the group. The convergent and mutually reinforcing behaviours of group members lead to the establishment of a shared representation of the group, i.e., the group identity.

> (Sandel and Johnson 1983: 131)

While this may sound like an almost too-obvious or too-easy goal with which to begin, the level of disorganization, isolation, fragmentation and distortion in some long-term patients' relationships with the people around them is quite a formidable reality that must be challenged; furthermore, if the patients can come to feel like part of their group, and can internalize the group's identity, this shift into relatedness can be of enormous therapeutic benefit to both themselves and to the other group members (Sandel and Johnson 1983: 133).

Further goals for DMT groups with long-term patients resemble those general goals for outpatients: improvement in interaction and the carefully managed externalization of feelings through movement, followed by their examination and containment by the group. While it is true that 'unconscious fears and fantasies can find expression in the symbolic images created to accompany the movement' (Sandel and Johnson 1983: 134), the use and interpretation of symbolism with long-term patients is less of a focus than is the case in higher functioning outpatient work. Instead, participation in the group process and engagement on a movement level are more immediately of benefit to the patients. Additionally, interpreting or processing the symbolic material that emerges in such groups must be done with extreme caution, and must be done clearly, immediately and simply, very soon after the movement behaviour has occurred; long-term patients are less able to recall the movement section of the group 20 minutes after it has happened, and so discussion of behaviour often cannot be left for the closure discussion (Liebowitz et al. 1989: 5). This does not mean that long-term clients are unable to use movement symbolically, but only that when it does occur it must be processed more rapidly. A recent article noted that as clients 'learn the language of movement, they become increasingly able to articulate feelings and explore interactions in a way that they may never be able to conceptualize and talk about' (Higgens and McLean 1990: 11). This comment describes well the manner in which it is the movement process itself that generates the most powerful therapeutic process for this patient population; later on the words can follow movement experiences, and lead to further understanding once the essential initial interpersonal learning and expression of emotion have taken place on the nonverbal level. It is useful to recall that not all experiences from the DMT group need to be verbally processed; sometimes, for long-term patients, the movement experience alone is enough. Ideally, the therapist can articulate for the group what they see happening on a movement level, such that the patients can begin to be aware of their behaviour, and come to be able to interact with others more verbally and to reflect on their feelings using words.

Practical considerations

The considerations for setting up a group with long-term patients are very similar to those described in Chapter 6 for outpatients, so they will not be repeated here. It is useful to have a co-worker, preferably one who will be available for quite a long time; long-term groups function best if they continue for periods of six months to a year or more, and a change in co-worker will disrupt the flow of the group's life. If practicalities make changes in co-worker necessary, the group must be prepared several weeks in advance. The ability to keep the DMT group room and the timing of the group as consistent as possible for the entire life of the group is crucial, because with long-term patients a predictable and safe environment is important if therapeutic goals are to be achieved. Because the therapist must work very hard to create the sense of a group, all efforts at keeping the room, membership, time of meetings, and co-worker consistent are crucial. Susan Sandel notes that the group's identity, for itself and for other staff, is so fragile that the therapist may fear that if one ceased to exert energy by gathering patients, preparing room, reminding other staff, and offering the relentless assertion to all that the group does exist, nobody would notice. Many nascent groups would simply disappear. The future of the nascent group is dependent on whether the therapist, despite this realization, continues his/her efforts, or allows the group to dissolve.

(Sandel and Johnson 1983: 133)

CASE ILLUSTRATION

Initial discussion

In the early stages it is helpful to inform the patients of the aims of the group in a manner that lets them know what is expected of them: explaining that it will use movement and music as a way to get up and around and activated, and to learn how to get along with others, or to let out or express some feelings by using movement is a good place to begin, depending on the level of functioning of the clients. Obviously, clients who are living on their own in the community could understand an explanation similar to that described for adult outpatients. For hospitalized patients, explaining the difference between the DMT group and OT (occupational therapy), or ward-based activities, and the expectation of regular attendance rather than voluntary or drop-in attendance, is important.

At the beginning of each meeting of the group, the members in turn say something about how their week has been, perhaps saying one positive thing that happened, and one negative thing, and rating their week out of 10. This highly structured form of interaction is consistent with verbal group therapy approaches which note that 'the use of structured techniques, such as the "go-'round", role playing and homework assignments increase involvement' (Kahn 1984: 150). If patients are asked periodically if they can remember the ratings that other members of the circle gave to their week, a memory exercise can be incorporated into the initial discussion.

Members have varying abilities to contribute to the initial discussion, but they make quick gains from month to month if the structure is consistent. The following examples are taken from a group run by the present author which was part of a rehabilitation and resettlement programme for hospitalized patients who were soon to enter community care. The age range of the patients was from 30 to 80 years, with an average age of 55, and an average length of hospitalization of between ten and thirty years. The majority of the group, including Jeff, Alice, Ruth, Bill, Debbie and Mike, suffered from chronic schizophrenia. Additionally, Ruth often had periods of severe psychosis punctuated by paranoia and violence; Debbie had delusional phases; and Alice and Paul often suffered depression in addition to their underlying schizophrenic illness. William, the oldest member of the group, might have been described as personality disordered, and there was some question as to whether he had been committed to a mental institution as a result of some criminal trial, though this was not clear from his admission records which dated just after the Second World War. Lewis had been diagnosed as suffering from severe obsessional disorder, and George had some neurological damage and intellectual impairment. All of the group members were seriously 'institutionalized' and were thought by staff to be passive and dependent on continual care, though it was thought that half the members could make an attempt at living in assisted accommodation of various types. The group, with ten members and a co-worker, was probably slightly too large: the group had been constituted from members of a reminiscence group run by two occupational therapists. Out of fifteen members of this group, it was expected that about half of them might be interested in DMT; when ten of the fifteen expressed an interest, it seemed unfair to turn any away. In practice, on average eight patients attended the group, with two absent due to either illness or inability or unwillingness to come to that week's group.

Typical things which emerged in the initial structured discussion in a group that had been running for about a year included: Jeff's complaints about the change in nursing staff over the weekend, mixed in with imagery from scary movies he watched on TV; George's reporting that he had been taken on a shopping trip to buy some fruit and to cook a meal with the occupational therapists; and Lewis's detailed, day-by-day account of his meals, his activities at the patients' lounge, and his worries that the nursing staff on his ward disliked him, or were going to leave soon, because they could no longer stand the pressure of work. Alice usually said she was fine, and had nothing else to add, and Ruth often said the same, though she would say she 'had been a little under the weather' if she was entering or recovering from a psychotic phase.

Paul never said anything unless questioned, whereupon he would say that he had done nothing at all except sleep and watch TV; this could be challenged by other members who had been on ward or occupational therapy outings with him, but altogether he preferred to have his hat over his eyes and respond to direct requests for information. It was important not to prod too much, and was interesting that he almost always gave his week an abominably low rating, even if he acquiesced and admitted to other members' telling that he had had some treats, or had a new set of clothing or a haircut, or had been relatively well off in pocket money and cigarettes, or had won 'a few bob' on the illicit underground off-track betting network purportedly run by some patients from the canteen. Debbie, the youngest member of the group still had her family involved with her, whereas the majority of the patients had lost touch completely with their relatives; her concerns were about whether she would find a community home near her parents, and she often reported shopping outings with her family.

Robert had a very hard time curtailing his conversation from his very circumstantial speech that would flood the group with confused details of fragments of conversation with nurses, his physical ailments related to his arthritis and palsied arms, mixed in with bits of news he had read in the paper and conversations he had with his brother in the early 1960s when he was committed to the hospital against his will. Mike, the highest functioning member, reported his activities in the outdoor working party, which some of the specially designated maintenance staff ran for patients who wished to earn some money doing outdoor work around the grounds of the hospital; this was consistent with his well-turned-out appearance, and his maintenance of daily routines in his life. Bill, who was often cantankerous and blustery, always had something to say about the weather, or about imagined misdemeanours or the other members' behaviour towards nurses on the wards. William usually reported that he was tired, and when he was moved to a ward for geriatric patients he said that coming to the group was the only time in the week when he didn't feel old; he gave astonishingly accurate and detailed comments about the state and progress of the plants and trees in the hospital gardens, which he could see from his window, over the course of spring, summer, autumn and winter.

In addition to each person's turn, the group also addressed issues in common, such as outings, or things that affected each of them. These included: their choice of area in which they were to be rehoused, and their relative degree of preparation for that; their fears or hopes for life outside the hospital; and their memories of old staff members and 'the grand old days' in which the hospital had had an adjoining working farm, had run weekly social dances, gala balls and annual fancy-dress dinners – times when the hospital had a cricket and football league, and when the total number of patients had been over two thousand, rather than a few hundred. Some of the patients were very aware of how changes in nursing policy and general mental health planning were changing their lives, and others were almost oblivious to changes on this level unless it affected them in a concrete way, such as by increasing or reducing their financial benefits or clothing allowance, or by altering their meal schedule.

The dance movement therapist must be careful to give each patient about the same amount of time, to curb too talkative members and encourage withdrawn ones (without being too pushy about it), and to model effective modes of verbal and nonverbal interaction. If patients appear dissociated, or are clearly not listening, this may be pointed out gently by saying, for example, 'Oh, Bob, did you hear what Jeff said? Did you say you went to that cookery group as well?' It is also good to be a little humorous, once one knows the patients well enough. One day, Paul fell asleep during the initial discussion, and other members had a chuckle over this; the following week, as he sat with his hat over his eyes, the dance movement therapist asked if anyone knew, or could guess what colour his eyes were, which provoked great speculation and, eventually, proud smiles from Paul who in fact had very bright blue eyes (when they were open at least). This was a somewhat forced but effective way to bring the group's attention to the need for eye-contact in inter-personal interaction.

It is crucial to remember the age, physical condition and mental state of hospitalized patients, and not to expect them to be lively and bouncy, or to fulfil one's need to feel effective by covertly trying to get them to be physically more active than they wish to be. While one can model activity and engagement nonverbally, it is important that the dance movement therapist modifies his or her own nonverbal presentation to come down to the general level of activity of which the patient is capable and comfortable (Silberstein 1987).

Choice of music

A wide range of music is suitable for use with long-term patients, and it is probably best if it is chosen or suggested by patients themselves. Some generic pop music, such as the Beatles, or some folk music, classical guitar, or ethnic music is useful; the hospitalized group had a preference for orchestral music from the 1940s, such as that conducted by Mantovanni, Glen Miller, and others. If possible, the choice of big-band music that has some strong or identifiable rhythm is preferable to music that is too soporific or too slow to assist in getting people motivated to move. It is a good idea to make the patients aware of the fact that they will not be expected to dance to the music, but that it is there for background. It can be useful to ask the group to choose from a bunch of cassettes a tape that reflects their mood that day; the dance movement therapist can help the members discern at least whether they would prefer something gentle or lively, and thus gain a good clue about how to proceed with the warmup.

Extended movement warmup

Dance movement therapists working with long-term patients all stress the necessity and benefits of a specialized warmup. The aims of this are to prepare the patients to move in the process section. Choreographically derived warmups may aid in the reconstruction of body image, and they may aid the patients in developing a higher degree of self-synchrony, as defined by Condon, in which the patients' arms, legs, and torso appear to move together in a more integrated fashion (Christrup 1978, Condon and Ogston 1966). Part of the aim of using a long warmup is to use movement in a corrective or prescriptive sense, in a qualitatively different way to how it is used in the improvised or process section of the group; patients need to get to know new ways of moving, to undo gross distortions in body movement. This is undertaken in hope that it will have an impact on body image and body ego; that is, how they picture themselves in stillness and in movement, and in how they feel and behave (Schilder 1950).

If the patients are sluggish, or slow to begin, and are hinting that they want quiet, slow music, or if members of a subgroup say that they'd prefer to sit down and observe for the group rather than move, it is a good idea to begin the warmup while the members are still seated in their chairs. A warmup starting while seated might include such things as lifting feet off the floor by straightening the legs at the knee and then flexing and extending the feet from the ankles, making circles with the feet. This can move into making a walking motion on the floor with the feet, which can then involve the torso by rocking lightly from side to side while doing this seated walking. If the therapist initiates it, the patients are likely to try to follow, despite what might be their natural inclination to have a frozen or immobile torso

(Davis 1970, 1988). This walking, if used with the strong effort element of weight, as defined by Laban, can engage the patients in making stamping noises on the floor, which can also generate a group synchronous rhythm (Laban 1948, Schmais 1985).

This can be followed by crossing the legs, one side and then the other, in a rhythmic fashion. Then hands can be warmed up, by making a piano-playing motion in the air, by pushing or reaching forward, by flexing and extending the hands at the wrists, and then shaking them out. Then, using the whole arm to make a swimming-type motion, patients are encouraged to do a contralateral rather than bilateral movement of the arms in relation to the torso. Swimming backwards is good, as is encouraging a light twist through the back to look behind; often the use of the space behind the patient is lost from mental awareness, and from movement behaviour (Davis 1970, 1988).

After this, a tensing and relaxing of the shoulders is useful, as it encourages an awareness of held tension and encourages diaphragmatic breathing. Some dance movement therapists do specific breathing exercises, which is fine, but patients' tendency towards hyperventilation and dizziness must be carefully checked; if they are proceeding with a warmup, it is not usually necessary to do any additional breathing exercises. As a final warmup, the group members can be asked to lean over and curl up as small as they can while seated, and then release into being as wide as they can, as in a yawn and stretch. This narrowing and widening in the horizontal plane, as well as growing and shrinking in the vertical plane, and bulging and hollowing in the sagittal and diagonal planes are all elements of carving or shaping the space, which have developmental correlates, as described by Judith Kestenberg, and which relate to Laban's effort–shape (Kestenberg 1975, Laban 1948, Bartenieff 1980). The inclusion of different movement exercises derived from choreographic and developmental body movement systems extends the patient's expressive range of movement, reconstructs a body image based on developmental experience, and mobilizes, reintegrates, motivates and helps to organize the patient's nonverbal presentation in space and time.

Movement can continue in twisting side to side, encouraging the patient to 'look at the person next to you', which is used again to counteract the immobile or one-unit torso that patients may have, as described by Davis's work. One favourite warmup suggested by patients is to touch their own body parts in a rhythmic sequence, while naming them, in order to organize the body parts. After a while it is good to get patients to lead this part of the warmup, in which they touch their own feet, ankles, shins, knees, thighs, hips, waist, chest, shoulders and head. It is interesting to see which parts are consistently missed or mislabelled by some patients, and how at each successive repetition they become more aware of themselves, and how the arms, legs and torso are related to one another in space. Nurses and psychiatrists watching videotapes of long-term patients before, during and after DMT groups comment on how patients appear so much more alert and alive after the warmup phase of the group, in contrast to the slow, listless, slumped-in-a-chair posture they may assume on the ward.

The warmup continues with the dance movement therapist asking everyone to stand up, and, once chairs are moved away, some rhythmic walking or stamping is undertaken, as is twisting at the waist. Such movements as slow marching, stepping forward and backward into and out of the circle, turning round, bending at the knees and swinging, reaching up, down, side to side and forward and backward are all undertaken fairly slowly, and repeated four or six times, with verbal encouragement towards group synchronous movement. After this, virtually any neutral movement that serves to get the patients ready to move is acceptable; one needs only to be wary of introducing too many movements that feature effort–shape combinations unique or favoured by the dance movement therapist: the present author's preference for spatial multi-focus using the sagittal plane (exemplified by stepping into the circle and reaching forward) was invariably copied by George during his own turns in the shared leadership, presumably in his simple attempts to 'do the right thing' and please the dance movement therapist.

Shared leadership

Once the patients are warmed up, the group can proceed using the shared leadership format. The following examples occurred during the shared leadership section of a group which had been meeting weekly for over nine months. At this point the group was probably functioning in the manner described by Sandel and Johnson as 'gestation':

> the slow development of relatedness occurs concurrently with the therapist's ambivalent struggle to maintain a conception of the group. The group may eventually move to a plateau of functioning, depending on the stability of the group's membership and leadership. At this point, most of the group's activities become ritualized.
>
> (Sandel and Johnson 1983: 134)

The dance movement therapist turned to Bill, who immediately did a very disorganized imitation of touching various upper body parts in a lightning speed tapping rhythm; he used the effort of quickness, but in a way that was not quick with a rhythm, but quickness 'coming out of nowhere' (Davis 1970). This made it jerky, and hard to follow, so the dance movement therapist suggested that he name the parts as he did the movement; this narrowed down his scattered automaton movement into a touching of the shoulders and head, followed by shooting the arms upward, and saying, 'Up!' Mike asked what part (of the body) the 'up' was supposed to be, and Bill looked perplexed. The student nurse ventured 'the soul?', whereupon Debbie laughed and waved her arms behind her, while the group tried to continue following Bill, but were probably following the dance movement therapist's version of Bill's movement. He said 'Pass', and the dance movement therapist said, 'Fine, that was good'. There is some debate as to how much positive reinforcement, if any, should be used with patients; it is a matter that each dance movement therapist must decide.

Jeff, the next in the circle, did a rapid rowing motion, going backwards with his arms, making his elbows fly back in a jagged way, which, had it continued, might have threatened to give George a black eye. The group followed the rowing movement but Jeff was moved back so that he could not hit anyone unintentionally. The dance movement therapist and the group continued to repeat Jeff's movement, and the therapist asked what the group could be doing with this gesture, in an attempt to elicit an association or an image. Ruth said 'rowing' and Mike said 'punching!', and there was general laughter from the group. Jeff stopped abruptly and touched his pockets, as though searching for cigarettes. He seemed oblivious to the presence of anyone else in the world, let alone in the group, as he stared straight ahead. The dance movement therapist said, 'OK, Jeff, will you pass to the next person?' He looked over at her, somewhat annoyed. Bill, standing in between, said, 'Get on with it', and the dance movement therapist tried to catch Jeff's attention to say 'pass' to the next person. He stepped back out of the circle about two feet, but remained somehow connected by proximity at least, so the dance movement therapist provided the transition by saying, 'Great. OK, pass to William then.' William did a militaristic set of jumping jacks, which everyone followed very seriously; his status as oldest member of the group was very much respected. He stood at attention and stared ahead of him at the end, and then said, 'pass, pass'.

Physical closeness

Everyone was still, waiting for George to go next, but just then Jeff started doing a few jumping jacks. George was nudged by Lewis, and he then did his usual stepping forward into the circle, reaching forward with extended arms, and giving a big grin. Everyone followed, happy in the correct expectation that George would do this movement, as he did in virtually every single group for the entire eighteen months! The dance movement therapist suggested, by using her voice in the same rhythm, that the group try to do it all together, by saying, 'So we're all stepping in . . . and reaching . . . and then out again.' Most of the group managed to do this, which increased the eye contact enormously, and made the group feel and seem very connected to one another. A few people who were unsteady on their feet, and not as adept at stepping backward out of the circle as into it, bumped into one another lightly and touched hands. This provoked more eye contact, made Ruth and Paul withdraw, and made Lewis hesitate and move his arms towards and away, with furious rapidity, while George, Debbie, Bill, Robert, Mike, Alice and the rest of the group stood huddled together in a jumbled way, with the outsides of their hands touching, and their shoulders fairly close together. The dance movement therapist suggested they move back, and the movement was initiated again by two members, dyssynchronously, but soon started up again in harmony.

It might be the case that the group was able to tolerate fairly well this non-sexual touch, and that it might have given some of the members a sense of mental as well as physical closeness. It did provoke some anxiety in Paul, and something similar in Ruth. Had the movement been a less rhythmic one that did not involve stepping into and out of the circle, it could have been awkward, in leaving members standing very close, touching hands. It seems that long-term patients initiate and can manage this form of contact more effectively than their higher functioning counterparts (Liebowitz *et al.* 1989). However, it is of the utmost importance that it does not get too intimate or sexualized, as these patients, like their higher functioning counterparts, need to find appropriate ways of satisfying their need for physical closeness and affection outside the group, rather than act these out during the sessions (Willis 1987).

The dance movement therapist suggested that the group step back and allow the next person to take his or her turn. Lewis went next, and did a strange twisting–walking motion while looking down at the ground, with his hands curled up, which involved right arm right leg, and then left arm right leg, done while twisting at the waist, and making a tense grimace with the lower half of the face. The dance movement therapist could only follow the spatial and rhythmic disorganization with difficulty, but few other members could, so it was simplified into a sort of hunched and tentative shuffle. The group walked in this way for a while, and Lewis became concerned about taking too long, when he sensed some members ceasing to follow, so Alice took over, and lifted up her arms, making a fluttering motion, and then bending over and trying to touch her toes, but reaching near her knees. The group groaned at this, but complied, and it was repeated. At this point Jeff came up, stood inches away from the dance movement therapist and mumbled in a very convoluted way that he couldn't understand why he couldn't see behind him, or even twist so that he could see someone coming. This happened several weeks after a patient had seriously assaulted another patient in the hallway, and the dance movement therapist noted the communication, thinking to take it up later in the process or discussion section, but sent him back to his place in the circle so as not to disrupt the turn-taking structure.

The student nurse went next. She bent at the waist and moved in a circular twisting motion with her hands on her hips. The group groaned and laughed at the difficulty, and most could manage either to bend at the waist with hands on hips and lean forward, or they could remain vertical and sway from side to side; the movement was too complex, because it occurred in too many planes for them to master at once. She passed over to Ruth, who extended her arm first to one side and then the other, in the manner of a farmer sowing seeds, or someone smoothing out water while standing in a pool. The group repeated this, and someone said 'hello', and the dance movement therapist suggested that all members of the group say hello to the person on each side of them. This amused Bill very much, and the group looked momentarily like a bunch of people meeting at a conference, rich in subgrouping, and smiling and nodding and eye contact, and making pleased noises, perhaps because they felt something in being recognized, and in seeing the person next to them as a person, with a facial expression, as opposed to simply sensing a moving blob of shape. Ruth made an elegant and polite 'pass' to Paul, who stood swaying with his eyes half-closed. He had to be cajoled into doing something; but he said he didn't want to, so we let it drop after getting him to say 'pass' to the next person.

Debbie came next, and bent forward and wiggled her posterior in the manner of a bunny rabbit doing the twist; she laughed maniacally while she shimmied. The entire group broke into loud laughter, and there were some 'oh noooo!' sounds from Ruth, Alice and Paul, and some appreciative imitations of her wiggling and giggling from Mike, George, Robert and William. Most of the group did a modified version of this slightly suggestive or provocative movement, and the dance move- ment therapist said, 'That's new and different!', which provoked further laughter from the group. Robert, next to her, said, 'Alright, alright then', and began to talk the group through what he wished to do for his turn, which seemed to be a swimming motion, combined with walking, but which he himself found very difficult. The dance movement therapist helped him to describe what he wanted to do, and then did this herself, which pleased him very much, 'Yeah, that's that, that's that,' he added in a proud tone. The group got into a spontaneous synchrony here, which was noted by the dance movement therapist who said, 'We're all doing this together!' This sort of unprompted high level of group synchrony was rather rare, and felt quite rewarding.

The group was stopped by Mike, who came next, and who was last in the circle, and stood at the dance movement therapist's right side. He suddenly clapped his hands loudly, quite close to her face, and gave a provocative grin. Half the group went silent, and the other half laughed anxiously, while Bill gave a wary murmur. Ruth said, 'No! I won't do that!', and Mike, who respected Ruth and was in fact involved in occupational therapy assessment of living skills with her, with a prospective view of their living in the same community home, quickly gave another movement which involved twisting at the waist and pulling his arms out in a smoothing fashion, which resembled, in shape if not in quality, Ruth's own side-to-side movement. Jeff asked if he could have a cigarette, and Alice sat down abruptly, and the dance movement therapist said, 'Okay everyone, we're following Mike, let's keep going for a minute more.' Jeff returned to his place and shuffled and the rest of the group carried on. Mike stopped, and the rest of the group looked either around them or at the dance movement therapist for a clue on what to do next. It was the therapist's turn, and she asked the group if they would like to do another turn around the circle, or use the stretch cloth. Most of the group said they could do another round, so another round was started. Before describing this, which featured the use of the imagery of animals and allowed for a controlled release of repressed anger, some comments about the dance movement therapist's function in the DMT group will be provided.

THE FUNCTION OF THE DANCE MOVEMENT THERAPIST

The description above cannot fully convey the experience of participating in the nonverbal atmosphere of the DMT group of chronic schizophrenics attempting to generate and follow their own improvised movement tasks. The level of general disorganization and dissociation that occurs is quite different from the usual nonverbal behaviours of a bunch of adults in a room who are engaged in a mutual task, such as described by Albert Scheflen in his nonverbal communications research, involving parameters like mutual focus of gaze, nodding, sequenced postural and gestural initiations and replies, spatial organization, cueing, and rhythmic alternations in stillness and activity, all of which constitute ordinary nonverbal 'speech' (Scheflen 1979, Scheflen and Scheflen 1972).

Instead, one is confronted with 'a profoundly fragmented, nonsensical, and chaotic human environment which borders on the nonhuman' (Sandel and Johnson 1983: 132). In this situation, the dance movement therapist is responsible for nonverbally reflecting, extending and clarifying the movement the patients give, as well as providing movement and verbal transitions between turn-takers, and between different sections of the group. The therapist provides the initial impetus for the group's activity, until the members can remember and initiate what comes next; when the patients cannot remember, the dance movement therapist must provide a sense of continuity and organization which, in many instances, is simply not there until the dance movement therapist acts as though it will emerge, or facilitates its realization. Amazingly enough, some order and interaction does develop, as week after week the group begins to be able to tolerate and expect to be able to give interactional behaviour to the structures provided, for example, by giving a movement, or associations, or information about their week, etc. This still requires encouragement and support to get more and more clear communication between members who, if left on their own, might not initiate anything but the most basic communication with others.

The provision of this function for the group is in part what constitutes the therapist being 'the container of the group identity' (Sandel and Johnson 1983: 133). The other aspect of being such a container is to be aware of and have a mental image of the group, which is communicated to the patients through the dance movement therapist's behaviour. This image can be kept alive (in the face of much contradictory evidence from group members) by discussing the group with other staff members, by theorizing, and by taking videotapes to a supervisor or by having a supervisor attend the group from time to time.

The dance movement therapist's containment of the group identity, in its initial and progressive stages, occurs 'on all levels, psychological and physical' (Skove 1986: 73). Verbally, as well as nonverbally, the dance movement therapist conducts herself or himself in a way that facilitates the highest degree of interpersonal relatedness possible for these isolated patients. The achievement of this group identity is tenuous, and is dependent on large amounts of repetition and keeping the group's rituals going; however, it if can be sustained, patients can gain enormous benefit from being contributing and receiving members of a group. It is imperative that supervision should know when the facilitation of structure is being used positively for the group, or when it may constitute a reinforcement of the institutionalized or compliant or dependent behaviour of the members (Liebowitz *et al.* 1989).

Countertransference stress

Much of the literature with long-term patients addresses the feelings evoked when working with these damaged and deprived clients. There is some controversy among clinicians in this area as to how the therapist's emotional responses should be used. Susan Sandel, noting her connection to the tradition of work with psychotic patients exemplified by D. W. Winnicott, Margaret Little, Harold Searles and Frieda Fromm-Reichmann, wrote that 'I experienced with equal intensity to my loving feelings, hate and murderous rage toward some patients in dance therapy sessions' (Sandel 1980: 27, Winnicott 1949, Little 1951, Searles 1965). This countertransference, or the dance movement therapist's feelings towards the transference material of the patient, is an emotional response to the powerful, preverbal distorted messages from the patients. Such evoked responses may be used therapeutically, because they offer a message from the patients' unconscious through the medium of the therapist's emotional responses. However, the sharing of such feelings, or interpretation of them, is a technical skill that can only be used safely after the dance movement therapist has had his or her own personal therapy, in order to understand the phenomenon of transference from a personal point of view. Furthermore, additional training and supervision by a qualified psychotherapist or psychoanalyst are of the utmost importance in endeavouring to use one's own emotional reactions to patients for therapeutic benefit.

Even if the dance movement therapist is not attempting to use his or her feelings to feed back to the patients the manner in which the patients are relating to him or her, the group members and their issues still give rise to emotional reactions in the dance movement therapist which mean that 'self examination, supervision and peer support are critical for the dance therapist who works in an environment where such countertransference stresses prevail' (Sandel 1980: 22).

The emotional reactions in the dance movement therapist include grandiose notions of rescue, feelings of having voracious emotional demands made by the patients, as well of feelings of hopelessness, dismay and confusion. Quite simply, due to the sense of hopelessness in these groups, therapists will often appreciate and overvalue even the smallest sign of organization or progress among patients (Sandel and Johnson 1983: 132). Further reactions to the loneliness and hopelessness of the group members are common, as Sandel and Johnson describe:

> Disgust and desires to physically harm people or to flee the group may be repudiated by grandiose rescue notions and intense feelings of involvement. The therapist experiences the group as extremely fragile. Omnipotent fantasies may develop in the therapist that his/her slightest intervention could have overwhelming effects, for good, or more usually for bad. At other times the therapist may feel like a victim of the group at the mercy of its unresponsiveness to his/her efforts.
>
> (Sandel and Johnson 1983: 132)

It is important to note that these reactions are to the therapist's *view* of the group, to his or her own mental representation, and not acted out towards the actual group. As a reaction or response to patients' feelings of being lost and isolated, the dance movement therapist may have grandiose fantasies of glimmers of their recovery. It is crucial not to develop unrealistic expectations about the patients' abilities (particularly when they are entering community life), but rather to convey a realistic attitude of positive hopefulness for improvements in the patients' functioning.

It is important for the dance movement therapist to have supervision and support to deal with his or her own feelings of omnipotence that can develop. Omnipotence is defined as 'the therapist's feeling of having great power, authority, or effect on the patient, that is, the power to use his or her charismatic qualities or techniques to effect change' (Sandel 1980: 22). While it is important to have some hope for patients, it is essential that these be realistic and not merely a reaction to the patients' low self-esteem and self-estimation.

Dance movement therapists must be especially wary of acting on their counter-transference feelings unknowingly, as Susan Sandel explains:

> The schizophrenic patient's voraciousness can be especially overwhelming for the dance therapist because the therapeutic context permits greater physical intimacy and acting out of transference issues than other treatment modalities. These characteristics, while advantageous in establishing empathetic relationships with regressed or seriously disturbed patients, create stress in the dance therapist who is struggling to maintain involvement without being devoured.
>
> (Sandel 1980: 28)

It is essential to be mentally prepared for the sessions and to be aware of the mental states that can be provoked in the dance movement therapist. A survey of dance movement therapists working with long-term patients found that respondents had experienced odd mental states that were felt to resemble those of their patients, and included such things as 'merging or focusing, fragmentation, loss of control, loss of direct focus accompanied by an increase in sensory input, and feeling ungrounded' (Skove 1986: 75). While this may be helpful in being empathetic with patients and in recognizing what is necessary in the context of the therapeutic interpersonal response to the group, it is essential that dance movement therapists use both movement-based and mental/emotional preparative and recuperative measures. Preparation might include remembering or looking at the previous week's session notes, being ready for feeling 'all over the place' in trying to manage the group's fragmentation, and being aware of those patients who evoke specific feelings. Recuperation might include discussion with a co-worker, some 'time out', and also some reintegrative movement experience, such as dance, yoga or relaxation, or the use of complex-structured rhythmic movement, along with grounding and centring techniques (Skove 1986). This nonverbal recuperation is necessary because the patient's confusion and illness are also manifested nonverbally; the dance movement therapist becomes intensely aware of this in endeavouring to mirror the patient's movement. In this 'kinesthetic empathy the essence of the patient's bodily tensions and how they are dynamically manifested are recreated [in the mirrored movement of the dance movement therapist] in various degrees' (Skove 1986: 72).

Despite the strong feelings that work with these patients can evoke, including feelings of dismay, disgust, apathy or hopelessness, and compensatory feelings of omnipotence or fantasies of rescue and recovery of the patients, the work can be extremely challenging and interesting, and long-term rewards are forthcoming as patients eventually will initiate spontaneous interaction, and begin to trust the group enough to allow some of their feelings to emerge.

Modifications in structure and technique

In keeping with the goals of containing and facilitating the group identity, such that the group members can come to internalize a concept of the group, there are certain modifications in the therapist's conduct which are useful. The first is the continual, relentless addressing of the group as a group, by using phrases like 'Let's all do this', 'What could *we* be doing?', 'Okay, *everyone*, let's do this together', 'What music does the *group* want today?', and 'How are we all this afternoon?' This obvious manoeuvre is more helpful than addressing individuals, and helps the group members get a shared sense of the 'we' that is vital for group functioning.

Additionally, the use of humour and a neutral and open manner are important. 'It is well known that psychotic patients will mirror fear that is manifested by the therapist. Similarly, the patient will be calmed by a therapist who seems relaxed and in good spirits' (Kahn 1984: 152). Additionally, redirecting questions that are addressed towards the leader onto the group as a whole, or onto other members, can facilitate members asking and listening to each other, and not only to staff members. If someone asks about the weather, or about a TV programme, or about which nurses are on which shift, or what day it is, the dance movement therapist can say, 'Does anyone else know what day it is today?' or 'Maybe someone else can help you answer this question' in order to facilitate interaction between group members (Kahn 1984).

For work with long-term patients, some modifications to the DMT group structure may be necessary; these consist of facilitating a structure that is safe and reliable, while allowing for small degrees of change. The use of a leaderless improvised format is generally not a good idea; these patients become anxious and disorganized unless a designated member or the dance movement therapist is clearly leading or facilitating the group. If spontaneous movement becomes too repetitive, imagery may be introduced to spur the patients on to new ideas; suggesting a slight modification to the shared leadership format can be useful, such as saying, 'Do any movement, or a movement that is like an animal, or a movement you've never done before, or a movement that shows how you feel about the weather today', as possible examples. Some patients may find the idea silly, or may not want to do a movement like an animal; this sort of thing is only possible if the patients are very familiar with the dance movement therapist and with each other, and are *never* forced or pressured to do something if they find it silly, embarrassing, demeaning or patronizing. Props can be extremely useful for facilitating interaction, in a similar manner to that described in the section on higher functioning outpatients. The long-term group may require more instructions on how to use props, and they must be introduced in a way that the members do not find intrusive or threatening, or feel that they are being asked to be childish, or transgress boundaries of conduct appropriate to their age, condition, or place in hospital life.

Some modification to the therapist's level of movement activity is also necessary. Most patients are physically quite out of shape, as well as suffering from minor physical complaints and the general state of health that comes from long-term institutional living, and so cannot be expected to engage in movement and dance as well as their non-psychiatric counterparts. Additionally, the patients' ages must be respected; their generational and cultural norms about the degree of expressive movement with which they will feel comfortable may differ from those of the dance movement therapist. The dance movement therapist must be sensitive to the level of activity of the clients, and modify himself or herself accordingly; 'a dance therapist who unwittingly gives in to his or her own movement needs can easily threaten apathetic or constricted patients' (Sandel 1980: 29, Silberstein 1987). The dance movement therapist, who usually has an emotional investment in movement and dance, must not presume that patients who do not wish to move (like Paul, above) are not getting anything from the group; it is important not to allow a patient's resistance, tiredness or disorganization to provoke 'anxiety about the curative effects of the medium' (Sandel 1980: 29). Just because a patient doesn't move as the dance movement therapist might wish, doesn't mean that the patient isn't making therapeutic gains; one is countering a great deal of apathy and passivity in getting the patient to move at all. Observing patients on wards will give a sense of how different the DMT group is to their usual or expected level of activity.

THE USE OF ANIMAL IMAGERY

As part of the modification in structure discussed above, the group undertook a second series of shared leadership around the circle. This time they opted for the choice to use animal imagery as a suggested framework, introduced by the therapist. In this instance, it allowed for a lot of release of anger and frustration, between two members, and possibly in response to anxiety that patients had about a recent assault of one patient by another that had occurred in the hospital. It was the dance movement therapist's turn first, and while trying to decide what animal to do, Mike offered suggestions of a cat or a dog. She did a kangaroo instead, using a full-body swing, and a very grounded thump on the floor at the end. She made a joke about herself hopping around, and was pleased with the synchrony the group showed as a result of stamping nearly all at the same time at the end of this clearly phrased movement.

She passed to Bill, who stood perplexed for a moment; he was then prompted to say an animal, so that we could do its movement. He flapped his arms up and down, and said, 'a bird, then!'. The group did this together, and the dance movement therapist asked where the group might be flying to. Mike suddenly said, 'Ireland!' Ruth said, 'Where?' and the dance movement therapist repeated the location. Paul piped up, mumbling at the mention of this, but could say nothing coherent. The dance movement therapist asked if he were Irish, but he said he wasn't. Lewis began to talk about terrorism, and said he always went to the west country, or Dorset, on holiday. Debbie giggled in a manic way, and Bill stopped moving, adding, 'that's it then'.

The dance movement therapist then prompted Jeff, who paused, and then started muttering unintelligibly as Mike suggested a dog again. He was trying to say the name of an animal, it seemed, but couldn't get it right. Finally the dance movement therapist, after offering elephant, hippo and anteater in response to his using his hand to indicate a horn on the head or a trunk, got it right with 'rhinoceros'. The group shuffled forward with their hands pointing from their foreheads in imitation of a horn, and adopting Jeff's posture and slightly malicious grin. The dance movement therapist asked Jeff if a rhinoceros would sneak around quietly, or if it would make a lot of noise, and illustrated both options in an attempt to elicit a richer quality of body movement. He increased the jabbing quality to his movement, as did the group. Debbie came forward and, while skipping lightly, attempted to engage the dance movement therapist in a dancing-type challenge or display of rhinoceros horns. She was amused when the dance movement therapist mirrored her hopping, and Debbie said, 'Will you bite me, or hit me?' She was assured that this would not happen, and skipped off happily. This might have been some replay of her arguments with her parents and ward staff about her transfer into the community; evidently she had become quite upset and struck out at one of the nurses. Perhaps she was replaying her angry encounters, along with feared reprisals. At this point William said he supposed rhinos would swim, or clomp through the grass, and, in the middle of this, Jeff abruptly stopped what he was doing and began to mutter aggressively at William. William stopped, and the dance movement therapist, noting that Jeff was not muttering anything about William, but was onto some internal monologue, nodded to William that Jeff had finished, and suggested George take his turn.

Mike proffered the suggestion of a dog again, and George made a barking noise and shuffled side to side. The group followed, and expanded the circle slightly. The dance movement therapist asked whether it was a guard dog, or a happy dog, or some other type of dog. Bob said it was 'happy, wagging his tail', and there was laughter about this. Bill repeated this exact phrase eleven times or so, and Robert got onto a story about a dog he had when he was a boy, addressing nobody in particular. Debbie came over to the dance movement therapist and tried to engage her in another paired movement, but the dance movement therapist resisted, and asked Bob to finish, which he did, and then passed over to William standing next to him.

William asked what we were doing, and it was explained that one could do any movement, or a movement like an animal. William pondered a moment, scratching his head, and then said, 'A tiger, there!' He put his hands out in front of him, and gave a convincing growl. The group took this seriously, and mirrored him very accurately. Some came forward a bit more, making more eye contact, and Mike made a mock lunge at Lewis, who withdrew, appearing happier when the dance movement therapist put up her hand to prevent Mike coming any closer than the three feet or so he was from Lewis. Mike was easily two feet taller than Lewis, and so no matter what he did, he looked quite threatening in stepping across the circle. William then sprang forward, jumping up, and the group followed, and again there was pressure to synchronize the movement, so it became an activity of landing on the floor, at the same time making a slapping noise of shoes against the linoleum. People looked tired, so the dance movement therapist thanked William, and he grandly passed over to Lewis.

Alice asked innocently what animal William would be doing, and William, looking confused, said he had done a tiger, but he thought his turn was over with. Lewis was hesitating wildly, and finally stammered that he would like to do a horse, perhaps, he thought, if nobody minded too much. Debbie said they went fast, and Lewis, doing a similar distorted walking to his previous turn, did a sort of hop, which Debbie turned into a three step gallop. Paul began to talk, and the dance movement therapist noted it was about Western movies on TV and said, 'Oh, Paul's just mentioned TV Westerns. They usually have horses in them, don't they?' Paul, amazed at this communication being picked up, made eye contact and gave a gracious smile to Ruth, who happened to be looking the other way; the dance movement therapist caught Paul's eye, gave a smile, and tried to encourage him to gallop on the spot, but he fingered his hat as a way of declining the invitation.

Mike had got some way across the circle to where Lewis was, and the dance movement therapist gestured him away. Lewis put his hands on his head as though in fear, but the dance movement therapist told him it was all right and he took his hands down, looking unsure. The therapist said it was Alice's turn next, and Alice, a sweet lady wearing a pink cardigan, often known to bring her knitting to the group, stood still, curled her fingers forward, raised her arms and bared her teeth (revealing a set of loose dentures), and gave a tiny but fierce growl. She stopped almost immediately, and said, meekly, 'A bear; a black big bear.' The awe-struck dance movement therapist thanked her, and said, 'Right everyone, Alice has done a great black bear, let's go.' She imitated Alice's movement and the group engaged in doing this, with the growl getting more integrated with the raising of the arms, in harmony rather than one after the other. Mike went for Lewis again, quite menacingly, and was clearly told to keep back a bit by the dance movement therapist standing in front of him a little and saying, 'Keep your claws in!' This made Bill laugh covertly behind his hand, and made Debbie giggle, but relieved Alice and William, who were standing huddled by Lewis. There was a great deal of general laughter and joking around as one or two members growled at the student nurse, who feigned surprise and horror, and Debbie giggled hysterically and growled at Paul, who had his eyes closed, and pretended not to, or perhaps didn't, notice this was happening. The dance movement therapist suggested that the group come together and do it one last time, which they did, all seeming to be very pleased. At one point in this sequence, the dance movement therapist noted that all the animals in this shared leadership format were becoming more alike; all being expressive of frustration or mock threat.

The student nurse took her turn next and did a monkey, which most found difficult but all found funny, especially Debbie. She passed to Ruth, who said quietly, 'A leopard'. She shuffled forward and raised her hands, which showed her red nail polish. She did not make a sound, which gave her movement a stalking quality. She walked quietly over to Mike and squinted at him. Bill said, 'Hah! Look out leopard!' and Mike smiled and turned his back on her, going out of the circle. Paul stood by blankly, Lewis looked at his shoe laces, Jeff scratched himself, and the rest of the group kept going, moving their arms slowly and quietly, also squinting. The dance movement therapist asked what leopards were like and someone mentioned the zoo, which prompted a discussion of the last time some of the group had been to visit a zoo. She further asked if they were graceful or scary or quiet, and Bob said 'Very scary', and Debbie said, 'Nice', while Robert mumbled about TV documentaries, addressing Paul, who was not listening.

It was interesting to see Bill, who had quite a pronounced Parkinsonian tremor in his arms and face, get quite a good sustained and smooth movement with his arms. When he was not using them voluntarily, his arms always looked very shaky; it gave a very different impression to see him using this lighter and less jerky movement; he looked more intent and purposeful. This turn seemed endless, so the dance movement therapist called it to a halt, and then mentioned it was now Paul's turn next in the circle. He said, 'No thank you', but Mike suggested he do a dog or a cat, and other members stopped and looked at him. The dance movement therapist said, 'Paul, people are giving you suggestions. Do you have a favourite animal we might try to do?' Robert said he could do an ape, and Paul turned this down. He then put his hands in his pockets, and in the manner of a country gentleman, put his hat up and began to whistle. The dance movement therapist, keen to take any participation by this member, said, 'OK, let's all whistle, then.' Most of the group put their hands in their pockets or by their side and the group whistled, tunelessly. There was general discussion of how difficult it was to whistle, and a yodel from Lewis, and laughs at the student nurse who could not whistle at all. The whistling ended in a haphazard way when the dance movement therapist stopped whistling to change the music cassette tape, which had finished. Evidently the group was dependent on the leader, rather than the initiator of the whistling. The dance movement therapist was a bit tired by this point, and asked whose turn it was. Debbie perked up and said it was hers.

She hissed, and did an odd arch backwards, like a cat with its back up. The dance movement therapist asked what sort of cat it was, and she said, 'A scardey cat, you daft thing!' The group did this all together; it was interesting to see people's facial expression involved, while hissing; it was a great contrast to the blank expressions many often wore. Mike went forward instead of jumping backwards and hissed at Lewis, and the dance movement therapist intervened and said, off the cuff, 'Let's not get too scared here!' Robert was talking about a cat, and Jeff tapped the dance movement therapist on the shoulder to ask if he could smoke, which was against the group rules; and while this was being clarified, George said he was tired and asked when tea was going to be served. The dance movement therapist said that the group was nearly finished, at which point Mike went for Lewis by stepping across the circle, and the dance movement therapist said 'This is peace here, not war' and clarified verbally that Mike was scaring Lewis by walking over to him.

It was Mike's turn. He seemed aware of the dance movement therapist's disapproval of his actions towards Lewis. He put out his fists and stuck out his arms, and said, 'Eeeeeaaww. A donkey.' The group laughed, possibly partly in response to the look of astonishment on the dance movement therapist's face at this very apt symbol for Mike, and his difficult behaviour that day in pursuing Lewis. She said, 'What's the thing about donkeys?' and Bill piped up, and sneakily said, 'Bloody stubborn!' Whether he was aware of this comment's relevance to Mike's behaviour didn't seem certain, but the other members found this amusing and engaged in walking forward, stopping abruptly, and putting out their fists. The dance movement therapist said, 'Are *people* stubborn sometimes too, maybe?' and Alice said, 'Yes dear,' followed by Robert really laughing at the joke rather than in response to some internal dialogue. Mike looked over at the dance movement therapist, as though for reassurance, and the therapist said, 'Well, maybe everyone is stubborn sometimes.' The group kept moving for a while, and it was apparent that they could each do this movement individually, but not together, and so the dance movement therapist suggested that they all reach together and do the sound of the animal, which they did. The turn had come back to her, and since she was aware that there was about 20 minutes of the group left, she asked if the group would like to finish with a few easy movements to relax. Bill hurried over, quite concerned, and said he hadn't had his turn yet, and he was reminded that he had done the first turn in the circle. The dance movement therapist (accidentally incorrectly) told him that he had done a dog, when in fact he had done the bird.

The group movement section concluded with some easy stretches, reaching forward, a stretch and a yawn, and some facial self-massage. After this movement-level closure, the group sat down for the discussion at the end, with the exception of Lewis, who continued massaging his face for a further four minutes before sitting down.

Closing discussion

The therapist asked if people remembered what was done that day, and the group remembered about half of the animals, and the jumping jacks. They were reminded by the dance movement therapist about laughing when wiggling (Debbie's movement) and it was pointed out that some people thought that was a bit embarrassing, to which half the membership admitted, while the others either could not remember or evidently found it somewhat titillating. Some dance movement therapists ask their groups to rate themselves from 1 to 10, as verbal psychotherapists suggest, in order to reward people who get a high rating for their contributions, and to find out what was right or wrong about low-rated members to encourage them to make the group more interesting for themselves the next time (Kahn 1984, Liebowitz *et al.* 1989).

Anger and annoyance

In this instance, the therapist commented that Mike and Lewis seemed to have been involved, at which point Lewis looked anxious and Mike looked rather sheepish. The student nurse raised her eyebrows, and the dance movement therapist asked how people managed things if they were angry or annoyed with people, which everyone was from time to time. Mike said 'It's his fault', and Lewis visibly cowered. Robert said, in a roundabout way, that everyone used to 'take the piss' and get upset with Lewis because, when they all lived on the same ward he didn't finish his dinner and everyone had to wait for their pudding or dessert. Lewis said he couldn't help being slow, and ventured an explanation that involved his early years at the hospital. The student nurse said she thought that it was good that Mike had been able to get annoyed but not hurt anyone, and Alice said, 'It was just a bit of fun.' The dance movement therapist ventured that it was okay to feel annoyed, but not okay to hurt people, and most of the group who were paying attention at that point agreed.

The dance movement therapist turned to Jeff and reminded him that he had asked her about not being able to see behind him. When prompted, he repeated the problem of not being able to twist easily at the waist, and not turn around quickly to see anything or anyone pursuing him. The dance movement therapist said, 'So the thing is you can't see what's coming up behind you?' and Mike added, 'That's how it happened, see, he got hit from behind.' It had to be clarified that the person in question was not Jeff, or someone from TV, but the actual patient (who was a friend of Alice's) who had been hit by another patient in the hallway, and had had to be taken to hospital with a minor head injury. It was clear that the patients all knew of the event, and the student nurse reported that the patient was now recovering, which relieved those who were concerned. Ruth (who was prone to aggressive outbursts when psychotic) said it was terrible to let that sort of thing go on, and that people just couldn't be safe on the streets any more. She gave examples from the recent TV news, and some that seemed to have happened ten or twenty years ago about random attacks on people. Lewis began to babble about being hit by his mother as a child, and Jeff lit his pipe, which was against the group rules. He was asked to put this out, which he did; and the dance movement therapist said that it seemed to her that people were worried about what happened to the other patient, and that Jeff was wondering if that could happen to him – if things could happen out of nowhere like that, and one could just be hurt by surprise.

The group quieted. Alice said she was often scared in the corridor, and Debbie said she didn't like going across from one building to the next. William muttered how awful everything was, and the dance movement therapist tried to reinforce that the patient's safety was not at risk, but that it was scary when people's anger got out of control and people hurt or hit people, but that on the whole the nurses and staff did and could help keep the patients safe, in addition to the patients trying to be more vigilant for themselves. A few members straightened themselves in their chairs at this sobering thought.

The dance movement therapist asked if there were any comments or questions or if anyone could rate the group out of 10, compared to other weeks. Paul said 'What weeks?' and George said, 'Is it tea yet?' and Mike added, 'Alright, six.' The dance movement therapist commented that it had been a lively group, and that people had got a lot of movement going when we did the animals. She illustrated the tiger, and the group rallied and came alive with interest and laughter, and she suggested that people all had some angry or mean or maybe scary or annoyed feelings inside them, that maybe came out when we did the animals. Alice smiled sweetly, Jeff did a boxing in the air with his fists, and Lewis said he didn't mean to make people angry, he couldn't help it. It was made clear to Lewis that other people's anger and upset were not his fault, and he was praised for understanding that sometimes his behaviour could irritate people, and for his efforts to try to change things. William said the weather was really beginning to annoy him, and Mike said he had to get going, so the issue was dropped for that day. The group were requested to help put away the chairs before going back to the ward for tea.

While it may seem that not a great deal happened in this group, the change from ward-based activity (or inactivity) is quite striking to an outside observer. The group were able to have moments of movement synchrony, notably using stamping rhythm, and express and safely release feelings of frustration and annoyance that often build up between patients and other patients, and patients and staff. The group did exhibit moments of group cohesion, and there was a sense of togetherness, which gained momentum as the session went on. Despite difficulty, Paul and Jeff were kept as part of the group though they had periods of total dissociation, and Paul was neither able nor willing to give ideas in movement, though his expression and character (in whistling and being the non-cooperative, avoidant member of the group) were accepted, tolerated and heard by the dance movement therapist and co-worker, and was felt to be important for group members, one of whom always noticed his absence and mentioned if he missed a session.

Common issues

On this particular day, anger and repressed feelings, as well as fears for physical safety in the hospital, were the primary focus. The group received the message that their anger and frustration were understood and were legitimate, though expressions of anger by hitting people (as the assault incident) or by blaming others (as Mike attempted to do with Lewis) were not acceptable ways of managing anger. Robert gained a lot by being curtailed, and Jeff, whom staff found often 'unreachable', did get a lot of his communications clarified and validated by the group. Though his membership always felt tenuous, he occasionally felt – and was certainly remembered by the group – as part of the group, despite gross deficits in social communication and masses of delusional muttering and confusion.

Mike gained a great deal in being of practical use to the group, in tasks like setting up chairs. Both Ruth and Alice gained respect for their kindness and the maternal atmosphere they created at times. All of the members benefited from being remembered and cared about by others, whether it was simply noting that someone looked smart, or had been to the hairdresser or barber, or that someone had done something amusing or interesting for the group.

In the early stages of the group some members lived on single-sex wards, and at that point it provided a valuable forum for getting used to mixing with the opposite sex. Gains can be assumed to be made by members' improved capacity to initiate, create and lead their own group movements. This was new for all the patients, and some said they liked not being spoon-fed ideas or themes, or treated like they 'can't do anything'. Additionally, though it is often not explicitly stated, loneliness and isolation are a problem for these patients, and the nonverbal group synchrony seems to alleviate this on a primary level at least.

Further issues that emerged in movement and discussion for this group were fears of the outside world, combined with desires to leave or remain at the hospital, and recollection or explanation to others about the incidents that led to their hospitalization in the first place. Some members, like Jeff and George, had no evident recollection of why they were in hospital, though Mike, Robert and William all shared their stories with the group after about fourteen months. The men were able to use strong movement, and to discuss their previous working lives and their experiences of serving in the war, which somehow gave them a measure of respect and regard that the younger members of the group (such as Lewis and Debbie) had not recognized before, and which altered both the student nurses' and the dance movement therapist's view of the patients.

Towards three-quarters of the way through the eighteen-month period in which the group was run, one of the members died, and the group, after a wobbly period of threatened dissolution or fragmentation, were able to discuss, very simply and not at extended length, their own fears of death, and wonderings about whether anyone would think of them when they died. The group survived a number of ward and staff changes and reorganizations of planning for community living, and members were able to express extremely negative and tentatively positive feelings about leaving the hospital, which they might otherwise have been unable to do in the context of expressing their feelings to other staff, all of whom were directly involved and invested in the resettlement programmes. Groups preceding holiday periods were predictably chaotic or flat, and there was some regression after breaks, and a return to more ritualized behaviour. The high value that the group placed on the activity was shown in the last day, when they organized, with the help of the student nurse, tea and cake for the last session (buying biscuits and sharing cigarettes from their meagre funds). They also told the student nurse and dance movement therapist that other patients were envious or curious about their participation in the group. It was hoped that they might be less fearful of making new relationships in community life, given their extended and generally positive experience of group DMT.

RELATIONS WITH THE INSTITUTION

Groups of this type cannot be run without cooperation and positive regard for the work by nursing, occupational therapy and psychiatric staff. Staff feedback was crucial, both in giving information on events in patients' lives, or changes in their mental state, and in receiving information, such as insights into patients, which emerged from the group. The opportunity to discuss emotional strains in working with deluded long-term patients was valued by ward staff, and sometimes a new way of handling a patient's particular problem emerged from these discussions between the dance movement therapist and nurses.

The resettlement team met frequently to discuss the group's progress, which was very useful for staff involved with planning, since they did not have much patient contact. These meetings also helped the dance movement therapist keep the group identity in mind, and reinforce the idea that these isolated individuals did function as a unit, at least from time to time. Staff who saw videotaped examples from the group were surprised at how much patients could initiate, when given the structure in which to do so, and some expressed interest in using exercise type warmups to precede their community and ward meetings, because it was seen to make the patients appear more focused and alert and more engaged in listening and speaking. Many became aware of how distortions in nonverbal presentation of their patients (seen on video) were a drawback in communication, and, once an awareness of things like eye contact, orientation and proximity were noted, some staff said they tried harder to get the patients to 'look a bit more normal' or look 'more with it' by initiating eye contact, using touches on the arm, and being more clear themselves in beginning and ending interactions with patients, rather than chatting while walking past, or standing behind a patient.

CONCLUSION

There is no doubt that running DMT groups for long-term patients requires persistence and a great deal of energy and optimism over an extended time period. The stresses are great in terms of the mental struggle to treat the group as a group, rather than a series of dissociated individuals. However, this conscious structuring and containment of the group identity, and a belief in its potential functioning, do pay off in the long run, as patients do make gains in interaction, self-initiation, and do share more of themselves with others and with the dance movement therapist, co-worker and nursing staff.

In working for extended periods with the same group of patients, it is possible to acquire a certain fondness, admiration and appreciation for these extraordinary people who have struggled for so long with quite debilitating mental illnesses, who have lived for several decades in mental hospitals, and who are courageously facing re-entry into community life. The task of running long-term groups is arduous but rewarding, provided that it is understood that 'supervision, personal therapy, and peer support from others who recognize these countertransference threats are critical for the dance therapist's own professional growth and self-esteem' (Sandel 1980: 31). As is the case with verbal group psychotherapy approaches, dance movement therapy can make a valuable contribution to the rehabilitation of long-term patients:

> through interpersonally focused treatment, patients may develop a greater capacity to achieve and tolerate closeness, and may begin to overcome the isolation, depression, and meaninglessness that has pervaded their lives.
>
> (Kahn 1984: 152)

Chapter 8

DMT in child and family psychiatry

INDIVIDUAL DMT WITH CHILD PSYCHIATRIC PATIENTS

In child psychiatry units the dance movement therapist will encounter children and adolescents with a wide variety of developmental, behavioural and emotional disturbances (American Psychiatric Association 1987: 39). Quite commonly, work in this area includes patients who have been sexually abused, as well as those suffering physical, emotional and psychological abuse or neglect. Children may or may not be in foster care while they are under the treatment of a child psychiatry team, and they are generally seen as outpatients. Child psychiatry clients may also include children whose parents are alcoholic or mentally ill, and who are therefore less well equipped to deal with the disturbances that their children may manifest. Most commonly, individual DMT with children is undertaken concurrently with monitoring and periodic therapeutic input of the child and the family by a child psychiatrist and social worker or educational psychologist. The child and his or her family may also be attending weekly or fortnightly family therapy.

A smaller percentage of child patients may be manifesting more serious psychiatric disorder, personality disorder, or possibly schizophrenia. There is some debate as to whether schizophrenia exists in childhood, and the diagnostic label is not often applied. In adolescents, outpatients or inpatients who have suffered sexual abuse, eating disorders such as anorexia or bulimia, as well as depression and early psychotic episodes are common. Conduct disorders, manifested in aggressive outbursts, truancy and violence, are also encountered. Recent studies illustrate that the prognosis for outcome of psychiatric disorders in children who receive treatment is good, with conduct-disordered children having the least favourable outcome, and emotionally disturbed children a promising outcome (Esser *et al.* 1990). Current studies also indicate that, given public concern about child sexual abuse, many abused children now being seen in child psychiatry units might previously only have been able to seek psychiatric treatment in adulthood (Bentovim *et al.* 1989, Shearer *et al.* 1990, Swett *et al.* 1990).

It should be mentioned that there is quite a bit of work being done using dance movement therapy with children outside the psychiatric setting, e.g. in mainstream and special education, and in community health and social services facilities. This work – with autistic, mentally or physically handicapped or otherwise emotionally disturbed or handicapped children who are not seen by psychiatric services – lies beyond the scope of this book, but is described in other publications (Kornblum 1982, Leventhal 1980, Payne 1991).

A child is usually referred to a child and family therapy or psychiatry centre by a general practitioner, teacher, social worker, or by his or her parents, foster parents, or guardians. The child is generally assessed by the psychiatrist and another team member, who may be a social worker, family therapist, child psychotherapist, child psychologist, community psychiatric nurse, play therapist, arts therapist, occupational therapist, or health visitor. If the child is thought to be one who would benefit from therapy, and if therapeutic resources are available, a short- or longer-term contract is usually made for the child to attend weekly individual therapy or group therapy, as part of the assessment and treatment plan.

DMT versus child psychotherapy

The aims of DMT with child psychiatry patients differ both from those of child psychotherapy and play therapy, though the aims of all three are, very broadly speaking, similar. In play therapy, a large number of toys are used so that the child can produce symbolic stories, which are interpreted by the therapist as indicative of the child's emotional difficulties or attempt to recover from trauma. The therapist may or may not choose to share his or her interpretation with the child. The stories are commented on by the play therapist, who supports the child's endeavours to make sense of his or her experiences. Play therapists often train initially as occupational therapists, and follow this training with two years of play therapy training.

In contrast, child psychotherapy, or psychoanalytic child psychotherapy, at least as practised by graduates of the training institutes of the Association for Child Psychotherapy in Britain, may be Freudian, Jungian or Kleinian in orientation. Their aim is to work in the transference, in order to effect a restructuring of the child's personality. The child may be seen two or three times a week over a period of a year or several years, and the treatment is therefore quite intensive. The child has the time and space to replay infantile and childhood interaction with the psychotherapist, who is trained to use his or her responses to the child as indicators of the child's inner world. The child may play with toys, a small number of which are provided, but the psychological relationship is the primary focus of therapeutic change (Gavshon 1989). The child psychotherapist has an extensive understanding of models of personality development, ego defence mechanisms, unconscious phenomena such as splitting and projective identification as described by Melanie Klein (Segal 1964). Child psychotherapy postgraduate training is five years or more in length, which allows for the psychotherapist to work in an intensive manner with a variety of children, many of whom suffer quite alarming levels of disturbance and deprivation (Boston and Szur 1983).

In DMT with children, the primary aim is to use movement as a symbolic communication of the child's current emotional difficulties. By understanding and addressing these difficulties, the child can better cope with his or her anxiety, and so reduce the level of behavioural disturbance (Delaney 1973). A second major aim is reflecting, mirroring and labelling the child's behaviour to encourage more appropriate interaction, and to begin to repair damaged parent–child relationships. Finally, DMT with child psychiatry patients focuses on movement experience as a way to repair body image and body ego (Goodill 1986, Leatherbee and Wood 1984). Furthermore, the dance movement therapist can assess the child's developmental body movement, and make hypotheses and observations on the child's psychological state based on the child's nonverbal behaviour (Kaplan-Westbrook and Sing 1988).

DMT is less intensive than child psychotherapy and usually functions as an adjunct to psychiatric, family therapy, education and social work input into a case. DMT is more focused on interpersonal functioning and may address primitive or preverbal psychological experience (Goodill 1987: 62). The interactional focus distinguishes DMT from play therapy: this is partly because there are fewer toys in the room, and because the dance movement therapist is sensitive to developmental aspects of the child's behaviour. In practice, the child's capacity to form a therapeutic alliance with the dance movement therapist, and to express his or her difficulties through movement and words (via metaphor or imagery), are central concerns in DMT with children.

Work with children using movement can be physically as well as emotionally exhausting; dance movement therapists must receive supervision and support from a qualified dance movement therapist in order to function effectively. After graduation, dance movement therapists may have supervision from child psychotherapists, to extend their understanding of disturbed children's psychological and behavioural dysfunction. In this respect, DMT with children is more accurately termed 'therapeutic work' (i.e. psychotherapeutically informed therapeutic work) than 'psychotherapy' proper, because of the intensity and duration of DMT work with child patients, and because of the relative length of the DMT training compared with that of the child psychotherapist.

In conclusion, dance movement therapists who work as part of a treatment team can provide important opportunities for therapeutic work with children for whom verbal communication is limited, or for whom conventional approaches are ineffective. The dance movement therapist working in a child psychiatry team can usefully help to sensitize other members of the team to the nonverbal elements of parent–child, or therapist–child, interaction.

Case illustration

This section will describe work with a 6-year-old boy who was seen in individual dance movement therapy for a period of nine months by the present author. 'Matthew' was referred by his GP, after his foster mother and teachers became unable to deal with his temper tantrums. He would throw objects around, hit out, and often inflict painful bites on his caretakers. He was an attractive child, of stocky build, with dark hair cut short and spiky, and green eyes. He was failing to make appropriate academic gains, and was disruptive at school and at home. His younger sister had recently disclosed to a teacher that she had been sexually abused by someone known to the previous foster carers, and, following a two-year social services and police investigation, the children were taken into long-term foster care with different foster parents with a view to adoption. Much of the therapy centred on Matthew's wish for the adoptive family to appear. Matthew's natural parents were unable to care for him and his sister, and they were assessed as being educationally subnormal. Social work rehabilitation of the parents was attempted, but was ultimately unsuccessful. As a result, both children had spent frequent periods in temporary foster care as infants, before being placed for adoption.

The sessions were held in a small consulting room, which contained a desk, three chairs and two cupboards. Toys were kept to a minimum; some dance movement therapists use no toys at all, because playing with toys can become a way to avoid interaction with the therapist, particularly if the toys are electrical or mechanical or if there are large number of them. This child was provided with a small box of his own toys, containing paper, coloured felt-tip pens, scissors, glue, some ribbon, a set of plastic Playmobil dolls about three inches in height, including a mother, father, two children and two grandparent figures, a set of plastic wild animal figures, and a set of farm animals of the same type, approximately to the same scale as the people, a few fences, also the same scale, and two cuddly toys, one a little rabbit with a cute expression and one a lion with a slightly ferocious expression. There were some hand puppets on the window sill of the room and three smallish Lycra stretch cloths and a wool blanket in a corner of the room. About three-quarters of the way through therapy he requested a large cardboard box in which he could sit, and some party balloons, which were provided.

Movement quality

In the first session, Matthew burst into the room, displaying an extraordinary lack of organization and integration in movement. He was quite ungrounded, in terms of the weight element, and was very indirect in space, being so multi-focused that he was chaotic. He used quickness in time, and only with difficulty could he do tasks that required fine motor coordination or care or patience, and therefore sustainment in time. He had a mixture of free and bound flow; his torso was held while his arms often flopped about. He was literally 'all over the place' and the confusion and exhaustion felt by the dance movement therapist was probably also a reflection of Matthew's own inner state.

Initial reaction

The first session consisted largely of a game in which he hid in the closet, and then behind the curtains. The dance movement therapist asked him if he might show his face, but he said 'No!'; he was giggly and nervous and was clearly anxious about being with an unknown adult in a room. He then began to make noises, which sounded like a phantom or a ghost. He was asked if he were a ghost, and he replied, 'Ooohhh. Mr Ghost won't come out.' He was then asked whether he was perhaps afraid of the dance movement therapist, to which he yelled, 'Yyyes! Mr Afraid-y ghost what's all scared.' This behaviour clearly illustrated not only his lack of trust, but his active fear of adults, whom he assumed would be mean to him. Several months later he said, 'Big people is all the same. NOOO good!' The dance movement therapist related this statement to other things he had said about his life, or which were known by the child psychiatrist and recorded on his file, and included issues like: the number of foster mothers and fathers he had had; the behaviour of the man who had hurt and upset his sister; and his belief that he was fundamentally too awful and unloveable for any parents to want to keep him.

Non-directive technique

After a few sessions, he slowly emerged, and took up the offer of helping him to understand how he was feeling and why he got angry sometimes. On the whole, the sessions were quite non-directive; his lead-in play was followed, and movement games or activities were not initiated; the dance movement therapist did not play with him unless he requested it. However, the dance movement therapist often verbally, or nonverbally, reflected his behaviour: for example, if he was unable to settle to a game, a comment was made such as: 'It seems you're not sure what you want to do today; what would you like to do first?' Sessions always began with his coming into the room and getting his little box of toys from the cupboard, and ended with summarizing what had been done in the sessions, while he sat with a drink of orange squash and a biscuit. These little beginning and ending rituals were important markers to enclose the session.

As therapy progressed, he made up stories, or fantasies, in which he would use the dance movement therapist, sometimes as an extra pair of hands, to paste, hold, cut or arrange something and, later, as a more cooperative person in his games. This indicated a shift in his relationship to the dance movement therapist; initially she functioned as an extension of himself, an object of convenience, and only later was valued as a helpful figure from whom separation was a sad and anger-provoking event. Being able to withstand his chaos was important; it took several months of simply reflecting to him that he seemed to be in a muddle, or in a mess about how he felt (about his current foster parents, and his previous foster parents and his natural parents, and his adoptive parents) before he recognized that he was being understood. He was gradually able to share his quiet, sad moments as well as his very direct and forceful anger with the dance movement therapist, which meant that he did not have to rush around in a disorganized way in order to avoid interaction and feelings.

He often played games of hide and seek, from which he would emerge, giggling. He was very upset if the dance movement therapist happened to be looking the other way when he emerged; somehow, being seen after a period of absence was a way of confirming that she was still holding him in her mind – a way of affirming his existence. The replaying of early mother–child interaction in movement is a common occurrence in DMT with individual children. Before holiday periods he would regress to being more disorganized, playing hide and seek, or being the ghost again. It would seem that, having found a figure who was able to manage his periods of destruction, sadness and confusion, he was not keen to separate from her.

Being dropped and being emotionally held

As therapy progressed, he was more adventurous in movement, and in asking the dance movement therapist to do things with him or for him. He went through a phase of enjoying jumping off chairs, or leaning forward and falling onto the floor. Sometimes he would give a warning, 'Mmmm gonna jump', but often he did not, so that he was barely caught in time. This sense of being in danger, of falling without security, seemed a good movement symbol for how he felt, being between foster parents and adoptive parents, and having been quite literally 'dropped' by his parents in the sense that they were unable to provide him with basic emotional or physical care. Many child psychiatry patients are often interested in falling and being caught, or running into a stretch cloth and being caught by that. It may be useful to think of this as a concrete movement illustration of an attempt to master what D. W. Winnicott conceived of as a primitive or infantile catastrophic anxiety about falling for ever, or falling to pieces (Winnicott 1958). This is related to a failure of the maternal caretaker to assist the child in feeling secure, or 'held' both physically and psychologically. The repetition of this game, and the intense satisfaction gained from the reliability of the therapist to catch the child, may therefore be behavioural support for Winnicott's conceptualization of personality development (Melville-Thomas 1988).

Low self-esteem

In one session, Matthew's fragile sense of self-esteem was revealed. He had been jumping, in a more focused way than in the previous sessions, which he associated with being strong. Suddenly, he jumped inside the blue plastic box which served as the rubbish bin. This did not seem an act of mischief, as he stood in the bin, looking very serious. The dance movement therapist asked him what he was doing in there, to which he replied, 'Me is rubbish too.' She attempted to correct this self-image by explaining that children who had been hurt by people often thought they were dirty, or bad, or ugly, but that this wasn't the case; it wasn't their fault that these things had happened, though they often felt responsible. He stared at the dance movement therapist for a while, and then began to talk about his previous foster home, where the foster mother had suffered a heart attack. He mumbled about his knowing why, and it seemed that he felt in some way responsible for the woman's illness. The dance movement therapist asked him if he felt that her illness had anything to do with him, and he told her quite seriously that he had done it (implying that he had killed her), and that's why they sent him (and his sister) away. The dance movement therapist clarified for him again that although the woman had been ill, it hadn't been his fault; it was something inside her, and not something he had done. She added that she was sure he wouldn't have been sent away. Children often have omnipotent fantasies in which they attribute external events to their own disavowed wishes or destructive impulses (Daws and Boston 1981, Segal 1964). In this instance, Matthew looked at the dance movement therapist, was quiet for a moment, and then jumped out of the bin, and said, 'Good things now', and sat down to find some crayons to make a picture. This radical shift from the serious to the frantic, and separation of nice versus nasty, was typical of his behaviour in the sessions, particularly those in which some past emotional problem was addressed.

Pretending to be dead

In another session, about three-quarters of the way through therapy and after adoptive parents had been found, Matthew had been telling the dance movement therapist that he had been on a day outing with his foster parents and their natural children, and he said they told him that he would spend next Christmas with his new mother and father. Then he proceeded to fall down onto the floor and pretend to be dead. In his hand he held a ruler which he pretended was stabbed into his stomach. The expression on his face and his stillness, in contrast to his usual highly active presentation, were a rather chilling sight. The dance movement therapist labelled his movement behaviour, saying that he looked very still, and might be injured. 'Noooo . . . dead!' he corrected. She expressed her sadness and concern, and wondered aloud how he had got injured, and if he maybe felt a bit dead sometimes, or a bit terrible about all the things that happened to him. He couldn't really keep a straight face, and started to giggle soon after this. He said, 'Better now', and got up and looked around the room for something to do next. The dance movement therapist wondered what sort of emotional death or injury he might be trying to communicate, or whether he was testing out the dance movement therapist's reaction to his being unwell. Much later she wondered if he was trying to tell her something about how he felt about the loss of his foster parents, to whom he was quite attached (and of whom he had been speaking a moment before his mock 'death') or perhaps something about the therapy ending, and his starting a new life with his adoptive parents.

It is difficult with children to know whether one's attempts at explaining feelings really get through. Often it takes some repeating of the idea, possibly at the next moment when the theme or issue emerges again, to be certain they have heard at all. Sometimes, several weeks after one has explained something, the child will repeat it, verbatim, even when one has been sure it hasn't been of use to the child, or one is convinced that the child did not hear it at all. For some children, one doesn't know if one has got through; it has, in such instances, to be assumed that a positive relationship to an adult functions as a 'corrective emotional experience'

(Winnicott 1958). This is particularly important for children who have been abused by adults in the past, and whose self-esteem is quite low, and trust in adults very fragile. Generally, if children feel the therapist understands something of their problems, their behaviour will lose altogether or diminish in its frantic quality, and they will interact more effectively, and get down to the business of playing out what is worrying them, in the hope that by repeating it, they might come to terms with their problem or experience. Often deprived children will yell or scream at therapists throughout the sessions; explaining to them that the dance movement therapist is listening, and that he or she can hear and understand what the children need, will usually reduce this loudness a little.

In a session near the end of the therapy, Matthew took the ribbon and some string and proceeded to knot and loop the chairs and desk together; he then wanted to tie the dance movement therapist's feet and hands to the chair. It seemed to her that he was trying to make connections between all the various things in the room, which was a contrast to his previously chaotic, fragmented and sometimes destructive use of materials. It is generally not a good idea for dance movement therapists to allow themselves to be tied up with string, stretch cloths, or other objects; although the child may imagine that he or she has power over the adult, this must remain on the level of fantasy and not be allowed to be the real situation, otherwise the child will become anxious at being given so much power. Furthermore, it is necessary to ensure the physical safety of the child, as well as that of the dance movement therapist. In addition to not tying up the dance movement therapist, usually the only rules are that the child should not hurt himself or herself, the therapist, or wilfully damage the room and its contents. In this instance, the dance movement therapist chose to verbalize the behaviour; it seemed he was trying to secure things, and tie them down, and she used her feeling to offer the idea to the child that: 'Perhaps you would like to be able to keep me here, because you don't want me to go away.' This brought a dark glance from Matthew, and he began to tighten the string around the chair in which the dance movement therapist was sitting.

Taking the child's worries seriously

In another session, when he knew that he would meet his adoptive parents quite soon, Matthew announced that he was in a 'bad bad mood'. He began to tear some drawings he had in his box, and he tore up a paper that had both his name and the dance movement therapist's written on it. He took the scissors and said he wanted to cut some of the dance movement therapist's hair and throw it out of the window. He threw the chair cushions and stretch cloths around the room, haphazardly, but not too destructively. She asked if he felt that everything was all over the place, or in a mess, and he said he was meant to meet his new Mummy and Daddy, whom he termed his 'forever family' on Sunday, but now it wouldn't be until after that. The dance movement therapist found out later that it had been delayed by a week, but to Matthew this seemed an intolerably long delay. She said she could imagine how much he wanted to meet them, and that he must be very disappointed. He sat down in a corner, as far away from her as possible, and covered himself with a blanket, and curled up. Here, it is important to note that the role of the dance movement therapist is not to offer reassurance, but to take the child's feelings and worries seriously.

Narrated play

He then made the noise of a telephone, and said he was dialling 999. He asked for an 'ambleeeance'. The dance movement therapist asked if he needed rescuing, to which he replied, 'No!' in an annoyed voice. He then told her that she lived in Australia, and he was calling her on the telephone. She asked if she were really so far away from him, and he didn't reply, but peeked out from the blanket, as though to make sure she was nearby.

As was often the case, he would narrate a story, which would be enacted using movement. He put his head out from under the blanket and said, 'I'm all tired, like, 'cause I just came back from a long aventure; and then you come, and give me oranges, and squash and all chocolate cake, and that puppet over there [his lion he had thrown into the corner] and all presents like Santa Claus.' The dance movement therapist proceeded to mime out these actions, commenting that it must have seemed like he was on a very long journey until the forever family would come to get him, to which he replied 'long, long long', and hid the lion under the blanket with him. The dance movement therapist sat down not far from him, and said that she thought he might be wondering if his new Mummy would be feeding him and taking care of him, and wondering what she might be like. He looked over suspiciously, and hid under the blanket again, making noises pretending to eat and enjoy the imaginary food that the dance movement therapist had just given to him. It seemed clear that he was working on his anxieties about meeting his new adoptive parents, and enacting his good fantasies about them taking care of him. The fact that he had mentioned them in the session that day allowed the dance movement therapist to feel reasonably confident that verbal comments on the source of his behaviour were accurate; this was corroborated by some of his reactions, such as looking directly at the dance movement therapist, and continuing the story without correcting her.

Endings and leavetakings

About eight weeks before the end of the therapy, he requested that he be given a large box, and some balloons. He was very creative in using this box as a television set (in which he used his stuffed toys as characters and played out a drama of 'goodies and baddies'); then it became a rocket that would take him far away from everything, and later, with crayon designs, balloons and ribbon attached, it became a boat and then an airplane.

He demanded to be pushed around the edges of the room, while seated in his box, with the dance movement therapist playing the engine, or the navigator and the map reader, as well as the airplane repair crew in case of accidents and emergencies. He imagined that the plane was going to Australia, Disneyland, and to the area of England where he knew his adoptive parents lived. He was able to journey, in his imagination, to see the place where he would live, and be variously delighted and frightened by it, sometimes asking what the dance movement therapist thought about it, asking if it would be all right, and other times relieved that if he was afraid, he could fly (literally by moving backwards) to return to an imagined home base and the security of the sessions. Difficult as it was not to be reassuring to him, the fantasies that he had about big dogs and monsters and ghosts coming out of his new house, did enable him to master, to a degree, his fears about the possibility that his new parents might be abusive, or might reject him.

The box, as a container for him, distanced him from the dance movement therapist in nonverbal terms, which was a useful way of expressing his separation. During the last few weeks he was variously sad, or denying, or angry when the ending of therapy was mentioned. In the second to last session the dance movement therapist presented him with an illustrated story she had written about the therapy, which used a lot of his descriptions and symbolism: it described how he had arrived as a ghost who was afraid of the therapist, and had been angry sometimes but had survived this, and described his long wait and adventures in hoping for a forever family, adding that he could remember the therapy as a time of sorting out some of his feelings. This was intended as an adjunct to the life-story work he had done with his social worker. Often, if therapy is to be successful, it must address the issue of separation fairly intensively, as it is a major developmental task in a child's life (Bowlby 1988: 137).

Gains during therapy

In conclusion, the gains of therapy can be summarized by saying that, in movement terms, his behaviour had become slightly more organized, though he regressed in the last few sessions under the strain of meeting his new parents, and in the sadness and anger over the loss of the therapy time. He was able to make eye contact, and was able to orient himself in space to two or three activities instead of being all over the place. Primarily, he developed a relationship with an adult that was largely positive, which hopefully went a little way to repairing his lack of trust in adults, and his belief that he was just 'rubbish'. He was able to stop himself from biting the dance movement therapist on one occasion, and the fact that she survived his angry attacks made him aware that some adults could be stable figures for him in his memory and his day-to-day life. In this instance, work about his previous sets of foster parents, and sorting out an emotional narrative of his life, helped him to gain a sense of who he was and how he got there. In therapy with children, one often does a small piece of work, which is appropriate only to the specific developmental level at which the child is functioning, or capable of attaining. For Matthew, the arrival of caring, adoptive parents was ultimately therapeutic; in conjunction with an excellent social worker, and ideas gained from dance movement therapy with him, they were able to manage and understand his outbursts to the point that, five months after adopting him, his tantrums had drastically reduced in frequency and severity.

Issues around fear of adults, suspecting retaliatory attacks from them (presumably in response to the child's anger and frustration with them) as well as, and wishes for, affection and nurturance from adults, are common in the therapeutic relationship with disturbed children (Hopkins 1986, 1987). Other typical issues in this work are: dealing with the child's low self-esteem, guilt and confusion about past foster family breakdowns, as well as symbolic statements about being dead, being injured and being rescued. These children tend to provoke in the dance movement therapist the responses that they expect from the imaginary parents they form in their minds, constituted from past experiences or from compensatory fantasies. This means that the therapist has to deal with being an object of both enormous terror and tremendous affection. This necessitates regular supervision, either by a qualified dance movement therapist or by a child psychotherapist, as well as peer support, and possibly individual therapy for the dance movement therapist in order to be able to be clear about whose emotional issues are being dealt with in the therapeutic work. Finally, good and supportive working relationships with other child psychiatry team members and the social worker and parents or foster parents involved, help the ideas gained from the therapeutic work to be most usefully employed by the entire system of caretakers and professionals who are involved with the child.

DMT GROUPS WITH CHILD PSYCHIATRIC PATIENTS

This section will provide some theoretical background to DMT groups with disturbed children. It will also consider the practical aspects of group work, such as the selection of children for a group, appropriate space and equipment, the benefits of a co-worker, and the therapeutic aims. Similarities between overall aims of DMT and those of verbal child group psychotherapy will be mentioned, with specific reference to using the child's nonverbal behaviour to achieve therapeutic goals. These include facilitating emotional expression, improving relations with peers, repairing trust in adults, recapitulating family dynamics, and recovering from the trauma of abuse. The theory section is followed by a detailed case illustration which describes the material from a DMT group for children with various presenting problems including sexual abuse, physical abuse and neglect.

Group composition

Group members may be selected from a range of child psychiatry referrals, as described at the beginning of the section on individual child psychiatry. Groups are most useful for children with specific difficulties in relating to peers and to adults. Groups are suitable for most sexually abused children, provided they are not too withdrawn or fragile, and that they do not find sexualized behaviour of other children too threatening or upsetting. As described in the theory section in Chapter 3, many different types of group therapy theory approaches can be applied to DMT with adults, and the same is true for children. For example, some dance movement therapists may do therapeutic work aimed at dealing with the trauma of sexual abuse, along the lines of specialized groups described by the Great Ormond Street Team (Bentovim *et al.* 1989). This way of working may be appropriate to the institutional setting in which the child is seen, as usually a group is formed from a group of patients with an identified need. Time-limited groups which run parallel to the school term are useful; children may be able to deal with anxieties about coming together as a group if they know the group has a limited duration. A reasonable time limit would be twenty or thirty sessions, or perhaps a full school year, though groups can go on profitably for longer periods.

There are various theories on whether groups should be of single or mixed gender, with most therapists favouring a mixed group. Depending on the level of disturbance of the children, a good number of children to include in a group is four or five. This is because if the group consists of only three children and two co-workers, there tends to be one child pairing with each of the co-workers, and one child excluded. However, with more disturbed children whose aggressive or destructive behaviour threatens the group, two children and two co-workers may provide a useful beginning. Usually groups of children are about the same age, but it is helpful to have a slight variation in age, so that there is not too much competitiveness between the children. Similarly, an optimal group would be a mixture of higher and lower functioning children, with some extrovert and some introvert in their presentation. With a mixed composition, the group resembles a family rather than a bunch of competitive siblings (Reid *et al.* 1981: 35).

Practical considerations

It is necessary for the dance movement therapist to have a co-worker for many of the same reasons as described in adult work earlier in Chapter 5. Further reasons in child work include the fact that the co-worker can help physically contain the more disruptive children, or attend to a particularly withdrawn or tentative child. He or she can also provide essential information on the child's behaviour in other settings, and aid in the organizing of feedback to other agencies, transportation of the children to and from the sessions, and preparation for the group. The co-worker should be briefed by the dance movement therapist on what he or she intends to do with the group, the directive or non-directive tone to set, and how to participate by taking the child's lead, rather than directing or teaching the child. The co-worker is a useful second set of eyes who can see things that are easily missed in the lively activity of the group.

The group room must remain constant throughout the life of the group, and should be private, quiet, and not contain anything breakable. This physical security illustrates to the children that the intensity of their feelings can be contained, and their angry attacks survived (Reid *et al.* 1981: 59). In the experience of the present author, a smallish, carpeted room, containing little or no furniture, is most comfortable.

Props

Props can be introduced at various points, but toys should not become the focus of the group. The aim is to use individual and group movement behaviour to express feelings and build relationships with peers and adults. Having as many stretch cloths as there are children is a good idea; these can function for many things: blankets, tug-of-war ropes, batman capes, flowing robes, ghost costumes; they can be made into camps or tents to hide under; or be used to hold or swing a child in a hammock fashion, etc. One very long stretch cloth, three metres or more in length and one and a half metres wide, is useful, especially if it is large enough to enable the therapist and co-leader to hold either end of it and for the whole group of children to run into it and be caught, or bounced back gently.

In more structured groups, props to assist children to illustrate how they are feeling can be useful. In one group, children began, seated in a circle, to tell one good thing and one bad thing that had happened during their week, and then rated their week out of ten. A series of cards with clown faces on them, ranging from a big frown (0) to a big smile (10), with varying degrees of happiness or sadness in their expression, were used to help children get a concrete sense of how each of them felt in relation to the others. It also solved the difficulty of the children saying that they would rate their week 'minus a hundred' or 'two zillion trillion out of ten'. Although this was probably an accurate reflection of how awful or how happy they felt, it did not make it easy to summarize the state of the group, or compare group members' experiences. This introductory ritual often concludes with children trying to remember everyone's number – and so provides a good indicator of which children can really listen to others, and which are more egocentric, that is, seem to remember that everyone must be nearly the same as themselves.

Some children cannot share and compete for the props, or want to destroy them, which means that the dance movement therapist must ensure that things are not easily breakable; even very angry children get upset if they actually do destroy something that has been brought for the group's use. Depending on the inclination of the dance movement therapist, other props may be used – such as foam balls, large cardboard boxes, balloons, mural sized paper to do body outlines, soft or rough pieces of fabric, neon-coloured tulle or soft acetate cloth, masks, or other objects. Groups generally end with children being given a drink of juice while seated in a circle, enabling them, and the dance movement therapist and co-worker, to cool down. DMT with children is generally extremely active and energetic!

Rules about the physical safety of group members and leaders, and about the safe use of equipment, need to be clearly stated to the children, if not at the beginning of the group then certainly at the first appropriate moment. Understanding that they cannot hurt each other or the therapists, or damage the equipment, is usually enough in terms of rules, which should be brief and simple. It is crucial that the dance movement therapist and co-worker make the children stop and think about what they are doing when they are aggressive towards each other, otherwise a cycle of mindless and casual violence can infect a group. Children should be told to wear clothes that are suitable for physical activity, though gymnastics outfits are not necessary. Therapists must wear loose comfortable clothing, and are advised against wearing jewellery which may be pulled or broken in the course of catching, restraining, lifting, spinning, or otherwise physically interacting with a child.

Therapeutic aims

Aims of group DMT with children are consistent with those of child group therapy and structured group play therapy approaches which are predominantly verbal. Surprisingly little has been written on working with groups of children along psychodynamic lines, in either verbal psychotherapy or DMT literature, which may reflect the difficulty of the task. Children who have experienced their primary parental relationships as fraught with difficulty are sometimes hardly able to conceive of other children as separate people, let alone as useful allies or friends, or someone with whom it would be enjoyable to engage in interaction. In a sense, the task of the group is to get the children to feel like a group, rather than a few fragmented individuals, each wrapped up in a personal inner world. Teachers often report that disturbed children don't play, or don't know how to play, with each other. This describes the solitary activity, consistent isolation or brief aggressive contact in which such children are generally engaged.

The aims for group work with children include making gains in clarifying feelings that may lead to a change in behaviour. Psychologically, the group aims to allow the communications of the children to be heard, and response made to them – a model which closely resembles that of the sensitive caring parent the children have probably failed to find in their own home lives (Reid *et al*. 1981: 60). Repairing relationships with adults is a central task for abused children: gaining a sense that adults can understand them, can help organize their feelings, and contain their aggressive impulses is centrally important for those who have never experienced it.

Being held in the mind of an adult rather than dropped or ignored is something to which abused children respond gratefully. Many also need to experience the fact that when adults stop a child from doing things, they do so in the child's best interests, and not from a desire to punish or persecute the child. Dance movement therapists must be acutely aware of how they approach abused children in games; many will flinch or look frightened if approached too quickly, which illustrates in movement terms their expectation that adults mean to do them harm.

In groups, children will often attempt to divide the dance movement therapist and co-worker; they have little or no idea of a couple of adults cohesively or cooperatively acting in a situation, and the idea of adults being in relative harmony is often a new experience for children from violent homes.

Improving relations with peers is an important aim in group DMT, as it is to verbal work with groups of children. Acceptance by a group helps children's social adjustment to groups they will encounter later in school and working life. The group also recapitulates the family, and foster children, or children whose adoptive families have broken down, or those who feel they have been rejected, will often be assigned roles in a fantasized family in which they are appreciated and cared for. Through the reflective comments of the dance movement therapist and the co-worker, the children can begin to understand things about their behaviour which may have contributed to the breakdown of the family, or which mars their desire to relate to peers in a meaningful and successful way. Children can also replay family dynamics in a group which accepts and does not scapegoat, abuse or ignore them. Children are brutally honest about each other's behaviour, and, under the protective supervision of the therapist, the children can learn what it is about their behaviour that makes other children avoid them. Furthermore, groups of children with similar problems can help each child feel less socially isolated, less alone in his or her suffering, and less stigmatized, which is particularly relevant for sexually abused children.

Nonverbal dimensions in interaction

Perhaps the most important feature of DMT is that the dance movement therapist has a specialized training and sensitivity to the nonverbal element of the child's expression. Obvious though this may sound, it is a skill that verbal child group psychotherapists value and recognize. In *Child Group Psychotherapy: Future Tense*, the authors – two psychoanalytic child group psychotherapists – write that 'the nonverbal activity of the child gives access to his or her inner world. Asking children to express themselves verbally is like asking them to cure themselves' (Riester and Kraft 1986: 34–36). They underline the nonverbal dimension of therapy, adding that

> By making provision for nonverbal modes of communication that permit group members symbolically to test our understanding and acceptance, we create conditions that eventually make it possible for them to talk openly about their feelings and problems.
>
> Because we as therapists are fluent in verbal communication, we tend to assume that discussion groups will be easier to manage, or will produce deeper insights. In making this assumption, we forget that talk does not necessarily help us enter the inner world of the child, nor does insight directly address the developmental needs of children with serious deficiencies in ego development.
>
> (Riester and Kraft 1986: 35)

Chaotic movement

A major therapeutic aim of the group is to allow the children to express their feelings, fears and fantasies in a safe environment. As verbal group therapists have described it in their work, 'creative movement allows children to discharge feeling; repressed resentment and hostility can be discharged with impunity' (Riester and Kraft 1986: 15). This does not only mean the cathartic release of aggression, though this may be important also. The time to allow aggressive children to regress and show their vulnerable, dependent sides is an equally important form of emotional release.

Francizka Boas, in her early work at the Bellevue Psychiatric Hospital, noted that the children initially engaged in movement as 'mere self indulgence and chaotic behaviour', but after a period of discharging this energy they were 'able later to use the control and body quality gained through such experimentation for the formulation of fantasies' (Boas 1952: 261). This early chaotic phenomenon may be defensive, a sort of manic rushing about to avoid the anxiety that being in a group provokes, and to avoid feeling, as Esther Bick describes (Bick 1968). Riester and Kraft also note that

> The early behaviour of children in groups is usually helter skelter, children may fight, make demands, and be provocative and unreasonable. The acceptance of the feelings behind this behaviour, and the relative relaxation of rules (excepting those ensuring physical safety) makes the therapy situation one where the child's feelings are accepted, which in turn allows the energy to be canalized, and put to more purposeful behaviour.
>
> (Riester and Kraft 1986: 18)

It is important that the therapist be able to distinguish between the time when the group is spending its energy in a chaotic way – i.e. continuous movement is being used as a defence – and the time when the movement is being used therapeutically. It is probably the use of symbols (either through the use of spoken metaphor or expressive bodily gestures) that differentiates defensive from communicative movement. Furthermore, the phraseless and spatially fragmented quality of defensive movement can be seen and felt by the dance movement therapist, who has many hours' training in observing videotaped DMT with many sorts of patients. Finally, the feelings evoked in the dance movement therapist and co-worker, in a room full of chaotic children out of touch with their feelings, is often a clear indicator of what is happening for the group. Sometimes, if the movement material is very disturbing, and it appears that the child is actually *re-enacting* a traumatic experience rather than replaying it in the service of understanding it, a prop or toy may be introduced to provide some distance from the experience. Motor labelling, and describing to the child what is being done, may also help distance the child from the experience in order that it can be thought about, and its grip on the child's psyche lessened. Simply narrating what is happening, by saying, 'Everyone is running around all over the place' at least gives the child the sense that his or her chaotic state of mind is understood by the adults in the room.

The therapeutic aims of groups must be formed in response to the general types of problems children have, and in accordance with the specific issues that concern each new group of children. For example, with sexually abused children, some common general emotional issues might be: how to trust adults, and having boundaries (both emotional and physical) to protect oneself against the memory or the repetition of sexual abuse by an adult. Also, intrapsychic emotional issues may emerge, such as how to deal with the confusion, anger and excitement that are associated with the experience of abuse. Another goal is the reconstruction of an age-appropriate psychosexuality.

Aggressive behaviour

It is often observed that disturbed children are more chaotic and aggressive than children in mainstream schools who have probably not been abused. This fact relates to the child's previous experiences. How can abused children relate to others? Will they take on the role of the aggressor, in identification with their abuser, and therefore treat each new child they meet as an object of scorn to be kicked around aggressively so as to make themselves feel 'big' and in violent control of another? Or will they continually feel that everyone and everything is going to hurt them, that they are a victim and so be a waiting target, or someone who expects to be neglected, left out, or kicked around; someone with low self-esteem, not worth very much, and so easily swayed and taken advantage of by others? Perhaps the children will feel that they deserved to be abused, and that they therefore look for adults or other children who will hurt them or behave so badly or aggressively that they provoke vengeful attack from other children, or angry frustration from foster carers. Or will the children be completely unable to think about the experience of abuse, and split it off into some realm of unconsciousness, not to be unlocked? All of these are possible responses to the experience of sexual and physical abuse.

Clearly there are as many types of responses to abuse as there are underlying personalities that experienced the abuse. Each child responds to abuse differently. Other factors, such as whether the abuse was prolonged or took place in an otherwise loving relationship with a parent, or conversely was accompanied by neglect, are also important, as is the help the child receives once the abuse is disclosed. Many children feel responsible for breaking up their families, and, after disclosure and criminal charges, may lose the attention of social workers and therapists just when they need it most – when they need to reconstruct their fragmented lives, make sense of what has happened, and go on to new things (Melville-Thomas 1988).

It is important that a therapist, including the dance movement therapist, does not get involved in doing therapy with a child for the primary goal of getting a disclosure of the identity of the person who is supposed to have sexually abused that child. Police and social workers are keen to use therapist's knowledge of unconscious symbols, the trusting relationship he or she has built with the child, to gain access to information. Of course, if the dance movement therapist or other worker does receive a disclosure from a child, it must be taken to the psychiatrist or supervisor to discuss its implications. The dance movement therapist's role is to help the child deal with emotional disturbance, not to engage in disclosure work. The therapist can support and help the child through the period in which this work is being done by another agency, provided the therapist's role in the treatment of the child is clear to all concerned.

Working with sexually abused children is an emotionally and intellectually complex and exhausting process, and it is essential that the dance movement therapist is supervised and supported in this work. Most dance movement therapists working in this area acknowledge that personal therapy for themselves during the period of working with this patient group can help mitigate the emotional strain. Additionally, it is important that the co-worker be in sympathy with the overall aims of the group, so that the children perceive the dance movement therapist and co-worker as essentially in agreement about the expectations for the group. Therapy with abused children means that the children often regress, which can bring up very primitive infantile material. It is important that both dance movement therapist and co-worker are sufficiently aware of the infantile aspects of their personalities so that experiences of exhilaration, dependency, anger, rage and the intensity of both positive and negative feeling can enrich the group process rather than hinder it.

Case illustration

The following are a series of vignettes from a group, run by the author, with 7 to 10-year-old children. The group had four members, two girls and two boys (a fifth had been selected but had not been given permission by the courts to attend therapy). The boys, whom I shall call Brian and Paul, were aged 7 and 8, and the girls, Becky and Mandy, were 8 and 10¾ years old respectively at the time the group began. It was set to run for two school terms, and took place at a small special educational unit for emotionally and behaviourally disturbed children. The group was held in an interviewing room, emptied of furniture, with a one-way mirror and a video observation room behind this. The co-worker taught the children art, and was familiar with the children's classroom behaviour.

All of the children were in foster care at the time of the group. Brian was a thin boy with brown hair and large round blue eyes. He had been grossly neglected by parents who were not able to care for him; there was medical evidence to suggest he had been sexually abused by someone who was evidently known to the family. No criminal proceedings had been taken against the perpetrator of this abuse owing to lack of a clear disclosure or evidence. Brian was in long-term foster care and had developed a strong and positive attachment to his foster parents with whom he had lived for several years. Paul, a taller and stronger child, with red-blonde hair and green eyes, was in his third period of temporary foster care after his mother, who was prone to periods of mental illness, had requested that he be taken from her until she recovered enough to take Paul and his sister back to live with her.

Becky had been grossly sexually abused by her father, and presented as a dishevelled little girl with bright eyes hiding behind thick glasses; she was sorely lacking in confidence. After a period of three years in foster care, her ability to articulate her needs was markedly improved, and she and her sister were due to be adopted to a childless couple. She left the group in the middle of the second term, as it appeared that she was ready to be adopted sooner than had been expected. Mandy had been sexually abused by her step-father and had been taken into foster care at the request of her mother. She was engaged in disclosure interviews with a social worker during the first term of the group, which clearly upset her a lot, and meant that she was continually preoccupied with sexual issues and prone to a great deal of sexual acting out. In retrospect, she may have been a little too old for this particular group; she would break into wild, sexual dances in part imitation of pop videos she had seen on TV. The younger members of the group were frightened and fascinated by this, and attempted to imitate her movements as they thought this represented an entry into early adolescence. At the time of the group, Becky and Brian were also in individual therapy with a child psychotherapist, and Mandy received therapeutic input from a counselling psychologist as well as a social worker.

Beginning the group

This group met for an hour each week, and began with the children seated in a circle. This structure frequently broke down, with children rushing over to windows, banging doors, hitting walls, hitting each other and screaming, or jumping and leaping about wildly. It seemed very difficult for them to contain themselves once they knew the group was for movement; they wanted to get going. With great effort, the dance movement therapist and co-worker managed to get each child to say one good and one bad personal experience since the previous weekly meeting. They then rated their week out of 10, using a picture of a sad or happy clown painted on a card to illustrate this. Watching TV and going to the shops were high on the good list, and missing access with a parent or having fallen down or been punished for something featured on the bad list. Children were very reluctant, at first, to say that anything bad had happened to them during the week; they seemed to want to present great happiness and glee, as though to please the leaders of the group. Once permission was established to say sad or bad things (with a minimum of foul language) the children began to trust us enough to tell us about nightmares they had, or people whom they disliked or were afraid of.

Warmup

The group then proceeded with a directive movement warmup, led by the dance movement therapist. This movement warmup was directly focused on helping the children to master impulse control, and getting them weighted or grounded, particularly Brian and Becky. The warmup also aimed at reconstructing an appropriate body image, as well as enlarging movement range by using a sequence of changing qualities of movement derived from Laban's effort–shape choreographic system, as described in Chapter 4. The warmup also gave the children an experience of group synchrony and cohesion in both movement and feeling, which was something new for all of them.

The warmup sequence consisted of a number of things, including running as fast as you could and then stopping, in order to restore phrasing and self-control over endings in movement. We sometimes asked the children to say 'stop!' and 'go!' in this warmup, and, significantly, Mandy was unable to stop and wanted us to keep running until exhausted. This was typical of the way she used movement as a defence against thinking or feeling, and of how she lacked internal controls (Bick 1968).

The next part of the warmup was to go all floppy and then freeze. This aimed at reintegrating a whole-body rather than a part-body movement experience. For children who have been sexually abused, 'certain parts of their bodies may be given distorted importance and meaning' (Weltman 1986: 56). This leads to distortions in integrated movement, which whole-body exercises aim to address.

Another warmup exercise was swinging to a definite rhythm spoken by the dance movement therapist, such as 'swing, swing, *swing*' in order to get the children to use the effort element of weight. The children preferred 'stamp, stamp, *stamp*', which was a variation on this. Further warmups included touching body parts in a sequence, with a child leading the group, taken in turns. It was important that this be done slowly and thoughtfully enough not to turn into the well-known nursery school song 'head and shoulders, knees and toes', etc., the aim of which for the children seemed to be to do this as quickly and as thoughtlessly as possible. Accenting a different rhythm, and including such parts as ankles, helped avoid this. There were general giggles and obscenities when one boy did 'bottom' and 'thing' and stared at Mandy and Becky. We respected and clarified sexual difference, but tried not to make a fuss of it. There is always a danger that dance movement groups will provide an opportunity for sexual acting-out by the children, and this needs to be addressed directly and brought within normal limits rather than criticized, ignored or frowned upon, as might be the case in the classroom.

Finally, an effort–shape sequence was done, with narrowing, widening (horizontal plane), shrinking, rising (vertical plane) and advancing and retreating (sagittal or diagonal plane) being translated into 'be as wide as you can, as skinny as you can, as tiny as you can (curl up into a fetal position), as tall as you can (touch the ceiling), as full as you can, and creep back, or catch an imaginary beach ball', all serving as images to facilitate body movement in the horizontal, vertical and sagittal planes. The children showed their delight and surprise at mastering and experiencing these new movement sequences, at least in between their periods of running off, yelling and making fun of one another.

Modified structure in the process section

In terms of structure, this group always included a discussion, then the warmup, followed by a process section which attempted to get the children to participate in Chaceian shared leadership format, and address current group emotional issues.

This worked moderately well, though Mandy was sometimes unable to follow the movements of the other children, which led to the periodic collapse of this structure. In response to this, several times we put a stretch cloth down to divide the room into audience and performers, and allowed each child to make up a movement sequence that was variously referred to as 'starring in your own rock video' and 'doing your own dancing'. Innovations in structure in DMT for psychiatric patients (adults as well as children) in collaboration with dramatherapists is a new and interesting area that needs further study (Furman 1990, Higgens 1990, Johnson and Eicher 1990: 159).

On two occasions, after Becky had left the group to go to her new home and Mandy was away with 'flu, the two boys constructed their own games with the stretch cloth. The two sat or lay in it, with the dance movement therapist and co-worker each holding an end. They were rocked gently, and sang a song about being babies; then they demanded to be slid across the room while in the stretch cloth, hammock-style, which they called 'being in a fast car'. Another time they had the leaders hold the cloth between them as though it were a very low tennis net, while they ran forward into the net; they called this 'the bouncy game' or the 'catchy game'. It seemed that the presence of just the two boys alone allowed a more free structure in which they used the movement to stimulate fantasy and action, which the leaders could follow in movement and reflect in words. In general, keeping to any structure was difficult when there were four children in the group, but it did improve gradually, and provided a guided opportunity for interaction between some members, which otherwise would never have occurred naturally. For example, between Mandy and Brian, who completely ignored each other in the classroom and playground, the movement turn-taking structure allowed them to look at, mirror and enter into a nonverbal dialogue with another child.

DMT with children can take various forms besides the Chaceian one, depending on the degree of structure offered by the dance movement therapist. The degree of structure is a response to the children's level of disturbance, which affects their ability to control and contain their impulsivity, and engage in cooperative interaction. If DMT is to be therapeutic, rather than resembling dancing classes, there must be a creative forum in which the children can present and suggest whatever *they* like. Other DMT structures that are useful with children include: total improvisation (by addressing a theme, or solving a problem or task without planning), dramatic play, fantasy action, movement exploration, group synchronized rhythmic body action and pantomime which

> offers opportunities for working with half-danced, half-acted, imitations of real actions and events through experimenting with a mixture of impersonation, dramatic movement and dance using large bodily movements. It helps with establishing contact with reality and provides practice in the election of appropriate movements for expressing specific emotions or feelings.
>
> (Delaney 1973: 136)

In Francizka Boas's work with children she used a structure that she termed 'spontaneous dance'. She worked in conjunction with strong and steady percussive rhythms of drums and cymbals, and suggested animal imagery to children in order to 'stimulate and find expression for primitive and deeply buried fantasies, as well personal conflicts' (Bender and Boas 1941: 244). Boas wrote that spontaneous dance and music 'gives the individual the satisfaction of the expression of deep instinctual drives, of new inter-human contacts and of original aesthetic experiences' (Bender and Boas 1941: 244). She worked with music provided by a live accompanist or occasionally played by the children themselves, but on occasions where she did not use music, she noted that 'if there is no sound, space has to be filled with the dancer's thoughts, emotions and fantasies' (Boas 1952: 264). This parallels Alma Hawkins' view of music, which she sees as prompting movement that is not stimulated by an inner impulse, but merely by a predetermined rhythm to the music.

The use of music

In terms of groups with children, it is up to the dance movement therapist and co-worker whether they see music as an integral part of DMT or an accessory to it. In the group comprising Becky, Mandy, Brian and Paul, the music was not very helpful for a number of reasons: first, there was competition and argument over whose music would be played, then it was played so loudly that no one could hear what anyone else was saying, and the strong rhythmic pop music often took over the atmosphere of the group. However, in the very early sessions, moving (or jumping or hopping) together to a piece of music did serve to allow the children to have a sense of group cohesiveness, and lay the groundwork for their developing sense that they were not simply isolated individuals racing about at random, but could share in and enjoy synchronous movement.

Sexualized movement as a defence

However, and quite importantly, the music gave rise to Mandy half-imitating rock video dancing, but adding a highly sexualized and chaotic colouring, which in the end served as a sort of auto-erotic stimulation and so slipped into a wild, unthinking gyration that seemed almost 'autistic', so much in fact that it cut her off from the rest of the group. When she spoke about this experience of dancing, she described it as 'getting away and being blowed up'; it was clear that she was not able to use it to address how her experience of sexual abuse had distorted the development of her own sexuality and feminine identity, but rather, she was overwhelmed by sensation, such that thought or communication could not occur. The way she moved to the music did give clear illustration into the sorts of emotional conflicts she was grappling with; her body was literally fragmented, with the torso being sexualized and the rest of the body being haphazardly hurled about, disconnected from the centre. This sort of disconnected movement and emotional behaviour is consistent with observations and research into DMT with sexually abused children (Biggins 1989, Goodill 1987, Weltman 1986).

In terms of responding to Mandy's sexualized behaviour, we tried to accept and understand what prompted it, while not reinforcing it, and gently pointed out the other children's anxiety about the intensity of the movement. It was difficult to explain to her why such 'getting away' was not appropriate for the group, but she did gain some insight into the effect of her behaviour on others. Mandy's psychologist and the dance movement therapist had some fruitful discussions about her behaviour, in which the distinction between cathartic and defensive use of her 'dancing' and 'getting away' was clarified for the psychologist, who had assumed that the dancing was predominantly identification with the pop stars whom Mandy imitated. Mandy later became able to both regress and recapitulate phases of development to try to work through the traumatic experiences of sexual abuse.

Recapitulating traumatic experience in play

When Mandy and Becky were absent from the group, Brian and Paul elected to work without music, and this allowed a great deal of verbal imagery to accompany their movement, as well as better dialogue to be established about their movement behaviour, and the dance movement therapist's and co-worker's reflections and readings of what they were doing.

The group movement sessions allowed the children to explore emotional issues around aggression and sexuality, as well as to replay traumatic experiences. For example, in one group, from which Mandy was missing but the other three remained, Becky wanted to play a game in which she would be a baby. The leaders of the group, whom she labelled Mummy and Daddy, and Brian and Paul as her two brothers, would them come and get her from the hospital and take her home. This seemed to be about her imminent adoption, and whether she would be valued for herself or be seen as a baby whom the new adoptive parents would shape anew. She asked if her name would be the same, and whether she were a boy or a girl, and which was better. The group enacted her verbal fantasies in movement, using the stretch cloth to go and get her, and wrap her up. She often muttered to herself, 'Will it be alright?', 'Gonna be okay?'

Soon the boys regressed, and also wanted to be babies who were rescued, fixed up by the leaders, and carried in 'the green cot' which they renamed the green stretch cloth. The children shared the largest of the stretch cloths, and began to sing a mumbled version of 'rock-a-bye baby'. Here, they were replaying, in very concrete terms, an experience of nurturance, using the group leaders as stand-in parents. For most of them, care and nurturance in early life had been scarce, and this fantasy-movement sequence allowed for a symbolic gratification of early unmet emotional dependency needs. Themes such as nurturance, feeding, repair, renewal, rescue, fixing and the giving of gifts are common in work with deprived children (see, for example, Reid et al. 1981: 62).

The leaders imitated the rhythm of the 'rock-a-bye baby' song with their movement, and used motor labelling to comment on the children's responses to the fantasy in movement. Motor labelling is the application of the therapist's voice and words to the child's movement. Brian grinned and narrowed himself into the cloth, to which the co-worker responded, 'Are you sure you're safe in there?' Paul was wriggling and in danger of dropping out, which was labelled 'being a bit unsteady or unsure'. This in fact was an accurate reflection of his current emotional state during the period in which the social workers attempted to rehabilitate his mother, to see if he could be returned to her. Motor labelling is a way of responding to the child's movement, and what this may say about what the child is experiencing or expressing. One day Paul sang a version of rock-a-bye baby which included 'bock-a-bye baby', 'smuck-a-bye baby' and 'fuck-a-bye baby', all of which seemed to express the violence he felt had been visited upon him during a vulnerable period in his early childhood. The dance movement therapist expressed surprise and sympathy at this version of the story. He responded by covering his eyes and laughing.

Motor labelling, as a technique, relates in part to a process which the child psychiatrist and psychoanalyst Daniel Stern describes as affective (emotional) attunement. The child's behaviour in movement or gesture is reflected by the mother in another sensory channel or modality, such as her voice, or a noise she makes which matches the duration, rhythm, intensity and shape of the child's nonverbal behaviour. The net effect of this seemingly simple and commonplace mode of mother–infant interaction is that an 'intersubjective sharing of affect' is accomplished (Stern 1985: 141). Matching can be cross-modal, so that voice can be matched with movement by either child or adult; in this instance, the dance movement therapist and co-worker matched the rhythm of their rocking with the song of the children, which made the children feel that the leaders had understood them, and that the quality and content of their emotional expression had been appreciated. This was evidenced by the children's continuation of the fantasy and movement sequence, and the further emergence of movement behaviour on the related theme of being a baby, including being hungry, being fed, being abandoned, being angry, etc.

Stories and adventures

This sequence of the three babies and their various adventures continued from one week to the next, for quite some time. The dance movement therapist said aloud that Becky, Brian and Paul all knew what it was like to be a baby, and to be hungry, and to be rocked. At this, the children did startlingly accurate imitations of babies crying and needing to be fed. Each was handed, by request, an imaginary bottle, or dummy. Brian chose to suck his thumb instead. Here, as in most situations, it is important for the dance movement therapist to make comments on the *group as a whole*, considering the overall behaviour of all the group members, and the symbolic or thematic connections that are present. This focus on group process in the mind of the dance movement therapist has the effect that the children begin to sense that they are connected to others. It facilitates their cooperative behaviour, and aids in their forming relationships, since they are enabled to realize that other children may have similar experiences to their own. For the leaders of the group, trying to attend and respond to each individual child in the group in turn is fragmenting and tiring; it is the interconnected behaviour of the group and its common themes and responses that form the key to DMT group process as opposed to individual DMT.

Monsters

In the next session, the children played the babies in a cot (stretch cloth) again, this time choosing to be more quiet and enjoy being contained within the cloths, and being rocked. Becky then suggested that a big black thing might come into the room and frighten the baby. She got out of the stretch cloth, and sat on one side of the room, leaving Brian and Paul as 'the babies' suspended in the stretch cloth. She walked over to the corner of the room, paused, and then came forward and emitted a heavy, low pitched threatening growl. The two boys immediately screamed in terror as a reply. The dance movement therapist said aloud, 'Oh no! the babies are really scared!', which elicited further screams. The co-worker said 'It's not nice to be frightened of big things, is it?' Brian said 'big people!' and Paul (who had not been abused) added, 'big monsters!' Becky continued the narrative: 'babies sleeping, and then AAAH!', which she accompanied by kicking the two boys. We told her she couldn't hurt them, but the boys began to scream again, this time in an accurate imitation of pain. The dance movement therapist said, 'It seems like the babies are getting hurt, oh dear!' This sequence, or a close version of it, with tension building up and screams getting louder and more intense, continued. The breaks in between sequences allowed the co-worker to mention that this was a game, and that Becky was *pretending* to be a 'big black thing', reminding the children that the leaders were not actually allowing Becky to hurt the boys, but that she was only enacting a story. It is important to recognize that this regression to an earlier mode of functioning (being babies) is useful to the children if it helps them to digest earlier experiences; being 'babyish' in itself, without playing out relationship patterns or traumatic events, may become therapeutically counterproductive.

Becky then asked the leaders of the group to play the monsters – a request that was not granted. We did agree to make the low scream to cue the children, which in retrospect was not a good idea; the children went completely to pieces, and really screamed loudly and in a truly petrified manner.

Here, it is important to note that while disturbed children may be able, expertly, to provoke anger in the leaders of a group in order to replicate their experience of abusive parenting, it is important that the dance movement therapist and co-worker should not respond to this personally as they may unwittingly repeat the child's experience of being on the negative end of parental anger. Of course, if children are hurting another child, or themselves, or equipment, the dance movement therapist must not allow this.

It is important to understand the child's propensity to provoke anger in the therapist, but *not* to respond to it. Rather, the child must gain the sense that the therapist can survive the child's rage, that it is not going to make the parent/therapist spill over into violence towards the child, and that anger or frustration on the child's part are not going to drive the adult away. This is in part what is meant by the leaders of the group providing containment for the emotions of the children. 'Containment' here is used in the sense in which object relations clinicians and theorists, including W. R. Bion, employ the term (Grinberg 1975, Reid *et al*. 1981: 59). For example, Becky and Paul both believed (as did the boy described in individual DMT in the previous section) that earlier foster placement termination and breakdown had occurred because they had been angry or misbehaved. The lack of continuity in parenting and lack of emotional containment allowed them to erroneously conclude that their angry and destructive impulses towards parents had caused them to be sent away. For Becky, this cycle of parental changes inspired her to believe that she was ugly and unlovable. For Paul, it led him to think that his feelings of anger were truly catastrophic and unmanageable by *anybody*, and therefore angry feelings needed to be denied or forgotten, or attributed to someone else when they occurred.

It is important, then, that even in play the adult does not become what the abused child fears. Requests for the therapists to play the monster or 'the baddie', are generally best circumvented by the therapist to allow the child to be in control of the bad fantasy figures via the use of a prop or object or word. In one session, Paul asked the therapist to pull him off the chair in which he was sitting while they were playing a game of tug-o'-war. Knowing he would fall off the chair and possibly hurt himself, the therapist told him she wouldn't pull because it might hurt him. 'Hurt me', he demanded. He was puzzled, but did not push the issue when the therapist said she would not hurt him. Abused children's repeated attempts to provoke abuse or to tend towards self-abuse is a phenomenon that can perhaps be explained by the fact that they are still emotionally attached to the memory of parents or others who have hurt them, and they feel it is better to hang on to a parent, or a mode of relating that is harmful, than to have none at all. Additionally, by repeating a difficult relationship pattern in the therapeutic encounter, the child hopes to master the pain, difficulty and anxiety that accompany it. In this way, a great deal of interpersonal learning can be accomplished by children when they see that they can have rewarding, non-abusive relationships with adults.

The group continued to replay the sequence in which a large dark person or object came and frightened the babies. After replaying this sequence four or five times, the dance movement therapist reflected aloud that most of the children in the group knew what it was like to get hurt, and that it was awful, but that now they were in a safe place. This calmed them a little, and broke the trance-like spell of waiting to be terrified, and then screaming, which was being repeated for the sake of it, rather than to think about it usefully. During another replay of this 'being frightened' sequence the co-worker reflected that it seemed that being frightened was also a little bit exciting, with which Paul especially agreed. By this remark, the adrenalin and flooding of the emotional system of the children was addressed. It is interesting to note that, after this sequence, the tone of the group changed, and the three children, who had in the beginning of the sessions been carrying out various random activities, actually seemed quite united and cooperative in playing out Becky's fantasy. In this instance they all shared an experience, and heard that their fears and pain had been registered by the leaders, and so they felt understood. Children continually replay or rework experiences that have troubled them; sometimes they do this helpfully, and at other times without thinking. There is debate among people who work therapeutically with children as to whether such playing out of experiences needs to be connected to previous experiences, by verbalizing this to the child in the form of an interpretation. In the example above, either leader could possibly have said 'This might be like when you got hurt by your Daddy' to Becky. However, it seems equally valid to argue that the play experience is in itself intense enough, and as such may be reparative of trauma. Some verbal therapists posit that 'insight is frequently derivative and non-verbal and attained without the aid of interpretations and explanations. Self-knowledge is developed through experience with many different relationships' (Riester and Kraft 1986: 40).

Therapeutic gains

The case illustration above hopefully provides evidence that DMT fulfils an important therapeutic function in working with abused children, primarily because it addresses the psychophysical self (Winnicott 1988: 123). For example, in many instances, the children in the group inflict pain on themselves, by falling, or hurting themselves intentionally, or asking others to hurt them, or by constructing dangerous games, the outcome of which will be getting hurt. This is beyond the ordinary child's proclivity for such activity, and in this case shows bodily what the children feel psychologically. They feel that they are in pain, and that the environment, and relations with the people in it, are often perceived as persecutory or randomly hurtful as a matter of course.

The attention to the child's use of fantasy and movement experience gives interesting insights that may be lost if a therapist is too focused on the symbolic potential of toy figures or drawings. For example, in one session Becky jumped into a pile of stretch cloths, covered herself in them haphazardly, and said, 'This is the rubbish tip. I'm a junk baby, junk baby.' This expression of horrendously low self-regard was gained from her use of movement, and imagining the multi-coloured jumble of blankets as garbage. This further connected with Becky's whole emotional life, which was coloured by her early experiences of parents who felt she was defective and inadequate, and treated her as though she were.

In writing about the quality of physical attachment that parents and children display, and of its effect on the child's psychological state, the child psychotherapist Juliet Hopkins writes that, 'babies whose mothers are physically aversive have mothers who are also liable to be emotionally out of touch. The effect of physical rejection [of a child] cannot be considered in isolation from the effect of lack of emotional rapport' (Hopkins 1987: 7). DMT with disturbed children offers an excellent opportunity to replay and so repair the nonverbal dimensions of early relationships.

In conclusion, DMT with disturbed children offers a creative forum that can address nonverbal aspects of relationships, replay traumatic experiences through movement, and offer the possibility of a positive group experience. DMT can provide a useful adjunct to individual therapy and treatment programmes for disturbed or abused children, and may offer an appropriate medium to undertake group work, and repair or improve peer relations.

There remains a great deal to be done in this area in linking psychodynamic ideas with DMT. For example, D. W. Winnicott's conceptualization of the child's psychological struggle in development, including concepts such as 'holding' and 'falling forever' translate very easily into movement terms, and provide concepts with which to enrich the understanding of symbolic and imaginary play in DMT with disturbed children (Melville-Thomas 1988).

DMT WITH FAMILIES

Family therapy is a form of treatment available to children, adolescents and their families. An increasing number of dance movement therapy dissertations are being written in this area. Generally, dance movement therapists work as co-workers with a trained family therapist. They might see a family weekly for approximately 90 minutes over two or three consultations, and this may be repeated for up to a year or more. Family therapy is offered on an outpatient basis at a clinic and often forms a mandatory part of inpatient adolescent treatment. Family therapy may also form part of a rehabilitation programme for abused children and the children of alcoholic parents.

DMT, accentuating as it does the constantly changing dynamics of interaction, translates itself easily and valuably to work with families. Some clinicians point out the way that nonverbal behaviour between members of the family may illustrate unconscious conflicts, or disavowed qualities of relationships, such as verbally unexpressed hostility between parents (Skynner 1978: 123). As is the case with group therapy, there are a spectrum of family approaches which are based in a number of theoretical perspectives, including systems, structural, psychodynamic, psychoanalytic, developmental and behavioural theory (Minuchin 1974, Skynner 1978, Skynner and Cleese 1983).

The structural theorist Salvador Minuchin describes an ordinary family as one in which

> the couple has many problems of relating to one another, bringing up the children, dealing with in-laws, and coping with the outside world. Like all normal families they are constantly struggling with these problems and nego-tiating the compromises that make a life in common possible.
>
> (Minuchin 1974: 16)

Within family therapy there are a number of important concepts, including boundaries, hierarchical structure, conscious and unconscious processes, models and styles of communication.

Working with families means working on a number of levels. For example, the McMaster model of family functioning includes problem solving, communication, roles, affective responsiveness, affective involvement, and behavioural control (Walsh 1982: 115). The point in a healthy family is not that they conform to any particular standard or pattern of behaviour but rather that relatively healthy families are extremely flexible and have a large repertoire of behaviours to cope with problems, in contrast to a pathological family which demonstrates a rigidity and paucity of alternatives. The task of the therapist is to elicit new behavioural responses that will get a family 'unstuck' from unworkable interactional patterns that maintain the pathological psychological symptoms of one of its members. The adolescent or child who is referred for treatment to a child psychiatry unit is often one who is an 'identified patient' who embodies the family's collective problems, or one who is a scapegoat, whose symptoms mask unresolved family conflicts.

Case illustration

The following clinical example will illustrate how DMT can be used in conjunction with a psychodynamic model of family therapy. The referred patient was a young boy called Peter, aged 12. He was slim, with dark hair and a somewhat serious expression. The referral had been initiated by his stepmother, who was becoming very concerned that, although Peter was diabetic, he was not following either his prescribed diet or taking his insulin injections properly. In her view, he was endangering himself. Peter said he did not see what all the fuss was about, or why anyone should bother to worry about it.

The original family to which Peter belonged had just suffered a difficult divorce, and so the referred family was a reconstituted one, consisting of Peter, his father, his elder sister Ruth, his younger brother Raymond, and his new stepmother and her two young children, Mike and Danny. Peter had two elder sisters who had remained living with his original mother.

At the initial family interview, the family therapist and the dance movement therapist noted that the family had difficulty expressing their problems using words. There were long periods of uncomfortable silence that could not entirely be explained by resistance. Three of the boys – Mike, Danny and Raymond – produced small cars and began to race them on the carpet in a space in the centre of the room, around which the family were seated in a circle. These three boys all went to the same school and so all wore the same uniform, thus emphasizing their identity as a subgroup within the family. Peter's father reported that he and these three boys often enjoyed playing football outside in their backyard, whereas Peter often refused or declined to play with them. The family therapist asked the family to describe their attitudes to Peter's father's recent remarriage. Almost all of the children expressed a sense of relief and a period of relative optimism about the future. They explained that their current living situation was better than before, that it followed a difficult time, and a period of instability, during which their father had left home, and variously taken one or two of the children to live with him once he had met his new wife. Everyone except Peter participated in this conversation, and when he was asked by the family therapist for his views, he was silent.

The issue of Peter's not regulating his diet and insulin intake was raised by his stepmother, when she said that this same type of silence followed her attempts at communication with him. She felt that essentially it was Peter's problem, and she didn't want to be held responsible should anything happen to him. She said, 'I don't care if he bothers with himself or not, but I don't want to be blamed.' This clearly had an effect on Peter's sister Ruth, who glared at her stepmother and turned herself in her chair so that she had her back to her. She crossed her legs and folded her arms, in positional synchrony with Peter. Peter's father said that he didn't understand what the fuss was, and he couldn't understand why his new wife couldn't sort out an arrangement with Peter. This provoked a discussion in which the two parents expressed, probably for the first time, how very difficult they were finding it to reconstitute a new family and to agree on parenting strategies for their five children.

When Peter was asked for his view, he said he didn't really care if he fainted or died or went into a coma, it just didn't matter to him. This expression of affect provoked tears in his sister Ruth, and a look of dismay passed from Peter's father to his stepmother. Here, it was clear that Peter was expressing his pain and distress through his behaviour, by acting out his feelings of self-destructiveness and showing his depressed feelings. The session ended with a brief discussion of the differences between Peter's stepmother and his original mother. While most of the younger children were quite positive about their stepmother, and dismissive or quiet about their original mother, Peter remained completely silent. Only Ruth expressed positive regard for both her own mother and her new stepmother.

Movement tasks

In the next session a similar feeling of confused silence was present at the beginning of the meeting. In a discussion of the problems that had led the family to seek help, the dance movement therapist and the family therapist had agreed to try to use some movement with this family should they become stuck again. The dance movement therapist explained to the family that they might try an experiment in which each member in turn would construct a family portrait or family sculpture. They would each be allowed to place the family in any pose or position that they liked in order to construct a family picture of their choosing. The younger children asked if they could make a sort of family holiday snap of everyone on the beach, and with the family therapist's encouragement they did so. They arranged their mother and father standing together, as a pair of palm trees, while they put the rest of the children in their shade, eating ice cream. The dance movement therapist and family therapist stood on the other side of the room, leaning on chairs, while different members of the family arranged a portrait, or came out one at a time to observe the portrait or offer suggestions.

Next, the family therapist suggested that the stepmother take a turn at constructing a portrait. She put herself and her husband in the middle, with her two children on her right and her husband's children next to him on the left, with Peter furthest away. At this point, an interpretation was made on the significance of Peter being on the edge of the family picture, and a parallel suggested with his emotional position within the family grouping.

The dance movement therapist then suggested that Peter's father take a turn. He arranged the children by height and placed his wife at the head of the family in a long line with her arms outstretched, putting the youngest children closest to her. He said it was like a school or army photo, because of the line of differently sized people. He realized after a few moments that he didn't know where to place himself in the picture, and there was general laughter from the children at him 'forgetting himself'. This sparked off a discussion of the long overtime hours that he had recently been working and the children's complaints that he had been missing from a number of family activities and outings.

We then asked Peter to make a picture of the family. He made two small groups. He put his stepmother and her two children standing very close together on the left-hand side, and his father and brother standing together on the right. He said that, in his picture, Ruth was a sort of fairy who whispered messages from everybody to everybody. He enacted this by telling Ruth something, and Ruth walked in a floating style over to the parents and delivered a communication. The dance movement therapist and family therapist noted this with interest and commented that it seemed that Peter, who was not very communicative, had Ruth do his work for him. Ruth confirmed that she often told her stepmother of Peter's activities, and told off the younger ones if they were annoying Peter.

The family were very much energized and enjoyed this novel approach, which was a contrast to the long and uncomfortable silences of the first session and the beginning of the second. The father was quite amazed at his inability to 'find a place for himself' in his new family, and he and his wife discussed the difficulties they had had in agreeing how to be heads of this family, and the occasional discomfort of parenting each other's children. The dance movement therapist noted that without Ruth it would seem difficult for Peter to communicate with his new stepmother. She responded by saying that she often felt the conflict between taking care of her own two sons and seeing the family as a group.

The family therapist asked Ruth what sort of things she imagined she would be saying as the fairy go-between for Peter. She said very suddenly, 'I think he'd like to be out of the picture. I think he'd like to be somewhere else.' We presented this statement to the family for consideration, and after some brief talk by the younger boys of the possibility of Peter going away to join the merchant navy, Ruth suggested that Peter still missed their original Mum. With this, several tears rolled down her face, and she sat down. The rest of the family sat down also. At this point, the family therapist discussed the possibility that Peter's misuse of insulin and lack of care over his diet might be an expression of his sadness and incomplete mourning for what he perceived as the loss of his original mother, with whom the children had no contact. When questioned by his father, Peter agreed that perhaps he would have preferred to see his mother, but that he felt it would in a sense have been wrong to do so (given his father's overt disdain for her), and that it might be perceived as a betrayal of his new family. He then revealed that for many days he had in fact been walking after school around the area in which his mother lived, in the hope of a glimpse of his two other elder sisters with whom she lived. The family therapist said that for many children, particularly young teenagers, it was difficult to balance loyalties between their first family and their new stepfamily. This provided great looks of relief from Ruth, and some eye contact and looks of recognition towards the therapists from Peter.

Peter's father said that he doubted whether Peter's mother would be able to afford to take Peter back, and that he was still very angry with her and that he had just assumed that Peter felt the same. Peter voiced a complaint about the house in which he now lived, and compared it unfavourably in location and decor to the one in which his mother lived. His father then asked him whether he would prefer to go to live with his mother were this possible. His stepmother added that she felt she would understand it if he would rather go back to his own mother, and that although she might feel a little bit hurt, she would try to understand. Peter then said that he didn't feel part of this family because he wasn't young enough to be like the younger boys, Mike, Danny and Raymond, and he didn't really see much of Ruth because she was out with her friends.

A mood of more serious contemplation and concentration overtook the family. It became clear that the children had been suppressing their own feelings of anger and loss in the hope that this would please their stepmother. It was clear that there were still many unsettled feelings about the recent divorce, some of which Peter had been expressing, seemingly on their behalf. The family therapist summarized the information gained from the family portrait exercise by verbalizing the pictures he had seen. The memory of this activity shifted the family's mood a little. Their gestures and postures became more animated, and they said that they enjoyed that part of the session in contrast to all the 'heavy talking'. The family therapist suggested that the family meet together during the week as a whole family, to see if they could recall the contents of the session, and report any further ideas any of them had about it, and the issues that emerged.

The family did not attend the third session, but later wrote to the clinic saying that Peter had gone back to live with his original mother once this had been arranged. In conclusion, it is clear that the combination of family therapy and dance movement therapy can be fruitful. The family were able to see themselves and their relationships in a new light. The family therapist felt he had gained a great deal of information very quickly, and that this family had been particularly able to make more use of this movement and visual mode than they could of strictly verbal communication. The use of DMT in family therapy is a potentially exciting field that will hopefully yield new ideas and new publications in the near future (Bell 1979, Dulicai 1977, Webster 1987).

DMT WITH ADOLESCENTS

Because work with adolescents is extremely challenging and needs to be undertaken with supervision – and usually late in the student dance movement therapist's training – a case illustration is not described here. What follows are some theoretical background comments on work with adolescents which may help the student prepare for co-working with a qualified dance movement therapist in an inpatient adolescent unit.

There is a minimal amount of information to be found in DMT journals or in general psychotherapeutic literature concerning work with adolescent groups, which probably reflects the difficulty of the task (Berkovitz 1986, Dunne *et al.* 1982, Sinason and Kirtchuk 1986). The developmental tasks that face the adolescent are formidable, and include issues such as separation from the family, the development of a personal and sexual identity, and the establishment of educational or employment goals. Disturbances in adolescence resemble those from both childhood and adulthood, but many are also unique to adolescence itself. Disturbed adolescents tend to provoke strong regressive tendencies in their caretakers, which means that structural and emotional boundaries are important for group work (Perinpanayagam 1987). Furthermore, confusions between expectations of adult level social interaction are combined with extremely primitive infantile emotional states, which makes facilitation of the adolescent DMT group an often dramatic and rewarding as well as exhausting and difficult experience.

Adolescents seen in psychiatric inpatient units are generally in some sort of emotional or familial crisis, or suffer from anorexia, or even a first psychotic episode in what may develop into full-blown schizophrenic or personality disorder as the teenager continues into adulthood. A large number are sexually abused, or are conduct-disordered. A recent study noted gender differences in aggressive and self-destructive behaviour, with females displaying greater internal aggression directed at the self, and males displaying aggression externally by acting upon the outside world in acts of violence or vandalism (Delga *et al.* 1989). Typically the adolescent who reaches an inpatient psychiatric unit has a long history of developmental and familial disturbance, and may have developed a self-identity based in difficult life experiences. For example, some anti-social children are thought to be externalizing feelings that they are essentially worthless, and unlovable, such that the entire world becomes a hostile environment against which they must rebel or which they must distrust and attack (Willock 1987).

Group work with adolescents needs to be carefully structured and managed in order that both the adult and the infantile elements of emotional functioning can be addressed. Adolescents are usually brimming with ideas, fantasies, imagination, political concerns, or anger: at society in general or as exemplified by teachers, parents and unit staff. Furthermore, they show extremes of sexual and affectionate feelings towards those around them. Interesting and effective therapeutic attempts can be made at using the seemingly random material which adolescents bring to sessions as a form of group free association or shared fantasy (Schaffer and Pollak 1987).

DMT with adolescents can follow a similar shared leadership Chaceian structure to that used with adult outpatients, though the material that emerges will reflect uniquely adolescent concerns. In the experience of the present author, issues around intimacy, aggression, sexuality, body boundaries, authority, and projection, or blaming others, as well as scapegoating, are paramount. Adolescent groups need to be managed carefully if tendencies to inclusion and exclusion and serious peer criticism are not to paralyse one or two group members. Generally, adolescents love to dance, and if this energy can be channelled into creative and spontaneous use of movement, rather than practising to go to the disco or nightclub, then movement can be an effective way of engaging a group. Physical safety and containment of adolescents is quite hard work, and requires a skilled and physically agile co-worker. Though it may take some time, the vulnerable and needy parts of even the most hardened street-wise adolescents can emerge through movement, as long as verbal comments or interpretations are carefully handled so that they do not inhibit the movement process by making the teenager too self-conscious and stifling the movement and emotional process.

In work with adolescents, it is possible to use movement and imagery almost exclusively, staying with material and developing it thematically, and perhaps not connecting it to other, real-life issues, but leaving it unanalysed as a creative experience. The issues may perhaps be allowed to re-emerge in verbal discussion at the end of the group session, or be taken up by nursing staff, foster parents, parents, teachers or peers. For example, a group of adolescents in foster care was fascinated by the imagery of being invaded, or poked into. They used bullfighting, slaying a dragon, being a vampire, and diving into a swamp as movement and metaphoric illustrations of how they felt. Two members of this group had recently disclosed sexual abuse, and several sessions later, when reminded of these images, concluded that they were coming to terms with what it felt like to have physical, sexual and emotional boundaries broken or transgressed.

DMT that uses novel structures derived from dramatherapy, or uses structured activities or equipment such as musical instruments or video, can also be useful in containing and channelling the considerable energy generated by a group of adolescents (Holmes and Karp 1991). Two recent excellent articles describing work of this type include the use of descriptive words, role play, structured fantasy, charades, and tasks in which adolescents take turns doing a TV talk show in which they are playing either an interviewer or themselves in five years' time (Furman 1990, Johnson and Eicher 1990). Departures from the use of DMT require support from the co-worker and the treatment setting, and are best attempted with close supervision from an experienced group facilitator or dance movement therapist.

CONCLUSION

The preceding chapters (i.e. 5, 6, 7, 8) have discussed the ways in which the format and structure of DMT can be used with a wide range of patients, from 5-year-old sexually abused children to 80-year-old chronic schizophrenics. The basic structure – which includes an initial discussion, a warmup led by the dance movement therapist, a shared leadership process section, the use of props and a closure discussion – can be used with most client groups. Groups not considered in this chapter include: groups for staff (which should not be led by the dance movement therapist working in the unit, but by an outside dance movement therapist who facilitates a single or a series of groups), groups for elderly patients, or groups for the homeless (Ginsberg 1991). Finally, also of interest are groups for mothers and children on 'at risk' registers, where there are concerns about physical, sexual or emotional abuse, in which special attention would be paid to interaction between the mother and child, and the manner in which the infantile aspects of the mother are managed in the context of her role as a parent.

While not suitable for everyone, DMT, like the other arts therapies, occupational therapy or psychotherapy, has a fairly wide range of clients for whom it can be beneficial. In work with this range of client groups, whose characteristics differ quite widely, the use of patient-directed improvised movement provides a unifying element, as does the facilitation of patient-initiated and created material which provides the therapeutic focus of the group. Furthermore, in addition to the very practical goals of encouraging interaction which are achieved through movement, DMT with psychiatric patients enables the careful expression or externalization of feelings, many of which are disavowed or unconscious. The human unconscious as such is a universal phenomenon, and so work with adults and children is not as widely disparate in emotional content as might be thought, though certainly it is in terms of behaviour and appearance. With adults, children and teenagers, 'the dance therapy group allows for a controlled regression in that people can re-experience repressed and disassociated feelings which are then valued and accepted by the group' (Schmais 1985: 27). Finally, the movement and verbal symbols that arise in the creative and improvised context of the DMT session are, in a general sense, universal. Symbol and metaphor perform a therapeutic function in combining a sense of creative play with one of accurate communication of feelings. The next chapter sets out to provide theoretical background for the privileging of the role of symbol, image and metaphor in DMT in psychiatry.

Chapter 9

A symbolic approach to DMT

Both in theory and in practice, DMT is faced with the complex intellectual and practical problem of how to inform the art of movement with theory and methods derived from psychotherapy. Debates about how experience of the arts can be therapeutic or how verbal psychotherapy can encompass the aesthetic dimension are still current. Many dance movement therapists begin with a background in dance and performance, and so they stress the therapeutic value of creativity, and the value of artistic and choreographic form in lending meaning to the experiences of their patients. Other dance movement therapists, who may come from psychology, teaching, nursing or social work backgrounds, stress the parallels between verbal psychological processes and the nonverbal dimension of experience. In practice, it is generally the dance movement therapists' adherence to a particular psychological or psychotherapeutic framework, as well as their experience of dance and their DMT training, which shape and form the content of their therapeutic work.

The needs of the client group are also important in determining what sort of work will be undertaken under the broad spectrum of approaches known as DMT. For example, Jungian dance movement therapists often work with private patients, and sometimes with professional dancers or artists as clients; in this work there is a sustained focus on psychological and creative integration, on the use of archetypal symbolism to explore the psyche of the patient. Technically, the mover/witness model is often employed, and there is a great deal of freedom of structure. By contrast, dance movement therapists using psychodynamic ideas and working with damaged or disturbed psychiatric patients will have as their goals such things as body level reintegration, and improvement in interpersonal functioning of their clients. These, rather than the spiritual or archetypal goals seem paramount for psychologically disorganized patients, at least in the first instance.

DMT is still a relatively young field: just over forty years have passed since the work of the early pioneers, Marian Chace, Franciska Boas, Mary Whitehouse and Trudi Schoop, and only twenty-five years since the professionalization of DMT in the mid 1960s, with the emergence of the American school, including such figures as Claire Schmais, Penny Lewis Bernstein and many others described in Fran Levy's *Dance Movement Therapy: A Healing Art* (Levy 1988). In contrast to this early period of proliferation and excitement at its genesis, DMT is now entering a period of consolidation and is defining itself more fully as one of the arts therapies. Recent European and American conferences have stressed the need for research in DMT as well as for the development of agreed training standards.

The preceding four chapters have sketched a psychodynamically based form of DMT which, it is hoped, gives voice to the work of a small number of dance movement therapists who have adapted their American training and incorporated some of the ideas and methods of the British schools of psychotherapy, exemplified by Winnicott and Bion. This type of work is an extension of the existing tradition of dance movement therapy, which can be traced in writings from the *American Journal of Dance Therapy* and *The Arts in Psychotherapy* (Fried *et al.* 1989). The current literature in DMT is highly diverse and encompasses a huge client range, as well as a wide spectrum of theories of psychotherapy. It seems important at this stage in the development of the profession to consolidate rather than diversify in the area of theory and practice. Students in particular need to understand that what they are taught as effective practice with patients has its roots in a coherent theoretical frame of reference as well as clinical effectiveness. Given this as a question, and in response to Penny Lewis Bernstein's persistent demand for the articulation of theory in DMT, it seems productive to attempt to articulate an approach to DMT in psychiatry that is based in psychodynamic ideas and stresses the symbolic dimension of DMT. What follows are a few examples of the theoretical ideas on which the clinical work described earlier has been based. The primary goals for DMT in psychiatry, which were described in the theory and clinical chapters, will be mentioned briefly with reference to the systems of therapeutic ideas from which they were derived, or from which they can gain theoretical support.

BODY–MIND INTERRELATION

DMT takes as a fundamental premise the necessity for integration of bodily and mental or affective experience as a prerequisite for an improvement in the general health of the client. For psychiatric patients, the degree of their illness is often visible in their gait, posture, and movement restrictions and distortions in coordination and synchrony. Their subjective experience may be of a body which is numb, for a depressed client, or perhaps subject to distortion and about which delusory thoughts are held for the schizophrenic person. DMT addresses the problematic task of reintegrating the body and the psyche.

In *Human Nature*, D. W. Winnicott wrote that

There is no inherent identity of body and psyche. As we, the observers see it, the body is essential to the psyche, which depends on brain functioning, and which arises as an organization of the imaginative elaboration of body functioning. From the point of view of the developing individual however, the self and the body are not inherently superimposed, the one on the other, and yet it is necessary for health that such a superimposition should become a fact so that the individual can become able to afford to identify with what is, strictly speaking, not the self. The psyche gradually comes to terms with the body so that in health there is eventually a state of affairs in which the body boundaries are also the psyche boundaries.

(Winnicott 1988: 123)

DMT, then, is concerned with using movement and feelings to re-establish or replay this process of a superimposition of the self and the body. This is an inherently integrative process, one that facilitates the 'dwelling of the psyche in the body' (Winnicott 1988: 123). It is important not to lose sight of the fact that for most psychiatric clients there is very little offered that addresses the somatic component of mental illness.

Also, it is important not to take the idea of body–mind integration as a given, but to explore and recognize that there are a range of psychoanalytic and psycho-therapeutic ideas about the relation of the body and the mind. Judith Kestenberg and Bela Mittelmann, for example, understand bodily experience in light of the development of a psychosexuality, as conceptualized by Freud (Kestenberg 1975, Mittelmann 1954, 1957). Other writers, such as Paul Schilder, Francizka Boas and Felix Deutsch, explored the relation of the unconscious to bodily expression in a rather different way, stressing the role of the body as an ego, as a repository for fantasy, or as a revelation of unconscious communication and tied to the state of object relations (Boas 1952, Deutsch 1952, 1962, Schilder 1950).

ALLEVIATING ISOLATION

A fundamental goal for DMT with adult outpatients or long-term patients is quite simply to make contact, or to enable a few random and fragmented individuals to gain a sense of belonging to a group, and being connected with others. This goal has its basis in the theories of the psychodynamic psychiatrists Harry Stack Sullivan and Frieda Fromm-Reichmann, whose work was a major influence on Marian Chace. Furthermore, Irvin Yalom's views on group psychotherapy process owe a debt to this tradition.

Movement is an excellent medium with which to pull psychiatric patients towards social life and away from interpersonal isolated states. In Claire Schmais's view, movement facilitates this process, and later verbal associations enrich the development of the sense of relatedness. She notes that

Being a part of the dance by sharing and repeating simple steps and rhythms builds a sense of community, but it is not until people actively participate in each other's symbolic statements that group cohesiveness takes root.

(Schmais 1985: 29)

This process was clearly at work in the outpatient group which described them-selves on a journey going up a mountainside, in which they each took on roles as they might have in a band of travellers or in a reconstituted family; the movement gave rise to an imaginative experience in which members could join with one another. A similar process took place for the family described in Chapter 8; arranging the moving bodies of other family members into a position allowed each member of the family to understand something of how other members conceived of them all in relation to one another. While such an understanding may be immediately obvious to a dance movement therapist observing such a scene, it is important to recognize that attending to nonverbal dimensions of experience is a fairly unusual process for an outpatient client group. It is important to appreciate that the existential goals of alleviating isolation and connecting individuals to each other, to their families and to society are goals that are derived from humanistic, existential and psychodynamic models of the personality, as described by Freud, Sullivan, Yalom and Bion, and put into movement terms by Marian Chace, Claire Schmais and others (Bion 1961, Freud 1924, Karon and Vandenbos 1981, Sullivan 1940, Chace 1953, Schmais 1985). Such models of personality and conceptualizations of mental health belong to a specific tradition, and are distinct from models such as the transactional, ego-psychoanalytic, Gestalt, or others.

MIRRORING

The groups described in the previous chapters make extensive use of Marian Chace's technique of mirroring. This process has a parallel in mother–infant interaction, as Winnicott and the object relations school describe it (Miller *et al.* 1989). Perhaps a similar positive function can be attributed to the use of nonverbal reflection in the DMT group, as is hypothesized to occur between the child and the mother. Winnicott asked,

> What does the baby see when he or she looks at the mother's face? I am suggesting that, ordinarily, what the baby sees is himself or herself. In other words the mother is looking at the baby and *what she looks like is related to what she sees there.*
>
> (Winnicott 1971b: 131)

In DMT, the role of the dance movement therapist is to refrain from teaching or directing the movement, and instead to present to the group a nonverbal reflection or composite picture of itself. This has parallels in the verbal psychotherapy process of rephrasing, repeating or re-presenting what the client has just said. DMT, like psychotherapy, is not about 'making clever and apt interpretation; by and large it is a long-term giving back to the patient what the patient brings. It is a complex derivative of the face that reflects what is there to be seen' (Winnicott 1971b: 137).

Through this mirroring process, verbally and nonverbally, if it is done well enough, the patient will

> find his or her own self, and will be able to exist and feel real. Feeling real is

more than existing; it is finding a way to exist as oneself, and to relate to objects as oneself, and to have a self into which to retreat for relaxation.

(Winnicott 1971b: 138)

While this may sound like a difficult task, the immediate changes in appearance of a group of psychiatric clients in a DMT group engaged in mirroring each other do evidence some change; if the movement is spontaneous, and the atmosphere is supportive, perhaps DMT can offer a preliminary step towards the client gaining some authentic self-experience. DMT makes use of other nonverbal processes that are posited to be at work in the early formation of the personality taking place in the infant–caretaker relationship. Narrating the infant or child's bodily experience with words, or motor labelling, is one such process, the importance of which has been described by Daniel Stern (Stern 1985). For example, the boy described in individual DMT in Chapter 8 showed some variation in his nonverbal interaction with the dance movement therapist as his therapy sessions progressed; he moved from a detached and frightened stance to one that used eye contact and synchrony, later moving away from the dance movement therapist in movement synchrony as the task of separation was explored.

EXTERNALIZATION OF FEELING

Perhaps the most important thing that DMT can accomplish is the externalization of feeling through movement and its accompanying imagery. As Claire Schmais describes it,

the most important feature of symbolism is that it allows for psychic distance from private preoccupations. Once it has been structurally represented, an idea or emotion can be apprehended, contemplated, analyzed, or connected to other symbolic material. The symbol can shed light on old issues, articulate current concerns and anticipate the future.

(Schmais 1985: 32)

She contends that symbolism 'is probably the least understood and the most valuable process in dance therapy' (Schmais 1985: 31). The symbol forms a 'bridge between the patient's internal and external worlds' (Schmais 1985: 31). The symbols furthermore pull the particular suffering of the person in the group into a shared or universal image that can contain feeling.

The use of symbol

DMT, as an arts therapy can make full use of the dance movement symbol as a creative tool. The symbols and metaphors arise from the somatic and mental unconscious, and as such, 'metaphors are more likely than a purely intellectual statement to touch a human chord and arouse our emotions, and thus give us a feeling for what is meant' (Bettelheim 1982: 38).

Although the visual arts may seem more engaged in the formation of symbols and imagery, the process of psychomotor free association, as described by Boas and as illustrated most clearly by the outpatient group described in Chapter 6, is central to the DMT process in which movement, image and symbol are interrelated. Additionally, focusing on symbols and imagery may be clinically more safe, and appropriate to the level of training of most dance movement therapists than forays into transference interpretations. By staying with the metaphor or symbol, and perhaps not even connecting it back to its sources or inspirations from the client's day-to-day life, the group member can digest the emotional material which arises in the group at a level that is appropriate to their own mental state. Whereas the long-term patients in a DMT group could feel and see how the angry animals moved and how they moved together, the outpatient group was able to ponder and question their own use of aggressive imagery and relate this to their everyday lives.

The function and creation of symbolism is a complex process at the heart of theoretical debates on creativity, philosophy and linguistics, and engenders fundamental questions about communication, meaning and experience. In his study, *Neurotic Distortions of the Creative Process*, Kubie writes:

> Conscious symbolic processes are the tool by which we can communicate the bare bones of meaning to one another, by which we re-examine critically our own thinking, by which we group multiple fragments of experience into unified patterns of comparable or overlapping experiences, condense different units, rearrange them in logical or chronological categories and build abstractions from them. It is important to realize that without symbolic functions on the conscious level human psychological functions would be limited to the sensory and emotional recall of fragments of past experience.
>
> (Kubie 1958: 137)

The symbol allows entry into the realm of affect in a safe way for most patients, provided the free association used to create group symbols does not disorganize the client. In the therapeutic terms, DMT should aim to use the symbol to perform an integrative function for the client. Schmais notes that 'the metaphoric dance symbol can externalize the internal state. With verbal symbols we can label, classify, discuss and reflect on this internal state' (Schmais 1985: 27). To a long-term psychiatric patient, whose ability to analyse conscious feeling, action and thought is limited, the creative play of movement expression, which is symbolic in itself, perhaps combined with imagery given by the dance movement therapist or generated by the group, offers a chance to put emotional life outside the confines of self-preoccupation and out to a collective space of the group in which it can be examined and its power over the inner world of the client reduced.

This focus on using free association to generate symbols that are either simply externalized or are later analysed as a way of integrating unconscious feeling is rather different from the ego-psychoanalytic approach which seeks to resolve conflict or dissolve defences, or from a Jungian approach in which individuation through active imagination and revelation of the archetypes is a journey or goal.

All of these aims are legitimate; but it would seem that, particularly for psychiatric clients, work with imagination and movement, picture and gesture is an especially appropriate and clinically non-threatening focus for DMT practice.

If direct interpretations of the patient's unconscious feelings in the transference are not as possible as they are in the case of psychoanalytic psychotherapy, how are we to assist the psychiatric patient in dealing more effectively with his or her feelings? It seems possible in this context to privilege the role of the symbol. In group interaction, in the DMT process which progresses from movement to image or metaphor and then on to interpretation, it is possible to form symbols, images, metaphors, movements and gestures that communicate something of the patient's inner world. As Sandel and Johnson note 'since undifferentiated and fragmented stages of group formation can be readily represented in actions and spatial arrangements, and *unconscious fears and fantasies can find expression in the symbolic images created to accompany the movement*' (Sandel and Johnson 1983: 134). The fundamental aim of DMT in psychiatry, which is the clarification and reintegration of the patient's emotions, can be attempted by the use of the movement and symbol. The symbol of the unexploded bomb, or the angry animals, allowed long-term and outpatient groups to play with notions about their own anger and how to recognize it as well as try out new methods of managing it. The symbols of the ferocious tiger or the dangerous bomb, as well as the synchronous movement that accompanied them, allowed for a contained release of aggression. The use of the symbol of monsters to stand in for adult abusers in the children's group also allowed the children to explore some of their traumatic experience in a way in which speaking directly about the experiences would probably not have permitted.

While many dance movement therapists employ the use of metaphor and symbol in their work, few might be able to point to theories based in aesthetics and psychotherapy to say why this focus is useful. Understanding more about the actual process of DMT, as well as trying to marry psychotherapy theory with theories about creativity, enriches the understanding and the technique of DMT and might allow the creation of a safe and effective way to address the concerns of psychiatric clients.

PSYCHODYNAMIC CONCEPTUALIZATION OF DMT

Using the ideas of Freud, Winnicott, Bowlby, Bion, Yalom, Stern and others means that the psychiatric client's personality is understood in a particular way. For example, attending to issues around attachment and separation in the therapy sessions, or looking at how a group might show its infantile needs to be taken care of, or to depend upon the emotional strengths of the dance movement therapist and co-worker, are themes that are derived from models of the personality discussed by these writers. It is important to keep in mind that the so-called 'objective' reading of a client's behaviour is never free of a mass of theoretical assumptions made by the observer. It seems paramount that the models of personality development, psychopathology, and the therapeutic process are relevant, safe and useful for work with the degree of distress and disturbance encountered in work in psychiatry.

CONCLUSION

A limited focus, which stresses interpersonal functioning and the externalization of feeling, is probably more useful to the student dance movement therapist than an attempt to compare and contrast eight or nine models of personality development. As shown by the clinical examples, an understanding of the personality based in psychodynamic ideas allows for a clear understanding of the goals and aims that are possible for psychiatric work. Sandel, Johnson, Chace, Bernstein, Bruno, Boas, Fletcher, Silberstein, Stark, Schmais and others have shown, through their work in psychiatry, that a psychodynamic understanding can facilitate the development of techniques that address the specific needs of disturbed psychiatric patients and aid them in their struggle towards health and the management of mental pain.

DMT can make a useful contribution to the treatment of mental illness provided that the people practising DMT with any particular client group are sensitive to the special demands placed upon them, given the nature of psychiatric disorder. It seems useful to adopt fixed structures that are designed to contain anxiety and discomfort, and help the safe release of feelings that may be frightening or of which the client may be unaware. The structured introductory discussion, warmup, shared leadership, and the planned use of movement image and interpretation, followed by a closure discussion are all predictable structures on which the group members can rely.

Furthermore, focusing on whole group interpretation, rather than addressing specific interchanges between individuals, serves to make the potentially rich insights gained in DMT groups digestible for clients who may be receiving little or no other therapeutic input. Being sensitive to the hospital or outpatient system around the psychiatric client is crucial: the freedom to work intensely with strong affect is not available for the dance movement therapist in psychiatry in the way in which it may be for the person in private practice. The context of the patient's overall treatment plan must be considered if DMT is to be a helpful rather than an upsetting experience for the patient.

Lastly, interpreting symbol and imagery, by creating group scenarios, stories and narratives, seems to be a careful and safe approach for even quite distressed or disorganized patients. Respecting the power of creative processes such as free association and symbol formation means that sometimes the dance movement therapist must leave the emotional learning process at the level of metaphor or process. This means then that the clients can incorporate new emotional experiences and insights at their own pace. The student dance movement therapist should have experience of high-functioning or non-psychiatric groups, staff groups, and personal therapy to appreciate the specific demands of psychiatric work, in order to be able to gauge the use of DMT to an appropriate level for the patient group. The task that dance movement therapy sets for itself in psychiatry is a difficult one:

'We must allow the person to lose themselves in kinesthetic responses to their inner life and help them face the content of their thoughts' (Boas 1989: 25).

If the creative resources of the personality of the patient are to be nurtured by DMT, it is imperative that the dance movement therapists have supervision and support, and perhaps as well, go on to postgraduate seminars or study groups or trainings in a particular psychotherapeutic system which seems relevant to them and to their client group. As Susan Sandel has discussed at length, the stresses of working in psychiatry are numerous and of a different quality than in most other types of employment (Sandel 1980, Skove 1986). 'As dance therapists one must always be aware of one's own reactions to the (movement) happenings and be careful to avoid stopping some development because of fear or discomfort with the content' (Boas 1989: 27).

In conclusion, it is hoped that the ideas presented here will provoke student dance movement therapists and practitioners to consider the historical, theoretical and technical aspects of their work in the light of the special demands made upon DMT in its use in psychiatry. If DMT is to establish itself more fully in a health care system that demands consumer awareness, cost-effectiveness and clear and focused goals, the profession must seek first to discover and then to articulate exactly what makes it unique and successful. While the bright eyes, shy smiles, flushed faces, and extraordinary sense of new relatedness and insight that can be seen in a DMT group for chronic patients may be reward enough in itself, the profession of DMT as a whole, if it is to survive, must strive toward greater intellectual coherence, develop a clearer therapeutic rationale behind its techniques, and seek to make connections with other psychotherapies as well as other arts therapies. Finally, dance movement therapists must make links with other mental health professionals and solicit their criticism, advice and comment if DMT in psychiatry is not merely to survive but to grow and flourish.

Chapter 10

Movement profiles and diagnostic criteria

INTRODUCTION

The nonverbal dimension of mental illness is a complex and fascinating area of study that has exercised researchers in medicine, psychiatry, psychology, neurology, and cultural studies since the mid-nineteenth century. In this section, a very brief outline of some of the existing research will be provided, in order than an appreciation of the concomitant motor phenomena accompanying psychiatric illness can be gained. The focus of this chapter will be on schizophrenia because it is a major diagnostic group encountered in clinical work, and because most of the existing literature stresses this category. Unfortunately, there is a lack of movement-based literature on other interesting diagnostic populations such as borderline personality organization, narcissistic disorders, manic depression and schizo-affective disorder. There is a single-case study of a multiple personality disorder which found differing movement features within some of the personality subsystems (Kluft *et al.* 1986). Some existing literature about the arts therapies approaches and movement patterns common to the diagnostic categories of depression, sexual abuse and eating disorders will be considered here, as these categories are of clinical relevance, and are a recent feature of professional writing in DMT and arts therapies journals.

Unlike the rest of this book, this chapter may not appear to have direct clinical relevance for the dance movement therapist; however, it is hoped that an awareness of the subject will inform and enrich clinical observation. It is important to recognize, for example, that the paucity of expressive range of movement in a schizophrenic patient is not solely the product of psychological resistances and repression, but must be seen in combination with movement evidence of the neurological dysfunction that accompanies schizophrenia.

The data presented here alone will not enable the dance movement therapist to recognize specific features of a schizophrenic patient's movement. This is something learned during professional training, through specialized movement observation seminars using videotaped clinical examples. However, in so far as a richer understanding of schizophrenia may be gained by a familiarity with research perspectives on the nonverbal dimension of serious mental illness, the following will aid the therapist working in psychiatry. It is hoped that a glimpse of this research literature might instil a desire in students to undertake much needed Master's and Doctoral level research in this area.

SCHIZOPHRENIA

In Chapter 5, the diagnostic criteria for schizophrenia were described, and some of the general psychodynamic issues specific to the illness were discussed. In this section, a detailed description of the nonverbal dimension of schizophrenia will be provided, and will be considered from a number of perspectives, including that of neuropsychiatric and nonverbal communications research.

Neuropsychiatrists working in this area believe that movement-based research into schizophrenia 'holds the promise of advances in differential diagnosis, etiology, pathogenesis and treatment' (Manschreck 1986: 65). When considered historically, it is apparent that movement has been used to support a variety of current hypotheses about mental illness and its aetiology, most notably the view that schizophrenia is primarily 'organic' (i.e. neurological) or 'emotional' (i.e. psychological) in its origin. The late nineteenth-century German psychiatrist Emil Kraepelin called the illness *dementia praecox*, because he believed that the early deterioration of the personality observed in patients was a form of organic dementia, like the loss of mental capacities seen in old age (Kraepelin 1919). His Swiss contemporary, Eugen Bleuler (who was influenced by Freud), disagreed and renamed the illness 'schizophrenia' (from the Greek *skhizo* to split and *phren* mind), because he thought that, while there was a disconnectedness of the personality, a loss of mental functions did not invariably result (Bleuler 1950, Seeman *et al.* 1982). Both Kraepelin and Bleuler, like many of the early psychiatrists, including Kleist, Steck, Charcot and Maudsley, took great interest in motor abnormalities of their patients, which they meticulously observed and recorded (Rogers 1985: 221, Simon-Dhouailly 1986).

Historically, the specific motor disorders of schizophrenia helped behavioural and medical scientists to distinguish schizophrenia from related neurological syndromes such as neurosyphilis, encephalitis and epilepsy which also manifest motor abnormalities (Manschreck 1986). During the mid 1950s, when neuroleptic medication was introduced on a wide scale, there was a flurry of interest in the further motor abnormalities that appeared in patients during a course of such medication. Because of the almost ubiquitous use of such drugs in treatment, 'it has now become difficult to separate the long-term [movement] effects of the illness from those of its treatment' (Owens *et al.* 1982: 452). The problems which plague the question of whether movement abnormalities in schizophrenia predominantly relate to the illness itself or to the side-effects of anti-psychotic medication will be considered later in this chapter.

Current movement-based research into schizophrenia centres on hypotheses concerning the specific sites of neurological impairment in schizophrenia. The neuroanatomical localization of neurological signs in schizophrenia may ultimately aid in understanding the aetiology of the illness, which in turn might lead to the development of more effective treatment (Owens *et al.* 1982). In order for this to take place, however, 'better, quantifiable, reliable, experimentally useful, (ideally) laboratory-based techniques for motor performance investigation would need to be developed' (Manschreck 1986: 90). DMT, with its sophisticated descriptive language of nonverbal phenomena, could potentially play a contributory role in the development of knowledge in this area (Wilder 1987).

In addition to being of benefit to neurological investigations into schizophrenia, new studies which aim to integrate the sophistication of nonverbal communications research with knowledge from neuropsychiatry could yield further insights into the illness. Researchers might describe more accurately the specific types of psychological impairment seen in patients. This would assist them in closely defining and categorizing the subtypes of the illness that are thought to exist (Davis 1981). For example, it may be that researchers could distinguish patients whose deficits are primarily in interpersonal communications ability, and those who display a more intrapsychic form of pathology. Furthermore, movement might help to identify a more 'neurological' or debilitating subtype of schizophrenia (Rogers 1985: 231, Yarden and Discipio 1971: 322). Finally, it has been suggested that corrective movement programmes could play a part in the rehabilitation and treatment of patients (Günther and Gruber 1983, Weaver and Brooks 1964).

The descriptions of abnormal behaviour in schizophrenia formulated by Bleuler will now be delineated in some detail, followed by a consideration of psychiatric and nonverbal communications-oriented research in this area.

In the late 1890s, Eugen Bleuler spent a great deal of time working with, observing, and living in close contact with many patients in a clinic in what was then the small Swiss village of Rheinau (Bleuler and Bleuler 1986). He collaborated there with C. G. Jung who was a member of staff from 1900 to 1910, and the two corresponded with Freud, and discussed the psychodynamic life of schizophrenics (Jung 1958: 256). At this point in psychiatric practice, there was great interest in isolating subtypes of schizophrenia, and in determining what the prognosis, or course of the illness, was likely to be for particular subtypes. Bleuler developed four subtypes including the paranoid (marked by delusions of persecution), the catatonic (exemplified by patients with stupor, alternating with agitated or hyperkinetic movements), the hebephrenic (defined by early-onset of the illness and culminating in a loss of social functioning), and the simple, which described patients who 'become effectively and intellectually weaker . . . who appear stupid and finally show the picture of severe dementia' (Bleuler 1950: 235, Morrison 1974). In modern psychiatry, the most common diagnosis is now 'undifferentiated' schizophrenia (which most resembles the hebephrenic). This reflects changes in diagnostic trends, and a lessening of interest in discovering subtypes (Morrison 1974: 677).

For Bleuler, 'all motor symptoms of schizophrenia were dependent on psychic factors for their origin, and he repudiated attempts, such as those of Kleist, to suggest a cerebral basis for them' (Rogers 1985: 221). The fact that this was

Bleuler's guiding hypothesis is evident in the descriptive categories of symptoms, including the movement abnormalities he elaborated. For example, he described catalepsy, in which 'the persistently maintained forced posture suggests a state of muscular rigidity' (Bleuler 1950: 180). He wrote that cataleptic postures were 'not tonic muscular contractions in the real sense of the word. What has been described as such are complicated phenomena of primarily psychogenic origin' (Bleuler 1950: 180). Further movement categories included: stupor, brought about by 'generalized blocking, by intense inhibition (melancholic) of the psychic processes, by lack of affect and will' (Bleuler 1950: 184); hyperkinesis, or agitated movement; and mannerisms, which appeared as exaggerated or incomprehensible gestures. Other movement and behavioural features were negativism, in which the patients could not do what was expected of them, but might do exactly the opposite; and command-automatism and echopraxia, in which patients either automatically obeyed every suggestion or command they heard, or imitated fragments of other people's actions. Of this last phenomenon, Bleuler wrote

> Slightly confused, but often even completely lucid, patients imitate and echo, usually without thinking and also without any evidence of resistance, the various actions which they see in others: facial expressions, gestures, cries, words, etc. . . . I frequently saw a half-dozen plates flying through the air after one patient had thrown a plate off the dinner table. Cries and shouts are quite contagious; a single restless patient can easily provoke a whole ward. The bizarre gestures and stereotypies of one patient are imitated by other patients.
>
> (Bleuler 1950: 199)

One final and important symptom he delineated was that of stereotypy, which Bleuler found not only in movement, but in action, posture, speech, writing, drawing, thinking, and the desires of the schizophrenic (Bleuler 1950: 185). Bleuler described motor stereotypies in the patient's expressive movement, posture, position, affective expression, acts, and general behaviour. The differentiation of these elements and levels of movement analysis illustrates the level of sophistication of his analysis. He recognized that movement disorder could occur within the postural, expressive, positional, behavioural and instrumental subsystems or spheres of the patient's movement. This contrasts favourably with contemporary studies which are less sophisticated in their operational definitions of movement (Owens et al. 1982). Such studies may merely note the presence or absence of an abnormal movement, without describing whether the abnormality occurred during a voluntary instrumental action (such as picking up an object at the examiner's request), or during an interpersonal interaction, or whether the movement was self-related, or even whether the movement seemed spontaneous or involuntary in relation to what the patient might have been saying. Understanding whether the movement was self- or other related, or whether it was voluntary or involuntary, would possibly allow qualitative recording of movement abnormality, and comparison of patients whose pathology varied across and between these categories.

Bleuler further recognized that the movement pathologies of his schizophrenic patients were different from those of other forms of organic neurological impairment. He noted that 'choreal, athetotic and tetanic phenomena are entirely different from the motor symptoms accompanying schizophrenia. Neither can the movements of idiots be mistaken for catatonic ones' (Bleuler 1950: 445).

The motor abnormalities described by Bleuler were not only of interest in academic circles, they made a great impact on clinical practice as well. The early nineteenth-century psychiatrists were enlisted to catalogue carefully the symptoms and course of new cases in order that data on their outcome could be collated (Morrison 1974). For example, the standard form of psychiatric admissions records used in south-east England, dating from approximately 1904, include movement pathology as a category in the intake record of the patient's overall mental state.

The admitting physician was to diagnose the patients and describe their condition under the following eight headings:

1 *States of consciousness.*
2 *Apprehension of surroundings*: orientation; mistakes of identity; etc.
3 *Intellectual state*: comprehension; association of ideas; reasoning powers; memory of remote, recent and current events; fabrication; coherence; state of education; etc.
4 *Disorders associated with the special senses*: auditory; visual; gustatory; olfactory; tactile; and organic; hallucinations and their nature; illusions; delusions; development of; systemization; relationship to hallucinations; affective states or bodily conditions; etc.
5 *Affective state*: prevailing feeling; misery; undue happiness; affective deficiency; etc.
6 *Psycho-motor activity*: retardation; flow of ideas; rhyming; delirium; pressure and nature of activity; noise; restlessness; turbulence; destructivity; etc.
7 *Volitional states*: attention; morbid impulses (suicidal, homicidal, erotic, etc.); catalepsy; automatism; negativism; muscular rigidity; resistiveness; mutism; refusal of food; retention of urine, faeces and saliva; stereotypy and mannerisms; obsessions; doubt; employment; attention to personal needs; etc.
8 *Moral and sexual state*: religiosity, family affection; sense of right and wrong; truthfulness; criminality; eroticism; masturbation; lewdness; sense of propriety; unnatural habits; etc.

It is interesting to note that in this examination of the patient's mental state, movement behaviour is considered an integral part of the illness. Furthermore, in including the motor symptoms under the heading 'Volitional states', the assumption is made that at least the stereotypy, negativism, catalepsy, and mannerisms are to be classed as a disorder of the will ('Volitional states'), in contrast to the motor phenomena included under the heading 'Psycho-motor activity', which are evidently of a different nature.

Bleuler's theories concerning the relationship between the mental state of the patient and the observed motor pathology are also relevant here. He wrote that 'while in organic states of clouded consciousness, the difficulty in moving is probably part of the patient's general cerebral condition'. In contrast, he attributes limitations in the schizophrenic patient's movement as having another cause:

blockings and the influence of split-off complexes generally, often interfere with motility. Hallucinations, delusions, and autistic withdrawal from the environment also frequently do not permit execution of movements or reduce inclination to them.

(Bleuler 1950: 448)

His account of the movement disturbances, in which he employed Freud's concept of psychological 'complexes', anticipated the ideas of Wilhelm Reich by at least two decades. Reich primarily considered inhibitions of movement largely in terms of muscular armouring and defence mechanisms (Reich 1933: 340). There is probably a richer potential in considering movement disorder in terms of the complex, because of its wider explanatory value. A 'complex' is defined as an organized group of unconscious or partly conscious ideas that have great affective force, and are constituted on the basis of the interpersonal relationships of childhood history, which serve to structure all levels of the psyche; emotions, attitudes, adapted behaviour (Laplanche and Pontalis 1973: 72).

In his essay on the theory of schizophrenic symptoms, Bleuler concludes that the motor symptoms are primarily psychological in origin, but he leaves open the possibility that neurological changes could also be responsible. In 1908 he wrote:

According to our present state of knowledge all motor symptoms are dependent upon psychic factors for their origin as well as their disappearance. The motor symptoms which we have been able to analyze could often be explained entirely on a psychic basis. However, the possibility must not be excluded that somewhere within the motor apparatus alterations take place which produce a portion of these symptoms or, at least, create the necessary predisposition to them (consider, e.g., increased muscular irritability). As yet we have not succeeded in detecting any evidence of such changes and to demonstrate, for instance, primary disintegration of associations in motility.

(Bleuler 1950: 445)

In writing this, Bleuler echoed the sentiment of his predecessor in psychiatry, Griesinger, who wrote in 1857 that 'In mental disease, this motory side of the soul-life and the musculo-motory function are both altered in the same morbid manner' (Griesinger cited in Trimble 1981: 200).

Medication side-effects

The general view that schizophrenia has both neurological and psychological components in its aetiology and its motor manifestation seems a reasonable guiding hypothesis in examining the next major movement-based research into schizophrenia, namely that concerned with the movement side-effects of antipsychotic medication. When neuroleptics were introduced in the 1950s, and for some time afterwards, until the general features of their movement side-effects were recognized, abnormal movements in patients were sometimes misdiagnosed, or 'mistaken for the worsening of psychiatric illness' (Trimble 1981: 197). However, there are now identifiable and specific movement effects known to be the product of reactions to medication rather than part of the disease process. Recent writing indicates that, 'although it is sometimes difficult in practice to distinguish drug-induced effects from those associated with psychiatric illness itself, both have distinct characteristics (Manschreck 1986: 70).

Neuroleptics all reduce the transmission of the brain chemical dopamine, a neurotransmitter. The reduction of dopamine results in fewer hallucinations and delusions (Seeman *et al.* 1982: 43). Exactly how this works is not yet known. Since there is a balance in the brain between the neurotransmitters dopamine and acetylcholine, the use of neuroleptics to block dopamine frequently produces a relative preponderance of acetylcholine. It is this which is thought to be responsible for the motor side-effects of medication, and for which 'anti-side effect' medication is prescribed (Seeman *et al.* 1982: 47).

Approximately 39 per cent of patients manifest some degree of movement abnormalities in reaction to medication (Ayd cited in Trimble 1981: 201). The specific reactions known to be elicited by medication are called 'extrapyramidal reactions', and include: akinesia, akathisia, Parkinsonism, dyskinesia, and tardive dyskinesia.

In working in outpatient psychiatry, the dance movement therapist is most likely to see akinesia and akathisia. The most common disorder is akinesia, in which the patient's spontaneous movements are reduced, facial expression is minimized and there is a reduction of spontaneous behaviour. Sometimes this is accompanied by a complaint of fatigue, and the clinical picture may be mistaken for apathy or depression (Trimble 1981: 203). When working in a day centre doing DMT groups, the dance movement therapist should check with psychiatric nurses regarding the initial stages of a patient's treatment. It is easy to assume that the sluggish and sleepy-looking patient is 'down in the dumps', and to attribute this to an underlying emotional state, when in fact it is a generally transient medication effect.

Akathisia may be seen in long-term outpatients, who appear restless, and unable to stay still or sit down for more than a few moments. The patient is aware of the need to keep moving. It is important not to mistake this usually repetitive, purposeless movement for agitation.

Parkinsonism, which is also seen in long-stay patients, resembles non-drug-induced Parkinson's disease. There may be 'tremors, facial rigidity, poverty of movement, disturbance of gait and posture and drooling' (E. R. Squibb & Sons Ltd information leaflet).

In clinical work, the dance movement therapist may not see the more extreme manifestations of these movement disorders, because, where reactions occur, the patient will be prescribed drugs to counter these effects, known collectively as 'anticholinergics'. Rather, quite subtle manifestations of these extrapyramidal symptoms may be detected, overlaid with the movement disorders which constitute the underlying illness (Rogers 1985: 230). These include abnormal nonverbal interpersonal interaction, such as lack of eye contact, etc. (Rutter 1973). Although there is a wide range of descriptive language employed in psychiatric and neuro-psychiatric research studies, which makes comparison difficult, the most commonly reported forms of spontaneous (as distinct from voluntary) motor abnormality are 'clumsiness, or awkwardness, a postural disturbance'. The second most common were stereotypic and manneristic movements, followed by motor blocking (Manschreck 1986: 77).

Dyskinesia, or dystonic reactions, are not likely to be seen by the dance movement therapist. These reactions have a quick onset after initial administration of dopamine blocking drugs, and include repeated spasms of muscles, facial grimacing and distortions, and laboured breathing (Trimble as cited in Janssen Pharmaceutical Limited Pamphlet 1987). Tardive dyskinesia is less common, but may be seen in long-term inpatients. It is constituted by orofacial movements such as smacking of the lips, chewing-type movements, and increased movement of the lower limbs, including choreiform or athetoid movements in limb or trunk. 'Choreiform' movements are short jerky movements, which may be fine or coarse, and 'athetoid' movements are slow, writhing and twisting in quality (Manschreck 1986: 67).

A recent study sought to investigate the subjective awareness of involuntary movements in a group of middle-aged schizophrenic patients who were all rated as manifesting tardive dyskinesia on the Rockland Tardive Dyskinesia Scale (Caracci et al. 1990). Only 25 per cent of the patients were fully aware of their involuntary movements, 20 per cent showed partial awareness, and 55 per cent showed a complete lack of awareness. The authors found that patients' lack of awareness of their involuntary movements was significantly associated with a lack of awareness of their psychiatric disorder as a whole, and suggested that 'a common pathology of insight may be at issue' (Caracci et al. 1990: 297). They added that lack of awareness of illness and its associated involuntary movement was related to longer duration of illness, and that young patients, early in the course of their illness, were found to be more aware of their involuntary movements than older patients. Interestingly, the degree of awareness was not correlated with a greater degree of severity of tardive dyskinesia. Although it is not known exactly why patients are unaware of their involuntary movements, various explanations have been given, including: 'psychological denial, cognitive impairment, and anosognosia associated with right hemispheric dysfunction' (Caracci et al. 1990: 297). Those authors recommended more interactive procedures to obtain patients' consents in undertaking neuroleptic treatment. They noted that while schizophrenics, like many types of patients (or even their healthy relatives), have some difficulty retaining medical information, 'methods need to be developed that will enhance the insight of patients into their disabilities and allow them to participate more meaningfully in their own treatment' (Caracci et al. 1990: 298).

The question as to whether the abnormal movements of schizophrenia are due to medication or to the underlying illness is one that has interested researchers. Some studies, in which gross movement parameters were used, found no difference in the presence of abnormal movements in hospitalized schizophrenic subjects, whether treated with neuroleptics or not (Rogers 1985, Owens *et al.* 1982). However, more sophisticated studies indicate that antipsychotic medications produce many motor effects, and they may

> reduce *voluntary* motor anomalies intrinsic to schizophrenic disorder and may not modify the occurrence of certain spontaneous *involuntary* disordered movements, at least among chronic cases. Further research, preferably in drug-free patients, could be an important step to clarification and extension of knowledge on this matter.

(Manschreck 1986: 91 – my italics)

Additionally, recent studies which employ neurological testing have identified qualitative differences between movement abnormalities thought to be a product of medication effect, and those presumed to be the result of the underlying disease process. For example, some researchers have described the differences between stereotypy and tardive dyskinesia.

Table 10.1 Features useful in distinguishing stereotypies from tardive dyskinesia

Stereotypy	Tardive dyskinesia
Highly repetitive	Less repetitive
Often involves complex movements of muscles in their normal synergistic relationships	Usually simple movements
Often appears to be a fragment of action or pseudo-purposeful behaviour	Usually purposeless movements
Often involves contact between widely separated body parts (such as hand and head) or involves movement of the body as a whole	Usually involves movements limited to localized parts of the body such as face or hands
Tends to be more asymmetrical in distribution	Tends to be more symmetrical in distribution

Source: Lohr *et al.* 1986: 108.

Some researchers feel that making the separation of motor disorders due to the illness and those due to medication is an artificial exercise, particulary if the motor disorders of the illness are themselves regarded as representing cerebral dysfunction (Rogers 1985: 223). Most researchers agree that it is difficult if not impossible to separate the two sorts of movement, due to a lack of unmedicated schizophrenic subjects to study, and due to the difficulties in measuring, describing, and scoring movement abnormalities.

The lack of standardized measures and clear definitions of movement abnormalities has 'led to a fruitless conflict which clouds all studies in this area' (Rogers 1985: 223). For example, while one research project found that 'neuroleptics tended to reduce the number and/or severity of such [movement] abnormalities', another found that the withdrawal of neuroleptics increased 'healthy movement' (Manschreck 1986: 77, Wilder 1987: 88). This latter study noted that their findings might indicate that the decrease in movement abnormality could mean that they had inadvertently measured a form of extrapyramidal side-effect rather than an enduring characteristic of the underlying illness. However, had the description of the movement been more precisely defined in both studies, such contradictory and confusing clinical results might not have occurred. In this respect, it is important that movement descriptions be as neutral as possible, and not as theory-laden as the term 'healthy movement' implies.

Several psychiatric researchers in this area bemoan the lack of precise, qualitative, descriptive categories of abnormal movement features (Heinrichs and Buchanan 1988, Manschreck 1986, Yarden and Discipio 1971). However, this difficulty has not prevented researchers from proposing some interesting hypotheses concerning the correlation of movement abnormalities in schizophrenics with other features of the illness. Although the evidence is not conclusive, it would appear that the presence of movement abnormalities may indicate a poor prognosis for the course of the illness (Manschreck 1986: 91, Rogers 1985: 231, Yarden and Discipio 1971: 322). Interestingly, studies of infants born to schizophrenic mothers found that delays in motor development and impairment of motor abilities, especially in fine motor coordination, are detectable at an early age, and may be associated with later development of schizophrenia, possibly of a more severe form (Fish 1975).

Other hypotheses concerning the correlates of motor abnormalities in schizophrenia include the idea that patients with such abnormalities may constitute a specific subtype of the illness, in which neurological dysfunction plays a prominent role (Rogers 1985: 231). Some research suggests that the neurological signs found in schizophrenia are 'not random but are concentrated in the functional domains of sensory integration, coordination, and sequential motor acts' (Heinrichs and Buchanan 1988: 16). Furthermore, schizophrenic patients have more neurological abnormalities than patients with mixed psychiatric disorders and affective disorders. Several studies indicate that motor abnormalities in schizophrenia are correlated with formal thought disorder (rather than more affective disturbance), which 'suggests that they may have a common pathogenic basis' (Manschreck et al. 1982: 73, Heinrichs and Buchanan 1988: 16)

Despite these interesting findings, which may have an impact on thinking about schizophrenia for psychiatric and neuropsychiatric research, the promising potential of early movement observation has not been fully realized. This may be because, with the increasing use of verbal therapy approaches to mental illness in general, movement features are thought secondary to the illness. A further reason is the crucial problem of the 'paucity of useful performance measures for reliably defining the motor capacities of schizophrenic patients' and 'fundamentally, the absence of a model that could predict and explain the relationships between thought, will, emotion, and motor anomalies' (Manschreck 1986: 72).

A potential remedy for these theoretical and technical problems which beset movement-based investigations into schizophrenia would be the undertaking of interdisciplinary research, combining neuropsychiatric, behavioural and nonverbal communications perspectives. A brief look at some findings from non-psychiatric fields will illustrate the potential richness of such interactive research.

Theo Manschreck, a psychiatric researcher from Harvard Medical School, raises an important criticism of movement-based research when he notes that these studies are complicated by problems of definition and interpretation, and that only major or clinically obvious manifestations have been examined. He believes that 'little work has attempted to explore more subtle features, such as clumsiness or incoordination, or the impact of motor disturbance on skilled performance' (Manschreck 1986: 73). While problems of interpretation certainly do exist, description of subtle features has been attempted. A major figure in this area is Martha Davis, a nonverbal communications researcher and psychotherapist, who has been interested in movement patterns of severe psychopathology for over twenty years (Davis 1972, 1981).

Davis's work was influenced by the early nonverbal communications researchers Condon and Ogston, who analysed movement using models developed from structural linguistics. Their preliminary work on schizophrenic nonverbal communication pointed out that the patients did not display 'the consistent harmony between speech and body motion' or the high level of integration which is characteristic of normal behaviour in the non-psychiatric population. Instead, they noted 'a lack of self-synchrony' in the patient, which they described in one subject where 'the right arm and right leg appear at times to be dyssynchronous with the speech, head, and the left aspect of the body, including the left arm and leg'. They further noted that those aspects of the patient's body which were themselves synchronous *were* in interactional synchrony with the interviewing therapist. Though their samples were small, they noted that the chronic schizophrenic 'does not participate in the mutual gaze meeting pattern of normal interactants' (Condon and Ogston 1966: 343). Finally, they remarked on a lack of variation of head movement, and the rigid relationship between the head and the trunk during speech. Here, it is apparent that their operational definitions of movement are quite different from merely noting the presence or absence of abnormality. This type of research investigates patterning, both with respect to the patient's body parts and the rhythmic interrelation, as well as the patterning of interaction between the patient and the interviewer. This information was gleaned from masses of data that were generated when examining movement and speech behaviour recorded at forty-eight frames per second, with up to twenty-four body parts being coded per each forty-eighth of a second. While this type of research certainly answers criticisms of lack of subtlety in observations, it is still difficult to interpret patterns in a meaningful way. The primary focus of Condon and Ogston's work was to obtain comparisons between ordinary control subjects and psychiatric patients, and to generate descriptions of significant differences.

Davis's preliminary work on hospitalized patients, undertaken over twenty years ago, sought to investigate whether there were correlations between clinical features of the illness and movement qualities which the author operationalized in terms of Laban's effort–shape analysis (see Chapter 4). The increase in such features, she hypothesized, would indicate a worsening of the illness. The categories were elaborated initially on an intuitive basis, and a scale of eight factors was composed. These included: fragmentation, diffusion, exaggeration, fixed/invariant, bound/active control, flaccid/limp, and reduced mobility. The last factor, that of dynamic/vital, was considered an indication of health (Davis 1981: 28).

The definitions of these patterns are organized according to restrictions and uses of the body, spatial patterns, effort dynamics, and special composites of these. In contrast to psychiatric research which stresses voluntary motor performance of specific tasks, or the presence or absence of abnormality in a specific body region, the work of Davis and other nonverbal communications researchers stresses the *quality* of the movement, and patterning of body parts in space. Trained movement observers rated the patients before knowing their histories, and made psychodynamic interpretations of the patients' patterns based on some of the psychological correlates of effort–shape developed by Irmgard Bartenieff (Bartenieff 1980). For example, the bound/active control factor seen in eight of the twenty-two subjects in the 1970 study was found to be literally related to 'extreme preoccupations with control of feeling as well as fears of being controlled' (Davis 1981: 31). Several of the patients with diffusion, and flaccid or limp features were found to be most seriously depressed and suicidal. There has since been concern to isolate movement patterns in depressed patients which might indicate a propensity to suicide (Davis 1981, Fresko 1987). Perhaps the most interesting result of this study was the confirmation of Davis's intuitive reading of movement fragmentation as 'a facet and reflection of severe personality disorganization' (Davis 1981: 64). Fragmentation is a quality of movement which involves ten categories of qualitative description for its definition, and, like many of the items on the movement scale used in this early research, is hypothesized to be indicative of severe psychopathology.

Despite the self-confessed limitations of Davis's initial study (small sample, lack of adequate control group, lack of rigorous tests of observer reliability), this early work did illustrate the rich research potential of qualitative effort–shape based descriptions of movement abnormalities. The movement categories derived were found to correlate with clinical diagnoses, and were a source of psychodynamic interpretation of the patient's clinical state which registered fairly subtle changes in the patient over several weeks of videotaped assessments. In some respects the study extended some of Bleuler's early psychodynamic readings of movement, and foreshadowed Davis's later work on nonverbal dimensions of interaction in psychotherapy (Davis 1985).

Although much work remains to be done on the use of these choreographic notation-derived categories of movement in research, initial studies indicate that inter-rater reliability in trained observers is good. This applies to both psychiatric and non-psychiatric adult and child subject populations. The development of a video-computer package to facilitate training and reliability research in this area is in progress (Davis 1987: 19, Sossin 1987: 28).

The most recent version of Davis's work on psychopathology of body movement has involved modifications to the initial research, and may provide the refined and subtle analytical tools which would be of great use in psychiatric research (Davis 1991, 1988). Movement is observed and coded at different levels. For example, using Davis's Movement Signature Analysis (MSA) the observer hones in on a few selected movements for an elaborate microanalysis of each individual's movement style. Alternately, the observer can use the Movement Psychodiagnostic Inventory (MPI), a revised version of her earlier Movement Behaviour Assessment (MBA) (Davis 1988). The MPI was designed as an instrument for assessing severe psychopathology from body movement, and developed for research into the nonverbal dimensions of psychodiagnosis, and the effects of medication on body movement. The MPI involves scanning all of the client's movements for specific patterns of serious disorder or constriction. In contrast, Davis has also developed an instrument called Nonverbal Interaction and States Analysis (NISA) which considers both interactants equally, coding their positions, gesticulations and specific actions in a continuous record in order to monitor levels of involvement, state changes of each, and relationships between the pair (Davis 1991). The NISA is most relevant to research into the process of psychotherapy, and is interactive in focus (Davis 1985). Each method (the MSA, MPI and NISA) has a range of research and clinical potentials. Of most interest to dance movement therapists working in psychiatry is the MPI, some features of which will be described here in brief.

It must be noted that dance movement therapists wishing to use such a movement assessment in research may only do so in consultation with nonverbal communications researchers and trained observers and raters. The outline of the MPI which follows is of interest to mental health professionals who might wish to refine their observation of patients through an awareness of descriptive categories of movement behaviour, but is not intended to substitute as a training in movement analysis methods. It is important to note that the instrument must be used with caution given the preliminary stage of validation. While earlier versions of Davis's work have been used in research and by dance movement therapists in clinical settings for many years, validity studies are still in progress (Davis 1991, 1988, 1987, 1987b). Until research rigorously substantiates the rating categories, each item of the coding instrument should be regarded as a hypothesis.

The MPI is divided into subsystems of activity, which are an interesting and convenient way to begin to think about categories and units of movement which one may observe in an interview with a psychiatric client or patients. The MPI subsystems will be described below in brief, and include those for gesticulation, self-related movements, instrumental actions, orienting movements, head movements and position and postural movements. The gesticulation subsystem includes hand/arm gesticulations that accompany speech as well as gestures that may substitute for speaking, such as a shoulder shrug, or the 'OK' sign of the hand. The self-related subsystem includes repetitive actions of limb or trunk and forms of self-touch, including preening actions or fixing one's clothes or hair. The instrumental subsystem refers to functional activity occurring during the conversation, such as smoking a cigarette, drinking a cup of tea or coffee, or moving a chair into place. The orienting subsystem involves behaviours necessary for focusing on the other, such as watching the other as he or she speaks, or turning towards the other. Head movements are considered as they relate to orienting to the other person, and as they appear related to speech – for example, nodding in emphasis or, accompanying listening, shaking the head in negation. Postural and positional subsystems record the number and type of resting positions held during the interview. Davis notes that there is reason to assume that some individuals display motor pathology in only certain subsystems (Davis 1991). For example, no gesticulations or head movement accompanying half an hour of discussion in an interview is noteworthy; less than two gesticulations per ten minutes would be considered signs of impoverishment or restriction in a patient's communicative repertoire.

Within each subsystem, the presence of pathology can be elaborated using the qualitative and pattern descriptions. These describe *how* the person moves, and not *what* they are doing within each subsystem. This level of analysis focuses on the presence or absence of a pathological quality or pattern. Each subsystem has further qualitative features when used at research level. A brief summary of some of the qualities seen within subsystems is described below, in order to provide the reader with a preliminary insight into the complexity of description of movement behaviour, and should not be used as a rating instrument by untrained dance movement therapists or nonverbal communications research students.

Movement Psychodiagnostic Inventory: primary MPI coding

1 *Disorganization*

Does the observer notice any phases in which the movement is notably disorganized, fragmented, severely out-of-synch? This category, like those that follow, refers to qualities and patterns of movement – how the person is moving, not what he or she is doing. These are distinctions regarding the manner of performance and the qualitative and structural patterning of the movement itself. This category refers to patterns that are more than simply awkward or ungraceful. Simultaneous or sequential actions occurring in different body parts may be severely isolated from actions of the rest of the body; even the hands and fingers may be hyperextended and flexed at the knuckles in such a way that the fingers are disconnected from the hand and grasping is not integrated. The fluency and coherence of the movement may be broken up with sudden changes in direction 'coming out of the blue'.

2 *Immobility*

The items of this category are extreme forms of constriction and immobility. Normal conversational behaviour involves some head and facial movement, at least occasional position shifts, gesticulations, and some degree of shifting in which the trunk is engaged. Low mobility refers here to extremes of holding or inactivity of various body areas.

3 *Low intensity*

Normal movement shows instances of dynamic 'colour' such as strong emphasis, quick gesture, slow turn of the head, or a very direct action, etc. This factor refers to the virtual absence of movement dynamics or effort qualities (sudden, sustained, light, strong, direct, indirect) and the display of very neutral and unchanging tension patterns. (See Bartenieff with Lewis for a vivid description of 'effort' terminology for describing movement dynamics (Bartenieff 1980).)

4 *Low spatial complexity*

Ordinary movements display some projection into space and directionality and have some degree of sequence complexity. In contrast, the patterns of this category refer to movements lacking spatial complexity and projection, such as vague in and out changes or moves that display a fleeting projection into a direction and then become reduced to spatially vague moves or fall back to a rest position.

5 *Perseveration/fixed–invariant*

Movements are often repetitive. People may tap a foot for a long time or perform gesticulations up and down in long series. This factor refers to a special case of repetition: exact repetition in which there is precise duplication of the movement size, intensity, spatial path and body-part articulation. Highly repetitive motions are rarely performed with each phase exactly like the next in terms of emphasis, tension, size, direction, path, etc. Analogous to perseveration in speech, this category includes forms of exact repetition in motor performance, as well as cases in which the entire movement phase is strictly limited to one spatial axis or plane.

6 *Flaccidity or retardation*

Is there marked limpness, or giving in to gravity within the trunk at the end of gestures, or in the resting limbs? Flaccidity in this sense is very extreme, not simply looseness or floppy movements. It involves losing tonus and any degree of active tension or carrying of one's weight, which gives normal movement its elasticity and aliveness. Related but different are the items of this category dealing with motor retardation. The operational definition of motor retardation in this coding refers to movement phases displaying continuous slowness in the effort dynamic sense or to movements performed with such a low level of tension and lack of acceleration in every movement that the action has a very long duration.

7 *Diffusion*
This category refers to movements that are very vague, formless, and without clear definition, such as distinct beginnings and endings. This may be profound spatial diffusion in which you cannot discern distinct directions or paths, or dynamic diffusion in which the intensity runs on and on without crescendos, decrescendos or coherent sequences of emphasis and development. It also includes diffuse overlapping in which the person starts a new activity before ending the previous one.

8 *Exaggeration*
Are the gesticulations very large, full limb extensions throughout the phrase? If there are points at which the movement varies in size or changes to a smaller body part, it would not earn coding in this category. Also included in this category are actions that appear exaggerated, too large, intense and dramatic for what they are, such that they seem bizarre. Again, this has to be very extreme to be recorded.

9 *Hyperkinesis*
This category refers to movements that are performed very rapidly, one after another virtually without pause or deceleration in any phase of the action. It also includes the pattern in which a person makes a very high number of position shifts during periods in which she or he is not talking/gesticulating or engaged in instrumental, functional activities that require them.

10 *Even control/suspension*
In motion or stillness the body weight may be controlled, the person not giving into gravity or becoming momentarily freer in tonus or flow. This may be seen in mild forms as high degrees of evenly maintained tension or flow throughout the entire phase. High, evenly maintained flow throughout a phase can also be performed with minimal vigour, force, and sense of weight. At its most extreme, the movement may have a very even, weightless, surreal quality.

(Davis 1991)

It will be clear to professionals working with psychiatric patients, particularly long-term in- or outpatients, that Davis's work provides a rich descriptive language with which to describe movement phenomena which some patients manifest. Sometimes, in an assessment or therapy session, those working with disturbed patients may notice that their own subjective state is affected by the patient. This may be considered a countertransference reaction to the patient's verbal material, but cognitive and emotional reactions to patients also have their nonverbal dimension. Some patients are difficult to communicate with because their nonverbal rhythm, phrasing, feedback, signalling, and responses are distorted, which sometimes makes it difficult for the worker to feel that he or she has actually comprehended the mental state of the patient, or communicated clearly to the patient, or been as aware of the dynamics of the interview as they ordinarily might be.

It will be clear that a great deal of observational data is amassed when using a qualitative scale, and that gaining inter-rater agreement on items could be time consuming. However, this type of research may afford rich clinical and diagnostic insights. While stressing that they are hypotheses rather than research conclusions, Davis writes that chronic schizophrenia might be defined nonverbally by the presence of such serious pathognomic features within the categories of Disorganization, Immobility, Diffusion, Exaggeration and Perseveration (Davis 1988). An award-winning research project based on Davis's work was conducted by the dance movement therapist Vicky Nichols Wilder in conjunction with a National Institute of Mental Health study on neuroleptic medication. This study indicated that the interaction between underlying movement pathology and medication was more complex than had previously been assumed (Wilder 1987).

Furthermore, a symbolic level of interpretation of movement may also be attempted using qualitative description. This seems more usefully specific when movement is measured in the subsystems described above. Davis argues that 'if the pathology is evident only in the self-related movements but not in the communicative repertoire or instrumental actions, this suggests a patient who has rather successfully compartmentalized symptomatolgy and may function better than a patient whose pathology is evident in each subsystem' (Davis 1988). This type of data could be developed in further research with a view to choosing appropriate rehabilitation programmes for particular patients or possibly using movement in a corrective, as well as therapeutic way, as has been suggested by some authors (Günther and Gruber 1983, Lawler 1979, Lipshutz 1978, Weaver and Brooks 1964).

In a pilot study conducted by the present author using a scale derived from Davis's work, it was found that a patient's movement profile might alter significantly when the patient embarked on verbal material which was delusional, and return to a baseline profile once the topic of conversation was changed. The study pointed out interesting connections between the shifting structures in patterns of movement pathology which might have their analogue in linguistic disturbances posited to be a feature of schizophrenia. As has been suggested by some authors, movement material might prove a more efficient means to analyse the qualitative disturbances present in schizophrenia than the descriptions based in language alone (Maher 1972, Manschreck 1982: 69).

Despite the potentially rich insights into mental illness, such as schizophrenia, which may be gained from movement-based studies, there are still serious methodological problems in research in this area from both the nonverbal communications and psychiatric perspectives. If comparisons between research studies are to be made, standardized experimental definitions of movement need to be created. The type or subsystem of movement under study needs to be more clearly defined, whether this be voluntary, involuntary, spontaneous, interactive, speech-related, or any other defined category. Follow-up research is necessary on outpatient as well as inpatient populations to prevent the possibility of conclusions of research being confined to a neurological subtype (Owens et al. 1982: 459).

It is essential that movement must not be invoked to corroborate simultaneously a wide variety of disparate hypotheses about schizophrenia (such as psychodynamic interpretation, neurological signs, medication effects, interactional patterns, etc.), but rather, if it is to be a meaningful dimension in research, its use must be clearly delineated and applied carefully to the specific research hypotheses under scrutiny. Additionally, there is a need for less theory-laden descriptions of movement; movement must be described in relatively neutral language to avoid conceptual confusion and contradictory clinical results. Despite these methodological considerations, researchers in the area remain hopeful that, given further research funding, the opportunity to 'integrate clinical and laboratory dimensions of motor abnormalities may significantly extend our understanding of schizophrenic disorders' (Manschreck 1986: 92).

DEPRESSION

Depression is one of the most common forms of mental illness, and patients suffering from it are frequently encountered in outpatient psychiatry. The diagnostic criteria for a major depressive episode include: depressed mood, markedly diminished interest or pleasure in all (or almost all) activities, significant weight loss or gain, insomnia or hypersomnia, psychomotor retardation or agitation (observable by others, not merely subjective feelings of being slowed down or of restlessness), feelings of worthlessness or excessive or inappropriate guilt, diminished ability to think or concentrate, or indecisiveness, and recurrent thoughts of death (American Psychiatric Association 1987: 222).

Current research stresses that there are varying sorts of depression, whether these be a reaction to a psychosocial stressor (such as the loss of a loved one), or of a more biochemical nature (such as the hypothesized genetic predisposition to depressive illness (Gelman *et al.* 1987)). Clinically, depression may be mild, moderate, or severe, and in some cases may include psychotic features such as delusions or hallucinations. Generally, the prognosis for depression is better than that for schizophrenia. A substantial number of patients are able to reduce the frequency and severity of depressive episodes, when given medication and/or psychotherapy.

As is the case with most mental illness, there are varying theories about the aetiology of depression, including views derived from psychoanalysis, cognitive and behavioural psychology, social psychology, existential and humanistic psychotherapy, as well as biological psychiatry (Akiskal and McKinney 1975).

Psychoanalytic views express the idea that depression represents the introjection of hostility resulting from the loss of an ambivalently loved object, or a reaction to separation from a significant object of attachment (Freud 1915/1917, Malan 1989: 118, Spitz 1942). Psychodynamic writers note that almost twice as many women as men are diagnosed as suffering from depression (Brown and Harris 1978).

There is a very small amount of writing about the nonverbal dimension of depression, given that psychomotor retardation is an important feature of the illness. Perhaps this is explained by the fact that, when viewed superficially, the primary feature appears to be a *lack* of movement rather than a qualitatively different type of movement pattern (Waxer 1974). Furthermore, there are a large number of types of depression, making generalization difficult. However, movement inhibition takes many forms, and a more subtle and complex language of description may be helpful in delineating the type of movement restriction that is present. In his neuropsychiatric survey of abnormal movement patterns and diagnostic criteria, Trimble describes depression by saying that

> there is diminution of motor activity with vacant facial expression, diminished blinking and speech rate, and motionless, sometimes stiff, limbs. The angle of the mouth is drawn down, the muscles of the forehead are in constant contraction, and the eye gaze is down with diminished eye-to-eye contact. In stupor, the patient's activity is reduced to a minimum, with, however, the ability to react to external stimuli. In agitated depression, restlessness is observed with increased central and peripheral movements, jerking of the limbs and trunk, repetitive, often stereotyped, movements of the hands, the fingers of which may, for example, pick at the skin or be clenched together, or clench the arm of a chair. If severe, pacing may occur with the stereotypy of a caged animal.
>
> (Trimble 1981: 198)

In the Davis Movement Behaviour Assessment just described, the features of severe depression include a decrease in the amount of postural shifts while seated (i.e. position shifts involving the trunk) and a notable degree of Flaccidity or Retardation (often at the end of a gesture, the movement seems to peter out, or lose its dynamic colouring) and/or Diffusion with low vitality (Davis 1988).

In terms of effort–shape analysis, depressed patients often exhibit a neutral attitude towards the effort element of weight (Dulicai 1988). In DMT group warmups the patients may appear to have a floating quality, they do not appear 'grounded', or able to 'put their foot down' in stepping or stamping movements. Given that weight is correlated with assertion and sense of self, this restriction is consistent with a lack of sense of self, of numbness, and low self-esteem which may characterize the patient's mental state. The kinesphere (or sphere of movement, the size of the area of the extension of the arms and legs) is also reduced. The use of the space effort is restricted, there is limited complexity, and the body attitude is narrowed and retreating through the trunk, giving a withdrawn appearance (Dulicai 1988). Often the person is unable to use multi-focused attention in space, which parallels the oft-reported self-absorption and inability to concentrate or focus on events or persons outside.

A recent study examined interactional nonverbal patterns in depressed patients (Noebel 1990). As was predicted by the research hypothesis, 'depressed subjects were found to engage in less postures and gestures towards the therapist, less eye contact, and lower levels of echoing and interactional synchrony' (Noebel 1990: 132). The study concluded that nonverbal patterns in a depressed patient, through the effect they may have on others, may act to further reinforce and justify the individual's sense of isolation, helplessness and low self-esteem. In DMT with depressed patients, it is important to respect the quality of pace of movement, and not expect the patient to be able to mirror movements of other group members which require quickness or spatial complexity. It is interesting to observe such patients over a period of weeks in a DMT group. Sometimes the recovery of a rich and dynamic movement pattern can be quite dramatic.

In her early work, Marian Chace made some interesting observations on patients with agitated depression. She noted that 'the patient who is expressing depression in restless activity seems to feel no reduction of his anxiety in these repetitive actions' (Chaiklin 1975: 137). She did, however, note that these patients (who may have been unmedicated and may have consisted of a subtype of depressed patients with psychotic features) were often very responsive to movement, specifically its rhythmic aspects. She noted that both the agitated and the more slowed type of depressed patients often sought movement experience as a way out of their heightened awareness of bodily sensation (Chaiklin 1975: 136).

The nonverbal dimension of depression is worthy of further study and matches the conceptual and methodological sophistication of the investigations of the nonverbal phenomena that accompany schizophrenia. Anecdotal evidence and Master's level studies suggest that DMT may be effective in alleviating the isolation of the depressed patient (Poteat 1981). Furthermore, research that focuses on nonverbal interaction, such as that in psychotherapy sessions, might yield interesting insights into the intrapsychic and interpersonal dimensions of depression (Rutter 1973).

EATING DISORDERS

There is an increasing interest in the use of DMT as an adjunct to behavioural and verbal psychotherapy in the treatment of eating-disordered patients. Eating disorders include anorexia nervosa, which is defined by the patient's 'refusal to maintain body weight over a minimal normal weight for age and height; intense fear of gaining weight or becoming fat, even though underweight; a distorted body image; and (in females) amenorrhea (cessation of menstruation)' (American Psychiatric Association 1987: 65). In the second major eating disorder, bulimia, sometimes called bulimia nervosa, there are recurrent episodes of binge eating, a feeling of lack of control over eating behaviour, self-induced vomiting, use of laxatives or diuretics, strict dieting or fasting, vigorous exercise aimed at preventing weight gain, and persistent overconcern with body shape and weight (American Psychiatric Association 1987). The main feature of anorexia is severe weight loss, whereas with bulimia, body weight fluctuations may occur in binge–purge cycles.

Both of these eating disorders have their onset in early to late adolescence, and occur predominantly in females, with estimates of a prevalence in the population of one in eight hundred to one in one hundred females between the ages of 12 and 18. Eating disorders can begin in response to stressful life situations, and are more common among sisters and mothers of those with such disorders. About one third of eating-disordered patients are mildly overweight before the onset of the illness, and many are described as having been 'overly perfectionist, "model children" '

(American Psychiatric Association 1987: 66). The course of the illness consists most commonly of a single episode, with a return to normal weight, though the course may be episodic, and in some instances can be unremitting until the patient actually dies of starvation. Since follow-up studies indicate mortality rates of between 5 and 18 per cent in anoretic patients, intensive therapeutic efforts are made at the onset of the illness. Often an inpatient or outpatient adolescent psychiatric service offers a behavioural programme aimed at weight gain, counselling, family therapy, and individual psychotherapy for the anoretic or bulemic teenager.

Disturbance of body image is a main feature of these disorders; the person experiences her body weight, size or shape as 'fat' even when she may be emaciated; patients may be dissatisfied and preoccupied with their physical self and appearance (Bowden *et al.* 1989, Hartley 1989). Therapeutic efforts with eating disorders include methods aimed at addressing the body image problem: making drawings of the body (in the context of art therapy or used in isolation), videotaping, biofeedback and relaxation techniques are often employed alongside other verbal psychotherapies. It is clear that because of DMT's focus on the psyche–soma relationship, it may have a major contribution to make in the treatment of people with eating disorders (Burn 1987, Krueger and Schofield 1986, Shenton 1988, 1990).

There are a number of consistent aspects to the movement profile of eating-disordered patients, at least when described in terms of Laban's effort–shape notation and Irmgard Bartenieff's psychological correlates (see Chapter 4 for definitions of these movement notation terms). The movement profile includes the use of bound flow (often related to difficulty in self-expression), a limited use of the weight effort (correlated with a lack of sense of self), and a distortion of the use of space and time (Shenton 1990). Furthermore, Jessica Shenton's research found a predominance of oral rhythms (as defined by Judith Kestenberg – see Figure 4.1 in Chapter 4), which may relate to early infancy and issues of dependence upon the maternal object. Additionally, Shenton found splits in rhythm and effort qualities (exemplified by bursts of angry-type movement quickly followed by calming suppressive qualities) co-existing in the profile of an eating disordered research subject. This was hypothesized to be suggestive of serious internal psychological conflict (Shenton 1988).

In a brilliant article which combines a psychoanalytic approach with DMT, David Krueger and Ellen Schofield describe their work in combining verbal psychotherapy with DMT in short periods of intensive treatment (Krueger and Schofield 1986). They have developed an understanding of eating disorders in a psychodynamic framework drawing upon the ideas of Freud, Margaret Mahler, Hilda Bruch, Elaine Siegel and others (Bruch 1978, Freud 1923, Mahler *et al.* 1975, Siegel 1984). In their view, the disorder is one of

deficient self-regulation, using food as the most basic external source to attempt to supplement both a deficient internal regulator and a deficient integration of mind and body (or, even more basically, a concept of mind and body).

(Krueger and Schofield 1986: 323)

They note that eating-disordered patients rely on other people for their affirmation and esteem, and that the function of exercise and movement is often perceived by the patients as a way to experience themselves, as a way to feel real. They note that in an attempt to counter 'anguish at internal emptiness, boredom and deadness' the patient focuses on bodily experience (Krueger and Schofield 1986: 324). This particular aspect of their theoretical model bears some relation to the object relations psychoanalyst Esther Bick's notion of the 'second skin', which was discussed in Chapter 4. In this, the function of movement, muscular holding, and focus on the moving somatic self functions as a way to hold the patient together against an experience of psychic disintegration (Bick 1968).

Krueger and Schofield's clinical work revealed a common theme running through the early childhood experience of their eating-disordered patients, in which the children were 'perceived as an extension of the parents, or their desires, interests, and even of the mother's own bodily experience', such that a basic or core sense of self was not developed (Krueger and Schofield 1986: 324). Controlling food intake and concentrating on pleasurable or painful bodily sensations is used by the patients as a way to create a separate sense of body/self, to break out of a symbiotic relationship in which they function as an extension of the primary care giver.

Krueger and Schofield develop the view, following Winnicott's ideas on the function of mirroring, that

It is as if the mother is incapable of accurate, consistent mirroring, of reflecting the child's aliveness, special distinctness, and body and psychic boundaries. It appears the mother is unable to allow the child the opportunity for an autonomous, internally-directed origin of experience and action.

(Krueger and Schofield 1986: 325)

For the person with an eating disorder, this results in the lack of a nuclear sense of self, and instead means that the person is incapable of recognizing effects or bodily sensations. This may imply that those people have a disorganized and primitive sense of who and what they are, and how they experience their own emotions and those of others.

In seeing the anoretic or bulemic as deprived of a sense of self, they depart from the ego-psychoanalytic view of therapy which would seek to locate an early infantile conflict in the patient. Instead, they take the view that the patient has a deficit in sense of body and self, which must be developed, and rebuilt using specific DMT tasks, and focused verbal psychotherapy. Their therapeutic model concentrates on 'an integrated body and self image and leads to the evolution of the capacity to symbolize and play' (Krueger and Schofield 1986: 327). In the beginning of combined DMT and verbal therapy, the patient is directed to internal experience by relaxation, breathing and centring exercises, so that 'the body self becomes the container of the emotional self' (Krueger and Schofield 1986: 328). This is followed by a phase of therapy in which the patient and the dance movement therapist mirror each other's movement, pantomime-like, using the patient's small, initiated movements and their verbal associations. This process occurs within the empathetic relationship to the mind and mirroring body of the dance movement therapist. This mirroring is a clear example of the recapitulation of developmental nonverbal processes in aid of therapeutic growth. In the tertiary stage of therapy, the patients face a real mirror in the studio/consulting room, and move while observing themselves. This facilitates a shift towards recognition of a separate self, and movement towards individuation, which is a natural outgrowth of the previous stage in which the patient/dance movement therapist dyad performed the psycho-logical developmental function of the original care giver.

In addition to the DMT sessions, sometimes videotaped feedback is used as a further therapeutic tool to address the direct view of the entire body as expressed in movement, and to aid in establishing an accurate body image. At the end of each session, the patients are asked to express in a drawing what they experienced during the DMT session, in order to aid in remembering, concretizing, and objectifying the emotional and movement experience. These drawings allow patients and therapist to monitor progress, and form a point of connection between the verbal and dance movement therapist and the patients.

The use of drawings and videotape techniques to further extend the exploration, externalization, and redevelopment of body image is an interesting area of DMT and arts therapies practice. In fact, this process has historical antecedents in the 1940s and 1950s in the work of Francizka Boas (described in Chapter 2). She was inspired by Paul Schilder, the psychiatrist and psychoanalyst who developed the theory of the psychic function of the body image in *The Image and Appearance of the Human Body* (Schilder 1950). Boas, in addition to her highly innovative work with child psychiatric patients, also engaged in therapeutic work with dance students in her studio, which she termed 'experimentation with the dance'. After moving, she sometimes asked students to create a figure of themselves in clay, or in paint, wood, charcoal or chalk, to resolve a block (or a defence, or resistance) which was apparent in the dance, or to come to terms with an imagined or actual bodily disfigurement (Boas in Bender 1952: 275).

In Boas's view, this translation from one art form to the other allowed the student to 'be made more conscious of the audience outside . . . in order that the movement may be dissociated from self-indulgence and may attain a more direct release from the original tension' (Boas in Bender 1952: 275). Furthermore, by working with clay, the student could

> concentrate the pleasure sensation which had been distributed over her whole body in her hands and fingers, [and] she could free her fantasies and give them form in a medium removed from herself. It seemed that the sensuous feeling enjoyed while working with clay enabled her to formulate what she could not

express in her own body. Her dance movement began to change and she was better able to create in both media.

(Boas in Bender 1952: 276)

In the work of Boas, as well as that of Krueger and Schofield, the additional use of other visual media offered the possibility of externalizing the patients' symbolic statements about feelings, along with their bodily sources or concomitants.

This area of practice, in which a dance movement therapist and verbal therapist work closely together, or in which an art therapist and dance movement therapist might work together with a patient population, is one which offers exciting possibilities. New techniques could be developed in which specific therapeutic areas, such as body image, were explored, with the additional possibility of theoretical advances in the understanding of psychiatric illness such as eating disorder (Levens 1990). Work with people with eating disorders may form a potentially dynamic and fascinating area of DMT practice in psychiatry; DMT, with or without other arts therapies, may challenge technical and conceptual models of therapeutic work with eating-disordered patients.

SEXUAL ABUSE

Given recent controversies about the criteria for diagnosis and the problems surrounding children's evidence in legal proceedings, there has been a clinical interest in finding behavioural symptoms which might support or refute other indications that a child has been abused (Bentovim *et al.* 1989, Davies 1990, Glaser and Collins 1989, Laurance 1988). While it is crucial to remember that therapy must not be employed to gain disclosure information from a child, it is important that DMT make a contribution to therapeutic work with abused children, particularly given its focus on bodily experience and symbolic expression.

Social service and mental health professionals involved in treating and diagnosing sexual abuse use criteria developed from 'traumatic stress disorder' research. Children may exhibit disturbed behavioural signs during or after abuse has occurred. The characteristics of acute, chronic, or delayed traumatic stress disorders are as follows: flashback of the traumatic experience; withdrawal in the form of psychic numbing, detachment and estrangement and frozen watchfulness; a sense of heightened anxiety, including hyperalertness and nightmares; memory impairment, depression and irritability (Figley and McCubbin cited in Bentovim *et al.* 1989: 26). Further research by Arnon Bentovim and the Great Ormond Street Sexual Abuse Team indicates that children often manifest a pervasive loss of self-esteem and a failure of self-care, 'often appearing in ill-fitting clothing and caring poorly for themselves – hair, skin hygiene – despite living in a context that would not necessarily be associated with poor care and neglect' (Bentovim *et al.* 1989). Another common response in children is a triggering of psychosomatic responses, including a general regression to earlier stages of functioning, evidenced in wetting, soiling, self-comforting behaviour, clinging, or specific responses such as abdominal pain, hysterical fit, faint and weakness, illness behaviour, etc. Additional ways of reacting to abuse include sexual confusion and repetitions of sexual activities, as well as many emotional problems and sexualized behaviour (Bentovim *et al.* 1989: 27–31).

If sexual abuse is viewed as a traumatic event in the life of the child, it seems reasonable to assume that, as is the case with other types of trauma, the psychological and behavioural marks which such an event will leave on a child will vary significantly from child to child. This is because a number of issues are involved. These include: the age of the child; whether the abuse is accompanied with physical trauma; the duration and intensity of abuse; whether the family context negates and ignores emotional responses in children; and, finally, the character of the family, i.e. the way communications, feelings, closeness or distance, and the alliances between people are negotiated. The response to sexual abuse depends on the internal 'digestion' of the experience of the individual (given the underlying personality with which the child began) and by the way the family and social context processes it (Bentovim *et al.* 1989: 27). There is some evidence to suggest that intra-familial abuse with emotional coercion produces the greatest behavioural disturbance in children (Finkelhor cited in Weltman 1986: 49).

Dance movement therapists working with sexually abused children note that the effects on movement behaviour can be widespread, because in cases of sexual abuse, 'relationships are altered, self-esteem is lowered, sexual identity becomes developmentally inappropriate and interpersonally dysfunctional, and body image is distorted' (Weltman 1986: 64). Given this, both interpersonal and intrapsychically inspired movement behaviour are likely to appear to be affected. DMT work in this area examines the effort–shape profile of the child's movement, and endeavours to make psychodynamic interpretations based on these qualities (Biggins 1989, Goodill 1987, Spitzer 1990, Weltman 1986).

In her work at the Neuropsychiatric Institute of the University of California, Los Angeles, Marcia Weltman identified some characteristic movement profiles of abused children in her DMT work. These can be summarized by saying that three overall patterns could be seen. The first was one in which there was a disconnection from the torso, or centre. This was accompanied by slow, listless movement and a minimum of initiation in the chest and pelvic area (Weltman 1986: 58). This might possibly correlate with Bentovim's descriptions of children who cut off, repress, or deny the experience of abuse for long periods of time.

A second characteristic pattern was one that featured 'awkward gyrations from the torso' and was accompanied by movement qualities that were fragmented and stiff (Weltman 1986: 58). A lack of integration, giving the impression of being 'all over the place' as well as impulsive phrasing are movement descriptions which could further characterize this pattern. This language depicts more accurately the chaotic appearance of emotionally disturbed abused children that mental health workers often describe (Bentovim *et al.* 1989: 29).

A third pattern that Weltman described was one in which the child's movement behaviour was focused on the centre of the body, or the genital area, either in inappropriate self-stimulatory or sexual activity (also acted out with other children), or seductive gestures. This was accompanied by a body posture featuring a slight pelvic tilt, with the chest pushed forward (Weltman 1986: 59, 61). In one case this was found to correlate with a way of dealing with abusive experiences by repeating the sensation of abuse. Weltman writes that children often experience a sense of self-betrayal when their 'bodies responded to the sexual stimulation in ways that they did not understand nor wholly desire' (Weltman 1986: 56). The attempt to diminish or normalize inappropriate sexual behaviour is a difficult task with abused children who may use this repetitive behaviour as a way of working through the abusive experience, or who may use self-stimulation as a defence against feeling or thinking (Bick 1968). Furthermore, abused children seem certain that they must relate to adults in a sexualized way to obtain affection, and clarifying the differences between expressions of emotional closeness and sexual intimacy can become a major issue in DMT with such children.

The work of Sharon Goodill at Hahnemann University in Philadelphia confirmed many of Weltman's observations. Goodill writes that 'in the area of nonverbal behaviour, abused children can be overly intrusive with others, or very distant, not allowing another person easily into their kinesphere or personal space' (Goodill 1987: 59). She observed that sexually abused children sometimes cower or are startled, or may manifest increased tension throughout the body when they are approached by an adult, as though they expected to be hurt or invaded by them.

She described one child whom she assessed as having a

> body attitude with extreme tension, held in the upper body, chest, and shoulder regions, and almost constant narrowing in the torso. There was an ineffective use of the effort of strength (weight), especially in the arms. This was possibly reflective of the child's restraint, and his holding back from effectively expressing emotions, presumably his anger.
>
> (Goodill 1987: 61)

Goodill added Judith Kestenberg's psychoanalytical developmental perspective to her DMT assessments. For example, she described a seven-year-old boy, 'David', who had

> a) poor body boundaries, frequently invading others' personal space, and easily overstimulated by tactile experience of any type, b) poor spatial awareness, in that the only clear full-body activity was in lengthening and condensing the body in the low level (a pattern that is commonly seen mostly in children one year of age, and c) tension flow rhythms, as defined by Kestenberg (1975), that were erratic and reminiscent of those seen in children under the age of five. Also, David exhibited poor eye contact, eye blinking, and hand flapping gestures when anxious, most commonly in interpersonal situations. In combination, these factors formed the clinical picture functioning at an early developmental level in the areas of psychomotor performance and object relations.
>
> (Goodill 1987: 62)

This detailed observation, as well as those of other cases corroborate well the behavioural descriptions found in psychiatric and social work literature on sexually abused children. Goodill's DMT approach involves 'movement prescriptions' using Laban's effort qualities which facilitate the appearance of more developmentally appropriate movement profiles, and expand the child's expressive range. Furthermore, these effort–shape derived prescriptions reinforced the treatment goals of facilitating a sense of personal power and self-assertiveness, which is a feature of some rehabilitative therapeutic approaches with abused children, in which children 'Learn to say "No!" ' to potentially abusive adults.

It is obvious that movement profiles of abused children vary a great deal, as might be expected, given that each child will react differently to the trauma of abuse. There is potential for further research into this area, in terms of both the diagnosis and treatment of sexual abuse. Until studies using larger subject populations are completed, movement indicators for sexual abuse must remain at the level of hypotheses and anecdotal evidence. However, it is clear from case studies that DMT has a great deal to offer in providing a bodily focused therapeutic intervention for abused children. DMT may allow children who re-experience and re-enact their abusive experiences physically to work through their memories via bodily experience and associated fantasies (see Chapter 8 for an example of a DMT group for abused children). For abused children, psychological recovery from trauma may take place on a bodily level, both within themselves and in their nonverbal relations with others.

PROFESSIONAL STATUS OF DMT

Dance movement therapy is still a relatively young profession. Many liken its current position to that of art therapy a decade ago; it has established training programmes, and is now in the process of obtaining formal recognition from health, education and social services. DMT in Britain is presently expanding, particularly in the areas of adult psychiatry and special education, as well as in child and family psychiatry, geriatric services, and private practice. Within the National Health Service, dance movement therapists usually work on a sessional basis, and, like their colleagues in art, music and dramatherapy, work for occupational or psychotherapy departments, or as parts of arts therapies departments.

The Association for Dance Movement Therapy (ADMT) in Britain was formed in 1982, and has approximately one hundred members, including qualified dance movement therapists from the two postgraduate training programmes in the UK. The ADMT has recently adopted a professional code of practice, and is presently evolving criteria for professional membership. Within the last seven years, two MA level courses have been founded in Britain – one at the Laban Centre for Movement and Dance, London, and the other at the Hertfordshire College of Art and Design, St Albans – both of which have recently received accreditation from the Council for National Academic Awards (CNAA). There is also a Standing Committee on Arts Therapies, which is based at the City University, London, in which DMT plays an active role. Dance movement therapy is also expanding in Europe; the first annual European Symposium on DMT was held in 1989, and was attended by dance movement therapists from Holland, Germany, France and the Netherlands. There are plans to establish a European Association for Dance Movement Therapy, which will reflect the diversity of practice and training, while striving to foster cooperation in promoting DMT and establishing research networks.

The American Dance Therapy Association was founded in 1966, with Marian Chace as President. There are over two thousand members, and an annual journal is published. There are numerous postgraduate training programmes on the east and west coasts, and an increasing amount of doctoral research in DMT. Many dance movement therapists in the USA are qualified in education, social work or counselling, as well as in DMT. In 1984, the American Psychiatric Association's Commission on Psychiatric Therapies established that the psychosocial therapies (of which the creative arts therapies are a part) have significant value in the treatment of mentally ill patients, in both inpatient and outpatient settings (Fink *et al.* 1984: 776).

In summary, the last twenty-five years in America, and the last ten in Britain, have been extremely positive for DMT. That period has seen the formalization of training programmes and the application of this 'innovative therapy' (Corsini 1984: 533) to a wide client population, including an increasing number of those with mental illness. There is still some way to go in terms of establishing an extensive research profile on the efficacy of these therapies, though this is a problem that seems to be endemic to psychotherapy in general. Certainly, more needs to be done in terms of systematizing the principles and techniques that are being employed by dance movement therapists, particularly by those working in psychiatry. Additionally, the work of forming coherent and complementary relations with verbal psychotherapies needs to continue, so that the role of DMT in the treatment of mental illness can be more clearly established (Zwerling 1989). Recently, dance movement therapists have identified a need to disengage themselves from a reliance on explaining their aims and methods as parallel to verbal therapy approaches, and have felt a need to go back to the dance as a source of inspiration for their technique, as a counterbalance to what was felt to be too heavy a reliance on the theory of verbal psychotherapy (Levy 1988: 273).

The next decade will be an interesting one for the development of DMT, both practically and academically. Intellectually, it will be important whether DMT Master of Arts (MA) dissertations and doctoral researches follow existing social science and psychology frameworks, or whether they will shift towards the humanities for support of their approach. At present, the attempt of most postgraduate training seems to be to cover both sides, though rather thinly, which in my view may not be the most useful employment of postgraduate dissertation research. There remains a tension between measuring and evaluating the movement and therapy components inherent in DMT on the one hand, and articulating its relation to a humanities or arts-based frame of reference on the other. The crossover between DMT as a branch of psychological treatment and its utilization of theories of creativity and the arts has yet to reach a satisfactory intellectual synthesis. The question of the character of arts therapies research is now being hotly debated, and was the subject of a recent conference in London (Gilroy *et al*. 1989).

DMT is already moving into new areas of practice. For example, work is now being done with families (Bell in Bernstein 1984) and with sexually abused patients (Biggins 1989, Weltman 1986, Goodill 1987), as well as with victims of psychological trauma (Johnson 1987). DMT can be applied to such a range of new treatment populations because its clear reliance on movement as a way to reintegrate emotional experience remains constant, while adding existing psychological frameworks appropriate to work with these groups.

Dance movement therapy is no longer a profession in its infancy or childhood, rather it is a fully fledged young adult trying to find its place within a wide range of institutions, and solidifying its practice, while still striving for an intellectual identity. There have been enormous advances since the 1940s when a handful of modern dancers discovered that their art had an exciting and powerful effect when used therapeutically with those in mental distress. As the profession strives to gain maturity, it will need to balance carefully the many elements contained within it: the creative process, dance movement experience, and psychotherapeutic theory and method.

Information on DMT groups for psychiatric day centre staff

Groups that will be run by a trained dance movement therapist are to include approximately eight patients, and will require a nurse or occupational therapist as a co-worker. Groups will last approximately 90 minutes, and run once a week for sixteen sessions.

Dance movement therapy is one of the arts therapies which 'provides the possibility to organize behaviour, bring it to conscious awareness, examine behaviour's symbolic meaning, and clarify communications signals' (Schmais 1986).

The group begins with approximately 30 minutes' discussion in which patients are asked to speak briefly about how they are feeling that day and how their past week has been. This encourages a group identity and communication and concentration skills. Then the group, standing in a circle, chooses some music, and the therapist leads a movement warmup, similar to a light physical exercise warmup. The warmup focuses on integrating body movement, as well as motivating and mobilizing clients. The group then spends about 30 or 40 minutes doing improvised movement, in which clients are asked, individually, to lead the group doing any movement they wish, from a small movement of the hands to a whole-body action, such as a jump. Sometimes props such as Lycra stretch-cloths or sponge balls are used. The members make verbal comments or images to accompany the movement, and the therapist interprets these as signs of the group's functioning and interpersonal communication. The aim is to permit patients a safe way to explore their feelings (verbally and non-verbally), to assist them in organizing and understanding their behaviour, and to clarify issues that will assist them in dealing with their relationships and the tasks of everyday life.

As the groups will be composed of primarily schizophrenic and depressed patients, the aim will be to use the group movement therapy as a supportive environment which encourages more effective relationships and what might be called 'creative coping', rather than group therapy which seeks to explore an individual's emotional history, or his or her transference reactions to the group leaders. Interpretations are made about the behaviour of the group as a whole, not that of individual members, so that anxiety levels are lowered and clients can explore new ways of behaving in a group, and how to deal with feelings of anger, frustration, isolation and hopelessness.

Because movement is active and concrete, lower functioning clients can participate, even if their verbal skills and insight may be poor. Also, more articulate clients who may get lost in endless verbalization about problems find that doing movement helps them attend to here-and-now experience, and learn from experiences in the group. The fact that the movement is a product of the patient's own leadership contributions means that the patient's self-esteem is generally heightened by being a successful contributor to a group's created movement sequences. Patients report feeling more alert and less tense during group dance movement therapy sessions, adding that they 'can get their feelings out', and that they enjoy working at something active, in contrast to abstract discussion.

The contribution which dance movement therapy can make in the treatment of psychiatric patients has been recognized by the American Psychiatric Association's Commission on Psychiatric Therapies (see Karasu 1984).

Appendix 2

Parameters for child psychiatry DMT assessment

Some aspects of a child's behaviour which can be assessed include:

Body movement level

1 Body attitude
2 Movement qualities:
   Weight: degree of sense of self, assertion
   Space: ability to focus, singly or multiply
   Time: decision-making style, impulsive or considered
   Flow: degree of emotional restriction
3 Acquisition of developmental norms in movement
4 Ability to plan or phrase a movement
5 Degree of integration

Psychological/behavioural level

1 Nature of play
2 Potential ability to use imagination or fantasy
3 Apparent intellectual capacity
4 Social behaviour (e.g. degree of trust)
5 Degree of withdrawal or extroversion
6 Impulsive, aggressive behaviour directed at self or other
7 Indications of sexual/physical abuse

Relationship to adult

1 Degree of trust
2 Nature of expectation of adult's behaviour (threatening or helpful)
3 Cooperation
4 Ability to follow instructions
5 Ability to make use of assistance
6 Possible sexual acting-out

Relationship to other children

1 Ability to relate to children alone or via adult only
2 Cooperation, competitiveness
3 Verbal or physical communication
4 Aggression
5 Affection
6 Initiation of tasks, passivity versus activity
7 Possible sexual acting-out with peers or siblings.

Appendix 3

Addresses of training institutes and professional organizations

In the UK there are three colleges which offer formal training in DMT:

1 The Laban Centre for Movement and Dance,
   Laurie Grove, New Cross,
   London SE14 6NH

2 Hertfordshire College of Art and Design,
   Division of Arts and Psychology,
   7 Hatfield Road, St Albans,
   Herts AL1 3RS

3 Roehampton Institute of Higher Education,
   Roehampton Lane,
   London SW15 5PU

The British professional association for DMT can be contacted (by post only) at:

   The Association for Dance Movement Therapy (ADMT),
   c/o Arts Therapies Dept, Springfield Hospital,
   Glenburnie Road, Tooting Bec,
   London SW17 7DJ

The ADMT can provide information regarding membership and accreditation. A self-addressed and stamped envelope should be provided with any inquiry.

The address of the American Dance Therapy Association is:

   American Dance Therapy Association (ADTA),
   2000 Century Plaza, Suite 108,
   Columbia, Maryland, USA 21044

The ADTA can provide information about membership and accreditation, as well as about conferences and publications regarding DMT.

In Britain, there is a Standing Committee of Arts Therapies Professions, which has produced a booklet entitled *Artists and Arts Therapists: A Brief Discussion of Their Roles Within Hospitals, Clinics, Special Schools and in the Community* (with the aid of the Carnegie United Kingdom Trust). Copies of this are available from the Hertfordshire College of Art and Design at the address given above. The Standing Committee is based at the Fulbourn Hospital, Cambridge CB1 5EF, where they can be contacted by postal enquiry only.

References

Adams, P. (1986) 'Versions of the body', *m/f* 11/12: 27–34.

Akiskal, H. and McKinney, W. (1975) 'Overview of recent research in depression', *Archives of General Psychiatry* 22: 285–301.

American Psychiatric Association (1987) *Diagnostic and Statistical Manual of Mental Disorders (DSM-III-R)*, Washington: American Psychiatric Association Publications.

Arieti, S. (1976) *Creativity*, New York: Basic Books.

—— (1979) *Understanding and Helping the Schizophrenic*, London: Penguin.

Arieti, S. and Bemporad, J. (1980) *Severe and Mild Depression: The Psychotherapeutic Approach*, London: Tavistock Publications.

Balint, M. (1968) *The Basic Fault: Therapeutic Aspects of Regression*, reprinted 1986, London: Tavistock Publications.

Balint, M., Ornstein, P. and Balint, E. (1972) *Focal Psychotherapy: An Example of Applied Psychoanalysis*, London: Tavistock Publications.

Bartenieff, I. (1975) 'Dance therapy: a new profession or rediscovery of an ancient role of the dance?', in H. Chaiklin (ed.) *Marian Chace: Her Papers*, Maryland: American Dance Therapy Association.

—— (1980) *Body Movement: Coping with the Environment*, New York: Gordon & Breach.

Beck, A. (1976) *Cognitive Therapy and the Emotiona; Disorders*, New York: International Universities Press.

Bell, J. (1979) 'Family therapy in motion: observing, assessing and changing the family dance', in P. Bernstein (ed.) *Eight Theoretical Approaches in Dance/Movement Therapy*, Dubuque: Kendall Hunt.

Bender, L. (1952) *Child Psychiatric Techniques*, Illinois: C. C. Thomas.

Bender, L. and Boas, F. (1941) 'Creative dance in therapy', *American Journal of Orthopsychiatry* 11: 235–244.

Bentovim, A., Elton, A., Hildebrand, J., Tranter, M. and Vizard, E. (1989) *Child Sexual Abuse within the Family: Assessment and Treatment*, London: Wright.

Berkowitz, I. (1986) *Adolescents Grow in Groups: Experiences in Adolescent Group Psychotherapy*, New York: Brunner/Mazel.

Bernstein, P. (1972) *Theory and Methods in Dance-Movement Therapy*, 3rd edn 1981, Dubuque: Kendall Hunt.

—— (1979) *Eight Theoretical Approaches in Dance-Movement Therapy*, 2nd edn 1982, Dubuque: Kendall Hunt.

—— (1984) *Theoretical Approaches in Dance-Movement Therapy*, Vol. 2, Dubuque: Kendall Hunt.

Bettelheim, B. (1982) *Freud and Man's Soul*, London: Penguin.

Bick, E. (1968) 'The experience of the skin in early object-relations', *International Journal of Psycho-Analysis* 49: 484–486.

Biggins, T. (1989) 'An outline of a preliminary investigation of the nonverbal characteristics of sexually abused, primary school-aged, girls', unpublished M.A. thesis, Laban Centre for Movement and Dance, London.

Bion, W. R. (1961) *Experiences in Groups*, London: Tavistock Publications.

Birdwhistell, R. (1970) *Kinesics and Context: Essays on Body Motion-Communication*, London: Penguin.

Bleuler, M. and Bleuler R. (1986) 'Books reconsidered: Dementia praecox oder die Gruppe der Schizophrenien: Eugen Bleuler', *British Journal of Psychiatry* 149: 661–664.

Bleuler, E. (1950) *Dementia Praecox or the Group of Schizophrenias*, originally published 1911, New York: International Universities Press.

Boas, F. (1952) 'Creative dance', in Bender, L. (ed.) *Child Psychiatric Techniques*, Illinois: C. C. Thomas.

—— (1989) 'Origins of dance', in J. Fried *et al.* (eds) *A Collection of Early Writings: Towards a Body of Knowledge*, Vol. 1, Maryland: American Dance Therapy Association.

Boston, M. and Szur, R. (eds) (1983) *Psychotherapy with Severely Deprived Children*, London: Routledge.

Bowden, P., Touyz, S., Rodriguez, P., Hensley, R. and Beaumont, P. (1989) 'Distorting patient or distorting instrument? Body shape disturbance in patients with anorexia nervosa and bulimia', *British Journal of Psychiatry* 155: 196–201.

Bowlby, J. (1988) *A Secure Base: Clinical Applications of Attachment Theory*, London: Routledge.

Brown, D. and Pedder, J. (1979) *Introduction to Psychotherapy: An Outline of Psychodynamic Principles and Practice*, London: Tavistock Publications.

Brown, G. and Harris, T. (1978) *Social Origins of Depression*, London: Tavistock.

Brown, J. and Avstreih, A. (1980) 'Art and dance as treatment modalities', in A. Robbins, (ed.) *Expressive Therapy: A Creative Arts Approach to Depth-Oriented Treatment*, New York: Human Sciences Press.

Bruch, H. (1978) *The Golden Cage: The Enigma of Anorexia Nervosa*, Boston: Harvard University Press.

Bruno, C. (1981) 'Applications and implications of "Structural Analysis of Movement Sessions (SAMS)" for dance therapy', *Arts in Psychotherapy* 8: 127–133.

Burn, H. (1987) 'The movement behaviour of anorectics: the control issue', *American Journal of Dance Therapy* 10: 54–76.

Burns, J. and Brookoff, M. (1988) 'Body politics: image management in the presidential campaign', *Performance Studies* 8 (1), 5–7.

Callaghan, K. (1991) 'Movement psychotherapy with torture survivors', unpublished M.A. thesis, Laban Centre for Movement and Dance, London.

Caracci, G., Mikherjee, S., Roth, S. and Decina, P. (1990) 'Subjective awareness of abnormal involuntary movements chronic schizophrenic patients', *American Journal of Psychiatry* 147 (3): 295–298.

Chace, M. (1953) 'Dance as an adjunctive therapy with hospitalized mentally ill patients', *Bulletin of the Menninger Clinic* 17: 219–225.

Chaiklin, H. (1975) (ed.) *Marian Chace: Her Papers*, Columbia: American Dance Therapy Association.

Chaiklin, S. (1975) 'Dance therapy', in S. Arieti (ed.) *American Handbook of Psychiatry*, Vol. 5, New York: Basic Books.

—— (1977) 'Defining therapeutic goals', *American Journal of Dance Therapy* 1 (1): 25–29.

Chaiklin, S. and Schmais, C. (1979) 'The Chace approach to dance therapy', in P. Bernstein (ed.) *Eight Theoretical Approaches in Dance-Movement Therapy*, Dubuque: Kendall Hunt.

Chodorow, J. (1984) 'Dance/movement and body experience in analysis', in M. Stein (ed.) *Jungian Analysis*, London: Shambhala.

—— (1991) *Dance Therapy and Depth Psychology: The Moving Imagination*, London: Routledge.

Christrup, H. (1978) 'The effect of dance therapy on the concept of body image', in N. Costonis (ed.) *Therapy in Motion*, Chicago: University of Illinois Press.

Ciompi, L. (1980) 'Catamnestic long-term study on the course of life and aging of schizophrenics', *Schizophrenia Bulletin* 6: 606–618.

Clarkson, P. (1989) *Gestalt Counselling in Action*, London: Sage Publications.

Cohen, M., Baker, G., Cohen, R., Fromm-Reichmann, F. and Weigert, E. (1954) 'An intensive study of twelve cases of manic-depressive psychosis', *Psychiatry* 17: 103–137.

Condon, W. and Ogston, M. (1966) 'Sound film analysis of normal and pathological behaviour patterns', *Journal of Nervous and Mental Disease* 143: 338–347.

Corsini, R. (ed.) (1984) *Current Psychotherapies*, Illinois: Peacock.

Cox, M. and Theilgaard, A. (1987) *Mutative Metaphors in Psycho-therapy: The Aeolian Mode*, London: Tavistock Publications.

Dale, F. (1983) 'The body as bondage', *Journal of Child Psychotherapy* 9: 33–44.

Davidson, J., Zisook, S., Giller, E. and Helms, M. (1989) 'Symptoms of interpersonal sensitivity in depression', *Comprehensive Psychiatry* 30: 357–368.

Davies, P. (1990) 'Out of the mouths of babes', *The Independent*, Law Page, Friday 16 March, p. 17.

Davis, M. 1985 'Nonverbal behaviour research and psychotherapy', in G. Stricker and R. H. Keisner (eds), *From Research to Clinical Practice*, New York: Plenum.

—— (1987b) 'Steps to achieving observer agreement: the LIMS Reliability Project', *Movement Studies* 2: 7–19.

—— (ed.) (1987) 'Observer agreement', *Movement Studies*, Vol. 2 A journal of the Laban Bartenieff Institute of Movement Studies, available from LIMS, 31 West 27th St, New York 10001, USA.

—— (1988) 'Movement behaviour assessment: guidelines for use and interpretation', unpublished guide to video assessment presented at the Laban Centre for Movement and Dance Advanced DMT Observer Training, London.

—— (1991) *Guide to Movement Analysis Methods, Part I: Movement Signature Analysis, Part II: Movement Psychodiagnostic Inventory, Part III: Nonverbal Interaction and States Analysis*, unpublished guide for observation training used at the New York State Psychiatric Institute.

Davis, M. and Skupien, J. (1972) *Understanding Body Movement: An Annotated Bibliography*, New York: Arno Press.

—— (1974) 'Movement as patterns of process', *Main Currents in Modern Thought* 31: 18–22.

—— (1975) *Towards Understanding the Intrinsic in Body Movement*, New York: Arno Press.

—— (1978) 'Laban analysis of nonverbal communication', in S. Weitz (ed.) *Nonverbal Communication*, New York: Oxford University Press.

—— (1981) 'Movement characteristics of hospitalized patients', *American Journal of Dance Therapy* 4 (1): 52–71. Originally published 1970, *Proceedings of the Fifth Annual Conference of the American Dance Therapy Association* pp. 25–45.

—— (1982) *Body Movement and Nonverbal Communication: An Annotated Bibliography, 1971–1980*, Bloomington: Indiana University Press.

Daws, D. and Boston, M. (eds) (1981) *The Child Psychotherapist and the Problems of Young People*, London: Wildwood House. Originally published 1977.

Delaney, W. (1973) 'Dance therapy with emotionally disturbed children in a psycho-educational day hospital program', *American Dance Therapy Association Monograph* 3: 134–173.

Delga, I., Heinssen, R., Fritxch, R., Goodrich, W. and Yates, B. (1989) 'Psychosis, aggression, and self-destructive behaviour in hospitalized adolescents', *American Journal of Psychiatry* 146 (4): 521–525.

Dell, C. (1977) *A Primer for Movement Description*, New York: Dance Notation Bureau Press.

Deutsch, F. (1952) 'Analytic posturology', *Psychoanalytic Quarterly* 21: 196–214.

—— (1962) 'Body, mind and the sensory gateways', in *Advances in Psychosomatic Medicine*, New York: S. Karger.

Dick, B. and Woof, K. (1986) 'An evaluation of a time-limited programme of dynamic group psychotherapy', *British Journal of Psychiatry* 148: 159–164.

Dosamantes-Alperson, E. (1984) 'Experiential movement psychotherapy', in P. Bernstein (ed.) *Theoretical Approaches in Dance-Movement Therapy*, Vol. 2, Dubuque: Kendall Hunt.

—— (1987) 'Transference and countertransference issues in movement psychotherapy', *Arts in Psychotherapy* 14: 209–214.

Dulicai, D. (1973) 'Movement therapy on a closed ward', *Journal of the Bronx State Hospital* 1 (4): 150–154.

—— (1977) 'Nonverbal assessment of family systems: a preliminary study', *Arts in Psychotherapy* 4: 55–62.

—— (1988) 'DMT group supervision', unpublished lecture notes, Laban Centre for Movement and Dance, London.

Dunne, C., Bruggen, P. and O'Brian, C. (1982) 'Touch and action in group therapy of younger adolescents', *Journal of Adolescence* 5: 31–38.

Ellenberger, H. (1970) *The Discovery of the Unconscious: The History and Evolution of Dynamic Psychiatry*, 2nd edn, New York: Basic Books.

Espenak, L. (1981) *Dance Therapy: Theory and Application*, Illinois: C. Thomas.

Esser, G., Schmidt, M. and Woerner, W. (1990) 'Epidemiology and course of psychiatric disorders in school-age children – Results of a longitudinal study', *Journal of Child Psychology and Psychiatry* 31 (2): 243–263.

Feher, A., Nadaff, B. and Tazi, C. (1989) *Zone 3: Fragments for a History of the Human Body*, New York: MIT Press.

Fink, P., Levick, M., Hays, R., Johnson, D., Dulicai, D. and Briggs, C. (1984) 'Creative therapies', in T. B. Karasu (ed.) *The Psychiatric Therapies*, Washington: American Psychiatric Association.

Fish B. (1975) 'Biological antecedents of psychosis in children', in D. Freeman (ed.) *Biology of the Major Psychoses*, New York: Raven.

Fletcher, D. (1974) 'The use of body movement and body experience in therapy', *Therapeutic Process: Movement as Integration, Proceedings of the Ninth Annual Conference of the American Dance Therapy Association,* Columbia: Maryland.

—— (1979) 'Body experience within the therapeutic process: a psychodynamic approach', in P. Bernstein (ed.) *Eight Theoretical Approaches in Dance-Movement Therapy*, Dubuque: Kendall Hunt.

Foster, S. (1986) *Reading Dancing: Bodies and Subjects in Contemporary American Dance*, Berkeley: University of California Press.

Fraenkel, D. (1983) 'The relationship of empathy in movement to synchrony, echoing, and empathy in verbal interactions' *American Journal of Dance Therapy* 6: 31–48.

Fresko, T. (1987) 'A study investigating the movement patterns of non-psychotic suicidal patients', unpublished M.A. thesis, Laban Centre for Movement and Dance, London.

Freud, S. (1900) *The Interpretation of Dreams, Standard Edition*, Vols. IV-V, London: Hogarth Press.

—— (1905) *Three Essays on the Theory of Sexuality, Standard Edition*, Vol. VII, London: Hogarth Press.

—— (1915/1917) 'Mourning and Melancholia', *Standard Edition*, Vol. XIV, London: Hogarth Press.

—— (1923) 'The ego and the id', *Standard Edition*, Vol. XIX, London: Hogarth Press.

—— (1924) 'The dynamics of transference', *Standard Edition*, Vol. XII, London: Hogarth Press.

Fried, J., Katz, S., Kleinman, S. and Naess, J. (1989) *A Collection of Early Writings: Towards a Body of Knowledge*, Vol. 1. Available by post from the American Dance Therapy Association, 2000 Century Plaza, Suite 108, Columbia, Maryland, USA 21044.

Fromm-Reichmann, F. (1954) 'Psychotherapy of schizophrenia', *American Journal of Psychiatry* III: 410–419.

—— (1960) *Principles of Intensive Psychotherapy*, London: University of Chicago Press.

Furman, L. (1990) 'Video therapy: an alternative for the treatment of adolescents', *Arts in Psychotherapy* 17: 165–169.

Gavshon, A. (1989) 'Playing: its role in child analysis', *Journal of Child Psychotherapy* 15, (1): 47–62.

Gelman, D., Hager, M. Doherty, S., Gosnell, M., Raine, G. and Shapiro, D. (1987) 'Depression', *Newsweek* 4 May: 42–48.

Gilman, S. (ed.) (1976) *The Face of Madness: Hugh W. Diamond and the Origins of Psychiatric Photography*, New York: Brunner Mazel.

—— (1985) *Seeing the Insane: A Cultural History of Psychiatric Illustration*, London: Wiley.

Gilroy, A., Hoskyns, S., Jenkyns, M., Lee, C. and Payne, H. (1989) *Arts Therapies Research: Proceedings of the First Arts Therapies Research Conference Held at City University on 11 March 1989*, available from Dept of Music, City University, Northampton Square, London EC1V 0HB.

Ginsberg, J. (1991) 'In search of a voice: working with homeless men', *American Journal of Dance Therapy* 31 (1): 33–48.

Giovaccini, P. (1986) 'Schizophrenia: structural and therapeutic considerations', in D. Feinsilver (ed.) *Towards a Comprehensive Model for Schizophrenic Disorders*, Hillsdale: The Analytic Press.

Glaser, D. and Collins, C. (1989) 'The response of young, non-sexually abused children to anatomically correct dolls', *Journal of Child Psychology and Psychiatry* 30 (4): 547–560.

Goodill, S. (1987) 'Dance/movement therapy with abused children', *Arts in Psychotherapy* 14: 49–68.

Goodill, S. and Leatherbee, T. (1986) *A Primer for Assessment and Evaluation in Dance/Movement Therapy*, Philadelphia: Hahnemann University Press.

Govine, B. (1971) 'The use of movement as adjunctive therapy in the rehabilitation of psychiatric day patients', *American Dance Therapy Association Monograph* 1: 12–15.

Graham, P. (1986) *Child Psychiatry: A Developmental Approach*, Oxford: Oxford University Press.

Green, H. (1964) *I Never Promised You a Rose Garden*, London: Pan Books.

Greenberg, J. (1974) 'Me and Miss Chace', *Proceedings of the Eighth Annual Conference of the American Dance Therapy Association* 3: 1–22.

Griesinger, W. (1857) *Mental Pathology and Therapeutics*, trans. C. Lockhart, I. Roberston and J. Rutherford. London: New Sydenham Society.

Grinberg, L. (1975) *Introduction to the Work of Bion*, London: Karnac/Roland Harris Educational Trust.

Günther, W. and Gruber, H. (1983) 'Psychomotorische Störungen bei psychiatrischen Patienten als Mögliche Grundlage neuer Ansätze in Differentialdiagnose und Therapie', *Archiv für Psychiatrie und Nervenkrankheiten* (Archives of Psychiatry and Neurological Sciences) 233: 187–209.

Hartley, P. (1989) 'Body-image and self-image in anorexia nervosa', *British Review of Bulimia and Anorexia Nervosa* 3 (2): 61–70.

Hawkins, A. (1971) 'Work with patients', *Proceedings of the Sixth Annual Conference of the American Dance Therapy Association*, pp. 67–69.

Heinrichs, D. and Buchanan, R. (1988) 'Significance and meaning of neurological signs in schizophrenia', *American Journal of Psychiatry* 145 (1): 11–18.

Higgens, L. (1990) personal communication.

—— (1989) 'The diagnostic movement assessment of deaf psychiatric patients', unpublished M.A. thesis, Laban Centre for Movement and Dance, London.

Higgens, L. and McLean, E. (1990) 'Dance Movement Therapy with Psychiatric Patients in the Community', conference paper presented at *Arts Therapies Education: Our European Future*, held at Hertfordshire College of Art and Design 5–7 October 1990. Copies available by post from the Association for Dance Movement Therapy (ADMT), c/o Arts Therapies Department, Springfield Hospital, Glenburnie Road, Tooting Bec, London SW17 7DJ.

Hinshelwood, B. (1989) *A Dictionary of Kleinian Thought*, London: Free Association Books.

Hodgson J. and Preston-Dunlop, V. (1990) *Rudolf Laban: An Introduction to his Work and Influence*, Plymouth: Northcote House.

Holden, S. (1990) 'Moving together: the group finds a dance', *Group Analysis* 23 (3): 265–276.

Holmes, P. and Karp, M. (1991) *Psychodrama: Inspiration and Technique*, London: Routledge.

Hopkins, J. (1986) 'Solving the mystery of monsters: steps towards the recovery of trauma', *Journal of Child Psychotherapy* 12 (1): 61–71.

—— (1987) 'Failure of the holding relationship: some effects of the physical rejection on the child's attachment and on his inner experience', *Journal of Child Psychotherapy* 13 (1): 5–17.

Horowitz, M. and Weisberg, P. (1966) 'Techniques for the group psychotherapy of acute psychosis', *International Journal of Group Psychotherapy* 16: 42–50.

Johnson, D. (1987) 'The role of creative arts therapies in the diagnosis and treatment of psychological trauma' *Arts in Psychotherapy* 14: 7–13.

Johnson, D. and Eicher, V. (1990) 'The use of dramatic activities to facilitate dance therapy with adolescents', *Arts in Psychotherapy* 17: 157–164.

Johnson, D. and Sandel, S. (1977) 'Structural analysis of group movement sessions; preliminary research', *American Journal of Dance Therapy* 1 (2): 31–36.

Jung, C. G. (1923) *Psychological Types*, trans. R. F. C. Hull and H. G. Baynes, Bollingen Series XX, Vol. 6 of Collected Works of C. G. Jung, 3rd edn 1977. Princeton: Princeton University Press.

—— (1958) 'Schizophrenia', in *The Psychogenesis of Mental Disease*, trans. R. F. C. Hull and H. G. Baynes, Bollingen Series XX, Vol. 3 of Collected Works of C. G. Jung, 3rd edn 1977. Princeton: Princeton University Press.

—— (1965) *Memories, Dreams, Reflections*, A. Jaffe (ed.), C. Winston and R. Winston (trans.), New York: Vintage.

Kahn, L. (1984) 'Group treatment interventions for schizophrenics', *International Journal of Group Psychotherapy* 34 (1): 149–153.

Kaplan-Westbrook, B. and Sing, M. (1988) 'A psychiatric movement assessment scale with developmental considerations', *Arts in Psychotherapy* 15: 37–46.

Karasu, T. (1984) *The Psychiatric Therapies: The American Psychiatric Association Commission on Psychiatric Therapies*, Washington: APA Publications.

Karon, B. and Vandenbos, G. (1981) *Psychotherapy of Schizophrenia: The Treatment of Choice*, New York: Jason Aronson.

Kästner, I. (1988) 'The emphasis of creativity in DMT', unpublished M.A. thesis, Laban Centre for Movement and Dance, London.

Keitner, G. and Miller, I. (1990) 'Family functioning and major depression: an overview', *American Journal of Psychiatry*, 1128–1138.

Kendon, A. (1979) 'Movement coordination in social interaction: some examples described', in S. Weitz (ed.) *Nonverbal Communication*, New York: Oxford University Press.

Kernberg, O., Burnstein, E., Coyne, L., Applebaum, A., Horowitz, L. and Voth, H. (1972) 'Psychotherapy and psychoanalysis: final report on the Menninger Foundation Psychotherapy Research Project', *Bulletin of the Menninger Clinic* 36: 1–275.

Kestenberg, J. (1975) *Children and Parents: Psychoanalytic Studies in Development*, New York: Jason Aronson.

Klein, M. (1959) 'Our adult world and its roots in infancy', in *Envy and Gratitude and Other Works 1946–1963*, London: Virago edition 1988.

Klerman, G. (1984) 'Ideology and science in the individual psychotherapy of schizophrenia', *Schizophrenia Bulletin* 10: 608–612.

Kluft, E., Poteat, J. and Kluft, P. (1986) 'Movement observations in multiple personality disorder: a preliminary report', *American Journal of Dance Therapy* 9: 31–46.

Kornblum, R. (1982) *A Perceptuo-Cognitive-Motor Approach to the Special Child*, Harrisburg: Arts in Special Education Project.

Kovacs, M. and Beck A. (1978) 'Maladaptive cognitive structures in depression', *American Journal of Psychiatry* 135: 525–533.

Kraepelin E. (1919) *Dementia Praecox and Paraphrenia* (trans. R. Barclay), Edinburgh: Livingstone.

Kreitler, H. and Kreitler, S. (1972) *Psychology of the Arts*, Durham: Duke University Press.

Krueger, D. and Schofield, E. (1986) 'Dance/movement therapy of eating disordered patients: a model', *Arts in Psychotherapy* 13: 323–331.

Kubie, L. (1958) *Neurotic Distortions of the Creative Process*, 2nd edn 1961, Kansas: University of Kansas Press.

Laban, R. (1948) *Modern Educational Dance*, revised by Lisa Ullman, 3rd edn 1980, London: Macdonald and Evans.

Laing, R. D. (1975) *The Divided Self: An Existential Study in Sanity and Madness*, London: Pelican.

Laing, R. D. and Esterton, A. (1961) *Self and Others*, London: Penguin.

—— (1970) *Sanity, Madness and the Family: Families of Schizophrenics*, London: Penguin.

Lamb W. and Turner D. (1968) *Management Behaviour*, New York: International Universities Press.

Laplanche, J. and Pontalis, J. B. (1973) *The Language of Psycho-Analysis*, 2nd edn 1980, London: The Hogarth Press.

Laurance, J. (1988) 'Blaming the messenger', *New Statesman and Society* July 1: 12–15.

Lawler, S. (1979) 'Movement therapy as a therapeutic intervention in establishing object-relations and fostering the integration of deviant ego functioning in schizophrenic individuals', unpublished M.A. thesis, Antioch/New England Graduate School.

Leatherbee, T. and Wood, S. (eds) (1984) *A Primer for Theoretical Models in Dance/Movement Therapy*, Philadelphia: Hahnemann University Press.

Lefko, H. (1974) *Dance Therapy: Narrative Case Histories with Six Patients*, Chicago: Nelson Hall.

Levens, M. (1990) 'Borderline aspects in eating disorders: art therapy's contribution', *Group Analysis* 23: 277–284.

Leventhal, M. (1980) *Movement and Growth: Dance Therapy for the Special Child*, New York: New York University Press.

—— (ed.) (1983) *Graduate Research Studies in DMT 1972–1982*. Compiled by the Council of Graduate Dance/Movement Therapy Education. Philadelphia: Hahnemann University Press. Copies available from New York University Graduate DMT Programme.

Levy, F. (1988) *Dance Movement Therapy: A Healing Art*, Reston: AAHPERD.

Lewis, P. (1986) *Theoretical Approaches in Dance Movement Therapy*, Vol. 1, Dubuque: Kendall Hunt.

Liebowitz, G., Mees, P. and Stanton K. (1989) 'Dance/movement therapy with long term psychiatric patients', *Newsletter of the Association for Dance Movement Therapy* 8 (2): 4–8. Available from the Association for Dance Movement Therapy, London.

Lindner, E., Harpaz, L. and Samberg, S. (1979) *Therapeutic Dance Movement: Expressive Activities for Older Adults*, New York: Human Sciences Press.

Lipshutz, J. (1978) 'The effects of movement therapy on interpersonal interaction in the chronic schizophrenic group', unpublished M.A. thesis, Hahnemann University, Philadelphia.

Little, M. (1951) 'Countertransference and the patient's response to it', *International Journal of Psychoanalysis* 33: 32–40.

Lohr, J., Wisniewski, A. and Jeste, D. (1986) 'Neurological aspects of tardive dyskinesia' in H. Nasrallah and D. Weinberger (eds) *Handbook of Schizophrenia, Volume 1. The Neurology of Schizophrenia*, New York: Elsevier Science Publishers.

Loomis, R. and Loomis, L. (eds) (1957) *Medieval Romances*, New York: The Modern Library.

Lowen, A. (1976) *Bioenergetics*, New York: Penguin.

Macdonald, L. and Ochera, J. (1990) 'User's views of Doddington Edward Wilson community mental health service', Internal Report, Dept of Clinical Epidemiology and Social Medicine, St George's Hospital Medical School, London SW17.

McDougall, J. (1974) 'The psychesoma and the psychoanalytic process', *International Review of Psychoanalysis* 1: 437–439.

Maher, B. (1972) 'The language of schizophrenia: a review and interpretation', *British Journal of Psychiatry* 120: 3–17.

Mahl, G. (1979) 'Body movement, ideation, and verbalization during psychoanalysis', in S. Weitz (ed.) *Nonverbal Communication*, New York: Oxford University Press.

Mahler, M., Pine, F. and Bergman, A. (1975) *The Psychological Birth of the Human Infant*, New York: Basic Books.

Malan, D. (1989) *Individual Psychotherapy and the Science of Psychodynamics* London: Butterworths.

Manschreck T. (1986) 'Motor abnormalities in schizophrenia', in H. Nasrallah and D. Weinberger (eds) *Handbook of Schizophrenia, Volume 1. The Neurology of Schizophrenia*. New York: Elsevier Science Publishers.

Manschreck, T., Maher, B., Rucklos, M. and Vereen, D. (1982) 'Disturbed voluntary motor activity in schizophrenic disorder', *Psychological Medicine* 12: 73–84.

Mantegazza P. (c. 1925) *Physiognomy and Expression*, Contemporary Science Series, H. Ellis (ed.), London: Walter Scott.

Martin, E. (1989) *The Woman in the Body: A Cultural Analysis of Reproduction*, Boston: Beacon Press.

Mayer-Gross, W., Slater, E. and Roth, M. (1954) *Clinical Psychiatry*, 3rd edn 1969, London: Ballière, Tindall.

Melville-Thomas, R. (1987) 'When actions speak louder than words', *Therapy Weekly*, 2 April: 4.

—— (1988) Unpublished papers, DMT Child Skills Seminar, Laban Centre for Movement and Dance, London.

Miller, L., Rustin, M., Rustin, M. and Shuttleworth, J. (eds) (1989) *Closely Observed Infants*, London: Gerald Duckworth and Co.

Minuchin, S. (1974) *Families and Family Therapy*, Cambridge: Harvard University Press.

Mittelmann, B. (1954) 'Motility in infants, children, and adults: patterning and psychodynamics, *Psychoanalytic Study of the Child* 9: 142–177.

—— (1957) 'Motility in the therapy of children and adults', *Psychoanalytic Study of the Child* 12: 284–319.

Morrison, J. (1974) 'Changes in subtype diagnosis of schizophrenia: 1920–1966', *American Journal of Psychiatry* 131 (6): 674–677.

Naess, J. (1982) 'A developmental approach to the interactive process in dance/movement therapy', *American Journal of Dance Therapy* 5: 43–55.

Noebel, K. (1990) 'Movement interaction in depression', Unpublished M.A. thesis, Laban Centre for Movement and Dance, London.

North, M. (1972) *Personality Assessment Through Movement*, 1978 edn, London: Macdonald and Evans.

Orbach, S. and Eichenbaum, L. (1987) *Bittersweet: Facing up to Feelings of Love, Envy and Competition in Women's Friendships*, London: Arrow Books.

Owens, D., Johnstone, E. and Frith, C. (1982) 'Spontaneous involuntary disorders of movement', *Archives of General Psychiatry* 39: 452–461.

O'Brien, C. (1975) 'Group therapy for schizophrenia: a practical approach', *Schizophrenia Bulletin* 13: 119–130.

Pasch, J. (1982) 'Movement for older people', *2D Magazine* 2 (1): 1–6.

Payne, H. (ed.) (1992) *Dance Movement Therapy: Theory and Practice*, London: Routledge.

Perinpanayagam, K. (1987) 'Organization and management of an inpatient treatment unit for adolescents', *Journal of Adolescence* 10: 133–148.

Perls, F. (1973) *The Gestalt Approach and Eyewitness to Therapy*, California: Bantam Books.

Pesso, A. (1969) *Movement in Psychotherapy: Psychomotor Techniques and Training*, New York: New York University Press.

Polhemus, T. (1978) *The Body Reader: Social Aspects of the Human Body*, New York: Pantheon Books.

Poteat, J. (1981) 'Effort–shape patterns of depression', Unpublished M. A. thesis, Hahnemann University, Philadelphia.

Reich, W. (1933) *Character Analysis*, 3rd edn 1976, New York: Farrar, Straus & Giroux.

Reid, S., Fry, E. and Rhode, M. (1981) 'Working with small groups of children in primary schools', in D. Daws and M. Boston (eds) *The Child Psychotherapist and the Problems of Young People*, London: Wildwood House Ltd. Originally Published 1977.

Reister, A. and Kraft, D. (eds) (1986) *Child Group Psychotherapy: Future Tense*, American Group Psychotherapy Association Monograph 3, Connecticut: International Universities Press.

Rioch, M. (1975) 'The work of Wilfred Bion on Groups', in A. Colman and W. Bexton (eds) *Group Relations Reader*, Vol. 1, Sausalito: GREX.

Robbins, A. (1980) *Expressive Therapy: A Creative Arts Approach to Depth-Oriented Treatment*, New York: Human Sciences Press.

Rogers, C. (1951) *Client-Centred Therapy*, Boston: Houghton Mifflin.

Rogers, D. (1985) 'The motor disorders of severe psychiatric illness: a conflict of paradigms', *British Journal of Psychiatry*, 147: 221–232.

Rolf, I. (1963) 'Structural integration: postural release', *Journal of the Institute for the Comparative Study of History, Philosophy and the Sciences* 1: 1, England: Coombe Springs.

Rosemont, F. (ed.) (1981) *Isadora Speaks: Isadora Duncan*, San Francisco: City Lights Books.

Rowe, D. (1978) *Choosing not Losing: The Experience of Depression* (1988), London: Fontana.

Royston, R. (1989) 'Schizophrenia, genetics and analytical psychology', *British Journal of Psychotherapy* 6 (1): 50–61.

Rutter, D. and Stephenson, G. (1972) 'Visual Interaction in a group of schizophrenic and depressive patients; *British Journal of Social and Clinical Psychology* Febuary 1, II(I): 57–65.

Ryle, A. (1990) *Cognitive-Analytic Therapy: Active Participation in Change (A New Integration in Brief Psychotherapy)*, with contributions from Amanda Poynton and Bee Brockman, London: John Wiley & Sons.

Samuels, A., Shorter, B. and Plaut, F. (1986) *A Critical Dictionary of Jungian Analysis*, London: Routledge.

Sandel, S. (1980) 'Countertransference stress in the treatment of schizophrenic patients', *American Journal of Dance Therapy*, 3: 20–32.

Sandel, S. and Johnson, D. (1983) 'Structure and process of the nascent group: dance therapy with chronic patients', *Arts in Psychotherapy* 10: 131–140.

Sargant, W. (1957) *Battle for the Mind*, London: Pan Books.

Schaffer, S. and Pollak, J. (1987) 'Listening to the adolescent therapy group', *Group* 11 (3): 155–164.

Scheflen, A. (1979) 'Quasi courtship behaviour in psychotherapy', in S. Weitz (ed.) *Nonverbal Communication*, New York: Oxford University Press.

Scheflen, A. and Scheflen, E. (1972) *Body Language and the Social Order: Communication as Social Control*, New Jersey: Prentice Hall.

Schilder, P. (1950) *The Image and Appearance of the Human Body: Studies in the Constructive Energies of the Psyche*, 3rd edn 1978, New York: International Universities Press.

—— (1976) *On Psychoses*, L. Bender (ed.), New York: International Universities Press.

Schmais, C. (1974) 'Dance therapy in perspective', in K. Mason (ed.) *Dance Therapy: Focus on Dance VII*, Washington: AAHPER American Association for Health, Physical Education and Recreation.

—— (1981) 'Group development and group formation in dance therapy', *Arts in Psychotherapy* 8: 103–107.

—— (1985) 'Healing processes in group DMT', *American Journal of Dance Therapy* 8: 17–36.

—— (1986) 'Introduction to dance therapy', *American Journal of Dance Therapy* 9: 23–30.

Schmais, C. and Felber, D. (1977) 'Dance therapy analysis: a method for observing and analyzing a dance therapy group', *American Journal of Dance Therapy* 1 (2): 18–24.

Schoop, T. (1974) *Won't You Join the Dance? A Dancers Essay into the Treatment of Psychosis*, California: Mayfield.

Schoop, T. and Mitchell, P. (1979) 'Reflections and projections: the schoop approach to dance therapy', in Bernstein, P. (ed.) *Eight Theoretical Approaches to Dance-Movement Therapy*, Dubuque: Kendall Hunt.

Searles, H. (1965) *Collected Papers on Schizophrenia and Related Subjects*, New York: International Universities Press.

Seeman, M., Littman, S., Plummer, E., Thornton, J. and Jeffries, J. (1982) *Living and Working with Schizophrenia*, London: Open University Press.

Segal, H. (1964) *Introduction to the Work of Melanie Klein*, enlarged edn 1988, London: Hogarth Press.

Shearer, S., Peters, C., Quaytman, M. and Ogden, R. (1990) 'Frequency and correlates of childhood sexual and physical abuse histories in adult female borderline inpatients', *American Journal of Psychiatry* 147 (2): 214–216.

Shenton, J. (1990) 'Move for the better', *Therapy Weekly* Sept 13: 4.

—— (1988) 'A comparative study of professional ballet training and anorexia nervosa', unpublished M.A. thesis, Laban Centre for Movement and Dance, London.

Showalter, E. (1987) *The Female Malady: Women, Madness and English Culture, 1830–1980*, London: Virago Press.

Siegel, E. (1974) 'The treatment of depressive states during movement therapy', *American Dance Therapy Association Monograph No. 3*, 76–85.

—— (1984) *Dance Movement Therapy: Mirror of Ourselves: A Psychoanalytic Approach*, New York: Human Sciences Press.

Silberman-Diehl L. and Komisaruk, R. (1985) 'Treating psychogenic somatic disorders through body metaphor', *American Journal of Dance Therapy* 8: 37–45.

Silberstein, S. (1987) 'Dance therapy and schizophrenia: vision of the future', *The Arts in Psychotherapy* 14: 143–152.

Simon-Dhouailly, N. (1986) *La Leçon de Charcot: Voyage dans une toile*. Paris: Imprimerie Tardy Quercy.

Sinason, V. and Kirtchuk, G. (1986) 'The function of the new member in an adolescent group', *Psychoanalytic Psychotherapy* 1 (2): 63–78.

Skove, E. (1986) 'The psychophysical effects on the dance/movement therapist working with a schizophrenic population', *American Journal of Dance Therapy* 9: 67–82.

Skynner, R. (1978) *One Flesh: Separate Persons, Principles of Family and Marital Psychotherapy*, London: Constable.

Skynner, R. and Cleese, J. (1983) *Families and How to Survive Them*, London: Mandarin.

Sossin, M. (1987) 'Reliability of the Kestenberg Movement Profile', *Movement Studies* 2: 23–28. A journal of the Laban Bartenieff Institute of Movement Studies, available from LIMS, 31 West 27th St, New York 10001, USA.

Sparshott, F. (1988) *Off the Ground: First Steps to a Philosophical Consideration of the Dance*, Princeton: Princeton University Press.

Spitz, R (1942) 'Anaclitic depression: an inquiry into the genesis of psychiatric conditions in early childhood', *Psychoanalytic Study of the Child* 2: 313–342.

Spitzer, S. (1990) 'Adult survivors of father–daughter incest: a case study in dance/movement therapy', unpublished M.A. thesis, Laban Centre for Movement and Dance, London.

Stanton, K. (1988) 'Temples or prisons?', *Times Higher Education Supplement*, 3 June: 26.

—— (1989) 'Moving into action', *Open Mind* 41: 4.

—— (1991) 'Dance movement therapy: an introduction', *British Journal of Occupational Therapy* 54 (3): 108–110.

—— (1991b) 'Rebel by nature: an interview with Judith Kestenberg', *Free Associations* 22.

—— (1991c) 'Dancing your cares away', *Times Higher Education Supplement*, March 29, p. 29.

Stanton K. and Stanton, M. (1989) 'Martha Davis: non-verbal aspects of psychotherapy', *Psychiatric Bulletin of the Royal College of Psychiatrists* 13 (7): 374.

Stark, A. (1989) 'The use of verbalization in dance/movement therapy', *The Arts in Psychotherapy* 16: 105–13.

Steiner, R. (1931) *Eurythmy as Visible Speech*, reprinted 1984, trans. by Vera and Judy Compton-Burnett. Southampton: Camelot Press.

—— (1953) *An Introduction to Eurythmy*, New York: Anthroposophic Press.

Stern, D. (1985) *The Interpersonal World of the Infant: a view from Psychoanalysis and Developmental Psychology*, New York: Basic Books.

Stone, M. (1986) 'Exploratory psychotherapy in schizophrenia-spectrum patients', *Bulletin of the Menninger Clinic* 50 (3): 287–306.

Strauss, J. and Carpenter, W. (1981) *Schizophrenia*, New York: Plenum.

Suleiman, S.R. (ed.) (1986) *The Female Body in Western Culture: Contemporary Perspectives*, Cambridge, Mass: Harvard University Press.

Sullivan, H. S. (1932) *Schizophrenia as a Human Process*, New York: Norton.

—— (1940) *Conceptions of Modern Psychiatry*, 1953 edn, New York: Norton.

—— (1956) 'Therapy with schizophrenic patients', in *Clinical Studies in Psychiatry*, New York: Norton.

Swett, C., Surrye, J. and Cohen, C. (1990) 'Sexual and physical abuse histories and psychiatric symptoms among male psychiatric outpatients', *American Journal of Psychiatry* 147 (5): 632–636.

Szasz, T. (1974) *The Myth of Mental Illness: Foundations of a Theory of Personal Conduct*, rev. edn, New York: Harper & Row.

Trimble, M. (1981) *Neuropsychiatry*, Chichester: Wiley.

—— (1986) *A Study of Movement Disorders*, Wantage: Janssen Pharmaceutical Limited.

Ursano, R. and Hales, R. (1986) 'A review of brief individual psychotherapies', *American Journal of Psychiatry* 143 (12): 1507–1517.

Walen, S., DiGiuseppe, R. and Wessler, R. (1980) *A Practitioner's Guide to Rational-Emotive Therapy*, Oxford: Oxford University Press.

Walsh, F. (1982) *Normal Family Processes*, New York: Guilford.

Warner, R. (1987) *Recovery From Schizophrenia: Psychiatry and Political Economy*, London and New York: Routledge.

Waxer, P. (1974) 'Nonverbal cues for depression', *Journal of Abnormal Psychology* 83: 319–322.

Weaver, L. and Brooks, G. (1964) 'The use of psychomotor tests in predicting the potential of chronic schizophrenia', *Journal of Neuropsychiatry* 5: 170–180.

Webster, J. (1987) 'A comparison of functional and dysfunctional adoptive families: a nonverbal assessment', unpublished M.A. thesis, Hahnemann University, Philadephia.

Weitz, S. (1979) *Nonverbal Communication: Readings with Commentary*, New York: Oxford University Press.

Weltman, M. (1986) 'Movement therapy with children who have been sexually abused', *American Journal of Dance Therapy* 9: 47–66.

Whitehouse, M. (1979) 'C. G. Jung and dance therapy: two major principles', in P. Bernstein (ed.) *Eight Theoretical Approaches in Dance-Movement Therapy*, Dubuque: Kendall Hunt.

Wilder, V. (1987) 'Effects of antipsychotic medication on the movement pathologies of chronic schizophrenics', *American Journal of Dance Therapy* 10: 77–94.

Williams, M. and Waddell, M. (1991) *The Chamber of Maiden Thought: Literary Origins of the Psychoanalytic Model of the Mind*, London: Routledge.

Willis, D. (1987) 'Ethical and legal issues of touch in dance/movement therapy', *American Journal of Dance Therapy* 10: 41–53.

Willock, B. (1987) 'The devalued (unloved, repugnant) self – a second facet of narcissistic vulnerability in the aggressive, conduct-disordered child', *Psychoanalytic Psychology* 4 (3): 219–240.

Wilson-Hagen, B. (1988) 'A case study of an autistic girl in movement therapy', unpublished Master's in Creative Arts Therapy thesis.

Winnicott, D. W. (1953) 'Transitional objects and transitional phenomena: a study of the first not-me possession', *International Journal of Psychoanalysis* 34 (2): 89–97.

—— (1958) *Collected Papers: Through Pediatrics to Psycho-analysis*, London: Hogarth Press.

—— (1971) *Therapeutic Consultations in Child Psychiatry*, International Psycho-analytical Library No. 87, London: Hogarth Press and the Institute of Psycho-analysis.

—— (1971b) 'The mirror role of mother and family in child development', in *Playing and Reality*, London: Penguin.

—— (1986) *Home is Where We Start From*, London: Pelican.

—— (1988) *Human Nature*, London: Free Associations Books.

Wolff, H. (1977) 'Loss: a central theme in psychotherapy', *British Journal of Medical Psychology* 50: 11–19.

Yalom, I. (1970) *The Theory and Practice of Group Psychotherapy* 1985 edn, New York: Basic Books.
—— (1983) *Inpatient Group Psychotherapy*, New York: Basic Books.
Yarden, P., and Discipio, W. (1971) 'Abnormal movements and prognosis in schizophrenia', *American Journal of Psychiatry* 128, (3): 97–103.
Zeitlin, H. (1986) *The Natural History of Psychiatric Disorder in Children*, Institute of Psychiatry, Maudsley Monographs No. 29, Oxford: Oxford University Press.
Zwerling, I. (1989) 'The creative arts therapies as "real therapies" ', *American Journal of Dance Therapy* 11 (1): 19–26.

Name index

Subject index